Adverse Mechanical Tension in the Central Nervous System

Relief by Functional Neurosurgery

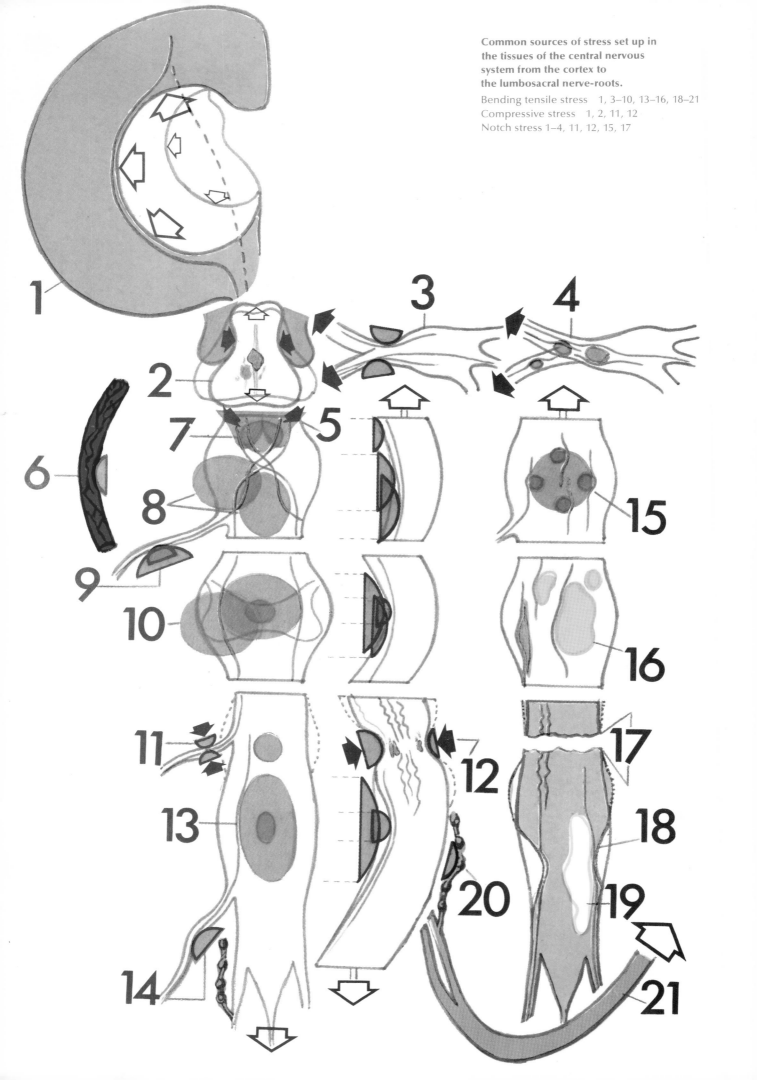

Common sources of stress set up in the tissues of the central nervous system from the cortex to the lumbosacral nerve-roots.

Bending tensile stress 1, 3–10, 13–16, 18–21
Compressive stress 1, 2, 11, 12
Notch stress 1–4, 11, 12, 15, 17

Adverse Mechanical Tension in the Central Nervous System

An Analysis of Cause and Effect

Relief by Functional Neurosurgery

BY **ALF BREIG**

ALMQVIST & WIKSELL INTERNATIONAL
Stockholm, Sweden

JOHN WILEY & SONS
New York, London, Sydney, Toronto

LRO JGJ

First published by

Almqvist & Wiksell International
Stockholm — Sweden
ISBN 91-2200126-3

in collaboration with

John Wiley & Sons, Inc.,
New York
ISBN 0-471-04137-8
Library of Congress Catalog Card
Number: 77-88852

Printed in Sweden by
Almqvist & Wiksell, Uppsala 1978

Foreword

After, in 1960, Prof. Alf Breig's book on Biomechanics of the Central Nervous System was published, it elicited increasing interest in the following years. This monograph presented not only a first endeavour to a systematic account of the biomechanical influences acting on the central nervous system under normal and pathological conditions, but also Breig's personal investigations formed a major contribution to the contents. A particular feature of Alf Breig's approach to the topic was his manner of visualizing the biomechanical mechanisms, which was perfectly adapted to the current techniques of clinical examination of disorders of the nervous system and its envelopes. Therefore it was of direct importance for the treatment of patients.

During my personal work in developing new techniques or modifying existing methods of spinal surgery I frequently consulted Breig's book and often was rewarded with worthful information. Many other authors, especially those involved in spinal surgery, have quoted from Breig's work in support of their own views.

The general recognition of the importance of Breig's contributions makes this foreword absolutely needless if it had not been written at Alf Breig's personal request, which I accepted with much pleasure.

The present book is the result of many years' experience, much thinking and meticulous investigation. Many illustrations reinforce the content of the writing. Whereas the first monograph was primarily focused on bio-mechanics of the spinal cord in health and disease and the hind brain occupied a secondary place, the pons–cord relations are, in the present book, intensively discussed, and much more attention is given to clinical and therapeutical aspects.

The author has in his own preface given an excellent survey of the lines of thought followed in his book, so there is no need to relapse in repetitions. The reader may encounter daring hypotheses such as those on the mechanism of the so-called cervical syndrome or on the pathomechanical influences on multiple sclerosis. They present a challenge as to their verification or falsification. On more simple matters the reader's opinion may differ from that of the author. Yet such differences in opinion are of minor importance as compared to the considerable value the author's contribution will have as an eye-opener towards a new important field of bio-mechanics.

In my opinion his work should not only be read by specialists in neuro-sciences or orthopedic surgery, but also by anaesthetists, whose activities regularly involve the positioning of defenseless patients, and last but not least by physiotherapists for reasons which need no further precision.

Henk Verbiest, M.D., Ph.D.
Professor of Neurosurgery
Utrecht University
The Netherlands

Preface

Since 'The Biomechanics of the Central Nervous System' was published in 1960 there has been an encouraging growth of interest in the topic. The investigation reported there was originally prompted by the observation on radiographs that flexion of the neck led to cranialward displacement of silver clips that had been clamped firmly on rootlets close to the upper cervical spinal cord. Interest was accordingly centred on the, previously undescribed, physiological deformation of the tissues of the spinal cord due to normal movements of the spine. In subsequent research the aim has been to investigate the effects that artificial deforming forces, applied to the spinal cord and meninges *in situ*, exert on nervous tissue from the brain stem to the conus medullaris and the associated cranial and spinal nerves. These effects have been studied macroscopically and microscopically, and with the help of photoelastic models.

The emphasis throughout this book is on the pathogenetic significance of tension. The primary source of meningeal and neural tension is the lengthening of the spinal canal on forward and lateral flexion. Normally, the soft tissues adapt freely to these skeletal movements; but in the presence of space-occupying lesions involving the spinal canal or located in the cord itself, and when there are sclerotic or fibrotic lesions that restrict the mobility or extensibility of nervous and meningeal tissues, the tension may be much increased. Even when the pathological lesion appears to be exerting an essentially compressive effect, the resulting deformation leads to a local increase in tension; it is the effects of this raised tension that appear to be of primary neurophysiological significance.

The clinical implications of this principle are manifest particularly in *cervical* spinal cord disorders that have arisen as the result of acute or chronic damage to the tissue—ranging from sudden trauma to degenerative lesions. The cervical part of the spinal canal normally undergoes greater changes of length during postural movements than do other regions, especially the thoracic. However, while tension is transmitted in both directions—to the brain stem and to the cauda equina—the pathological effects are manifested chiefly in the lower region.

Clinical evidence will be presented indicating that excessive tension in the cord may produce measurable changes in motor, sensory and autonomic function. These are accentuated whenever the cord is stretched, and may be reversed, and the symptoms relieved, if stretching can be eliminated and the affected tissues are kept relaxed. Even in the presence of irreversible myelopathic lesions, whether focal, sclerotic or space-occupying, the existing symptoms and neural function can be improved significantly by surgical measures designed to prevent over-stretching of the cord.

In the course of clinical enquiry over nearly two decades I have found that many neurological disorders in which no mechanical component has ever been suspected do in fact have their origin in tension in the nervous tissue; we are at present only just beginning to recognize the histological and neurophysiological sequelae of this tension.

To apply the fundamental principles to clinical problems, in particular the important one of securing relaxation of the spinal cord tissues, presented a constant challenge. But advance on this front was hampered by the wide gap between our knowledge of how the pathological forces are transmitted in the spinal cord and our imperfect understanding of the mode of action of those forces at the sites from which neurological manifestations emanate. While it has long been obvious that these have their origin in some form of distortion of the nervous tissue, the fundamental effects of the forces acting within the tissue network of the spinal cord remained obscure.

In order to examine more closely the relevant internal trigger mechanisms the biomechanical analyses were extended to the microscopical level. These analyses have shown that tension in the nervous tissue that gives rise to symptoms is characterized by focal deformation of its complex three-dimensional fibre network as seen in histological and microangiographical sections. It was evident that an important cause of functional disturbance both of the axis-cylinders and the blood-vessels lies in the reduction in their cross-sectional area resulting from tension. By slackening the nervous tissue the tension is relieved and the conductivity and circulation are restored. Surgical measures have been designed for permanent relief of pathological tension in the cord tissue in patients with chronic myelopathies and acute traumatic cord lesions. These methods are described and their potentials illustrated in a series of patients.

The work presented in this volume, being essentially one man's tentative approach to a new subject, has many shortcomings. The author hopes that the reader will forgive for these defects. At the same time, he would welcome criticism and proposals from readers so that the presentation can in the future be improved upon.

The publication of this book affords me the opportunity of recording my deep-felt appreciation of the contributions made to the manuscript by a number of British specialists in the respective fields.

I wish particularly to thank Duncan Troup, Department of Orthopaedic Surgery, The University of Liverpool and Spinal Research Unit, The Royal Free Hospital, London, for his revision of part of the sections on Thoracic Myelopathy and Pathodynamics of the Lumbar Spine; his lively interest in the work as a whole has been a welcome source of encouragement.

To Phillip Harris, Department of Surgical Neurology, Royal Infirmary, Edinburgh, I am indebted for his suggestions on the section Pons—Cord Tract Surgery; Beneficial and Adverse Biomechanical Effects.

I should also like to acknowledge the efforts of the following to present my ideas in a more readable form:

Peter W. Nathan, Medical Research Council: Neurological Symptoms Generated by Flexion of the Spine, and The Histodynamic Background to Neurological Symptoms Evoked on Flexion of the Spine. William G. P. Mair, Department of Neuropathology: Biomechanics and Pathodynamics of the Pons–Cord Tissue Tract. Edward P. G. Houssemayne du Boulay, Department of Radiology: Radiological Diagnosis of Tension in the Spinal Cord—all three at the National Hospital for Nervous Diseases, Queen Square, London.

To Professor William Blackwood and Professor Valentine Logue, also at the National Hospital, I should like to express my thanks for valuable criticism and stimulating discussions.

I wish, in addition, to acknowledge the great encouragement I have received from colleagues in North America, where my earlier book first received recognition.

To Professor Rudolf Hiltscher, Swedish State Power Board, Stockholm, I am grateful for his suggestions relating to the state of stress in elastic bodies and for making available laboratory facilities for the stress optical investigation.

The elaborate shape of this comprehensive volume is the result of close collaboration between Mr Victor Braxton and myself over a number of years. For his valuable contributions to the intelligible presentation in the English language of my mechanical concepts, the clarification of the terminology and the description of the preparatory and surgical techniques, I am greatly indebted to him.

For working facilities over many years at the Department of Pathology, South Stockholm Hospital, I am much obliged to Dr Bo Törnberg.

The histological preparation of the specimens was performed by Mrs Margareta Asplund and they were photographed by Mrs Karin Hallert. For photographic work from the outset I am grateful to Mr Nils Börje Nilsson.

I gratefully acknowledge the promotion of the investigation by Professor Bror Rexed, Director-General, The National Board of Health and Welfare, Stockholm, and the special arrangements for its completion made by the Board of the Karolinska Hospital, Stockholm. In this connection I would like to convey my sincere thanks to Professor Gustav Giertz, Professor Carl-Axel Hamberger, Professor Lars Leksell and Mr Carl Oswald Palmstierna.

For substantial grants towards the translation and editing of the manuscript I am greatly indebted to the Service Company of the Swedish Insurance Industry (FSAB) and in particular to its Director Mr Richard Schönmeyr for his personal involvement in this matter. For his sympathetic interest I would also like to thank Mr Per Boëthius, Director, Skandia Insurance Company, Stockholm.

A grant towards the costs of the translation has also been received from the Swedish Medical Research Council and The Axel and Margarete Johnson Foundation.

The publication of this book has ultimately been made possible through the generous support of The Sven and Dagmar Salén Foundation and the Service Company of the Swedish Insurance Industry (FSAB).

Finally, I should like to thank Mr F. Davids Thomsen, Director of the publishing house Almqvist & Wiksell International, Stockholm, and the staff of Almqvist & Wiksell Printers, Uppsala, for the personal interest they have taken in the production of this book.

Stockholm 1977

A. B.

Contents

Introduction

In order to examine the effects of the pathological forces that deform the soft tissues in the spinal canal a series of experimental studies were undertaken. Most of these have been performed on the cadaver. The pattern of deformation of the cord tissue when subjected to thrust and pincer forces was analysed histologically and microangiographically, with supplementary photoelastic analyses performed on models. In addition, detailed clinical observations were made on patients in whom the effects of pathological deformation of the soft tissues in the spinal canal had been relieved surgically.

During the course of these investigations new concepts of basic biomechanics and of neuropathology emerged and new terms have had to be coined. These basic concepts are outlined here at the outset.

Basic biomechanics

The spinal canal undergoes considerable changes in length between the extremes of flexion and extension,[1] particularly in the cervical and lumbar regions. The total change is of the order of 5–7 cm (12, 35), and is greater on the posterior than the anterior aspects. Similarly, on lateral flexion, the canal is lengthened on the convex side and shortened on the concave.

At its cranial extremity the spinal dura mater is attached to the circumference of the foramen magnum, and at its caudal end it is anchored to the coccyx by the filum terminale. When the trunk is fully flexed the dura is under tension, as is also the cord, and stretching occurs. Part of this tension is transmitted from the dura mater *via* the dentate ligaments to the pia mater, but by far the larger component of the tension is set up directly in the cord by virtue of its anchorage at its two extremities, namely the brain stem and the cauda equina.

From the biomechanical aspect the spinal cord therefore cannot be considered in isolation but must be treated as a continuous tract of nervous and supporting tissues, from the mesencephalon to the conus medullaris. This is referred to in this book as the *pons–cord tissue tract*, or simply the pons–cord tract.

The static and dynamic properties of the pons–cord tract constitute a self-contained biomechanical compartment. In extension of the spine from the neutral posture the axis of the spinal canal, and hence that of the tract, is shortened, and the tissue slackens and folds. When the neutral posture is assumed the tract recovers its original length, the slack is taken up and the folds are eliminated. In flexion, in which the length of the canal is increased, the tract is stretched elastically. During these spinal movements the axons and blood-vessels of the spinal cord undergo deformation similar to that of the cord as a whole.

Deformation of nervous tissues; its pathological effects

The concept of the effect of dynamic forces on the tissue elements is so fundamental and so comprehensive in its implications that it would appear justified to regard the relating field as a specific entity in medicine.

The term that would seem to suggest itself to designate this field is *histodynamics*. It may be defined thus: *A branch of medicine dealing with the effects produced on cell elements by the action of dynamic forces*. This is a general definition. But in the context of this book we are concerned primarily with the effects of *pathological* forces. Moreover, we are concerned exclusively with the *neurological* effects of these forces.

It is evident that during postural changes in the living subject the presence of unyielding pathological structures, whether located anterior to the pons–cord tract or within it, will result in incorrect loading of the nervous tissue and its abnormal deformation, particularly during the stretching phase.

Concerning pathological sources of deformation within the canal, it has been traditional to think solely in terms of *compression* of the spinal cord or nerve-roots. From the work reported earlier and from the new evidence presented here it is abundantly clear that this concept is too narrow. Even a demonstrably compressive force generates short-range axial *tension*. In a compressive brain or spinal cord injury the nerve-fibres and blood-vessels are not compacted (138), but stretched and torn apart. A typical situation in which local tension is set up in the cord is that where, during *extension* of the spine, it is pinched or clamped between the pathological structure and the canal wall. In most other pathological situations in which nervous tissue is deformed there is no firm opposing surface, the deformation instead being produced by the pathological structure impinging on the cord that is stretched due to *flexion* of the spine. The interstitial pressure is then raised (Figs. 77, 135, 136) and the blood supply is put at risk.

Tension is thus the pathologically significant force, whether generated by a pincer action, by local induration and deformation, or by a space-occupying lesion. Whether or not the tension leads to neurological deficit will depend on its magnitude and its duration of action.

The magnitude of the tension in the cord depends firstly on the anatomical factor of body posture, which

[1] 'Extension', in the dictionary sense, means 'the process of becoming longer'; but applied anatomically to the spine it has come to mean movement in the sagittal plane dorsally. In general, the latter usage is clear, but in certain passages where confusion might arise the phrase 'backward flexion' has been used. Similarly with 'flexion'; where it would add clarity, the prefix 'forward' has sometimes been added.

determinates the relative lengths of the spinal canal and cord. Under physiological conditions with the column flexed the cord is in a state of normal *pre-tension*.[2] On this will be imposed any tension of pathological origin. The total tension induced may well lead to neural dysfunction, and then the involved nerve-fibres in the cord or nerve-roots may be said to be *over-stretched*. The most significant consequence of over-stretching nerve-fibres is impairment of their conductivity.

A new approach to therapeutic management—functional neurosurgery

Ultimately, over-stretching due to a pincer or clamping action may lead to rupture of the intramedullary tissue. When nerve-fibres and their supporting structures are torn, the physiological tension set up during flexion of the column will lead to separation of the ruptured ends. Measures must be taken to prevent this separation, where possible, and otherwise to restore contact between the intramedullary wound surfaces so as to promote outgrowth of the axis-cylinders, and hence regeneration (136).

Conductivity and circulation can often recover by eliminating tension due to structures impinging on the cord and nerve-roots from without or to an intra-medullary unyielding lesion and hence to the constriction of the nerve-fibres and blood-vessels. This can be achieved without manipulating, disturbing or even inspecting the site of the neural lesion—simply by obtaining relaxation of the soft tissues of the spinal canal *in situ* (55), and maintaining it until recovery is established. To designate this aspect of neurosurgery in which the primary aim of treatment is to restore normal conductivity, the term *functional neurosurgery* is suggested—'functional', not merely in respect of the aim, but in terms of surgical technique.

Since the stress field in the nervous tissue differs in extent and intensity for unilateral or multilateral thrust and a bilateral pincer or clamping action, the two main deleterious mechanisms, the surgical countermeasures are also different.

To prevent flexion of the cervical spine when there is a risk of pathological tension and hence over-stretching of the nerve-fibres and blood-vessels, a brake may be inserted in the neck, an operation that has been designated *cervicolordodesis*. This procedure also prevents separation of intramedullary wound surfaces in the case of tissue rupture due to compression. It has now been employed in a score of patients for the relief of symptoms in various types of myelopathy and rhizo-pathy and to promote approximation of the intra-medullary wound surfaces after compressive cervical spinal cord injury.

To eliminate compression of the nervous tissues in the cervical canal by means of bilateral laminectomy it is mandatory to use a protective technique which avoids introducing any part of an instrument into the lumen of the canal and thus exerting even the slightest momentary pressure on the dura and cord. For this purpose the techniques of *protective bilateral laminectomy* and *protective arco-cristectomy* have been designed. The latter consists in sawing out only the upper rims of the laminae and then raising them carefully from the canal. This type of partial superior bilateral laminectomy maintains spinal stability; it is therefore recommended wherever it is practicable.

Presentation of the material

The aim of the book is to present the experimental and clinical evidence on which the concepts set out in this Introduction are based. This evidence can best be offered in visual form; the figures and their legends to a great extent tell their own story, while the text, in which full reference is made to the illustrations, is subservient to them.

Definitions

Elastic deformation.—Deformation that disappears on removing the external force(s) causing it.

Elasticity.—The property whereby a body, when deformed, recovers its configuration on removal of the deforming forces.

Plastic.—Capable of being modeled or shaped. Capable of being deformed continuously and permanently in any direction without fracture under the action of a stress equal to, or greater than, the yield stress.

Strain.—A change in length of a body and especially of an elastic solid produced by a force, the change being expressed as the ratio of the increase or decrease to the original length.

Thrust.—A pressure exerted by a body on another, especially a horizontal (transverse) pressure.

Viscosity.—The property of a substance whereby it may develop and maintain a certain shearing stress, which is dependent on the speed of flow, and then continue to offer constant resistance to flow.

The property of a solid whereby it may yield continuously under a shearing stress.

Yield stress.—The minimum shearing or normal stress required to produce continuous deformation of a solid.

---

[2] Theoretically, one should distinguish between tension set up during normal elongation and tension set up by a structure impinging on the dura and cord from the anterior aspect of the spinal canal—that is, a unilateral thrust. The latter might be labelled the *static pathological* pre-tension. On this is superimposed the physiological dynamic tension in the soft tissues on flexion of the spinal canal. To simplify the presentation the term *pathological tension* is used to cover both this pathological pre-tension and pathologically increased dynamic tension.

PART ONE
Experimental biomechanical analyses

Biomechanics of the pons–cord tissue tract

To understand the changes that the spinal cord undergoes when it is stretched and relaxed it is essential to be conversant with the morphology, physical properties and architecture of the various tissue components. Similarly, one must be aware of the changes in shape of the soft tissues lining the canal, the dura mater with the dentate ligaments, the root-sheaths and their attachment to the endosteum of the spinal canal, the disc tissue with its annulus fibrosus, the posterior longitudinal ligament and the ligamenta flava.

The fibres of the spinal cord are disposed in three patterns, namely, folds (35, 201), spirals (64) and a rhomboid network (33, 45, 164). In the last of these, which occurs in the pia mater, the stiff collagen fibres intersect in several planes to form a network of trabeculae (Figs. 16, 18). Through the opening up and closing of this network the nervous and glial tissues are able to undergo elongation and shortening without mutual displacement of the various tissue components. The forces involved in these changes of the cord are quite small; if a piece of cervical cord 7–9 cm long is placed on wet dura mater on the anterior aspect of the spinal canal it will lengthen and shorten on flexion and extension of the cervical spinal column to almost the same extent as when *in situ* (Figs. 3, 4).

Spinal cord tissue from which the pia mater has been removed has a mucous appearance, and during micromanipulation offers no resistance to small deformations, but behaves as a homogeneous fluid of low viscosity. It also displays the properties of plasticity and elasticity. Only when the tissue is subjected to greater tension, either in the axial or transverse directions, is there an observable tendency for elastic recovery. The elasticity of the nervous tissue is manifested as a visible retraction when the cord is transected in the flexed position of the column.[1] Under normal conditions the stretching of the cord and its tendency for elastic recovery are greatest in full flexion.[2]

When the body is supine and the spine is fully flexed the stretched pons–cord tract overcomes the effect of gravity and approaches the anterior aspect of the spinal canal or the base of the cranium (Fig. 10). Likewise, when the body is in the lateral position and the spine is flexed so that the thoracic section is raised from the table, the tract is elevated towards the upper aspect of the canal (Fig. 125 D). In extension of the spine, in any position of the body, the slackened tract sags on to the canal surface or the aspect of the posterior fossa that happens to be lowermost; while the cord comes into direct contact with the arachnoid and the dura mater of the canal, the pons and medulla oblongata sag towards the clivus, and make contact with it, only in the prone position. Because they are anchored, in any other posi-tion the pons and medulla oblongata can sag only towards the lowest aspect of the posterior cranial fossa and the foramen magnum, though, of course, they will not come into contact with it (Fig. 102).

The changes in shape of the dura mater and the ligamenta flava that occur, or are accentuated, in extension are still not completely understood. One obscure point is the effect of the cerebrospinal fluid pressure on the folding of the dura mater. As has been shown earlier, shortening of the spinal canal results in axial compression ('telescoping') and folding of all the soft tissues that are contained in it (35). During flexion of the spine from full extension the slight stretching of the soft tissues takes up the slack until, just when the neutral position is reached, the folds are eliminated.

In the cadaver some folding of the dura is observed in normal lordosis of the cervical spine. It would be of interest to know whether the folding and forward bulging of the ligamenta flava that occur in extension of the cervical spine produce folding of the dura and corresponding deformation of the subarachnoid space in the living subject. Whereas laminectomy and excision of the ligamenta flava of the cervical spine performed *intra vitam* with the body in the prone position do not result in folding of the dura because of the pressure of the cerebrospinal fluid (Fig. 142), in the cadaver such folding does appear; when the cadaver is in the erect posture, however, the folds are eliminated by the fluid pressure. In gas myelograms also no folding of the dura or forward bulging of the ligamenta flava has been observed when the cervical spine is extended (178). The folding in the cadaver in which laminectomy has been performed occurs at the same sites and in about the same way as if the ligamenta flava were still present. Experience from a large number of cadavers indicates that the deformation of functionally associated structures often displays an identical pattern. It would seem justified to conclude that the forward bulging of the ligamenta flava and the folding of the dura occurring in extension of the cervical spine are normal vital phenomena, but that the conditions under which they occur are eliminated by laminectomy; moreover, in gas myelography the phenomena may be concealed by the gas pressure.[3] In full extension of the cervical spine,

---

[1] Between its folding in extension and its incipient elastic tension in the neutral posture of the spinal canal the nervous tissue is under slight and growing tension ('low-tension phase').
[2] 'High-tension phase'.
[3] Immediately after injection of gas into the subarachnoid space the pressure raises steeply; however, after about 3 minutes it has decreased to its normal value.
Courtesy of T. Greitz, M.D., Dept. of Neuroradiology, Karolinska Hospital, Stockholm.

when the vertebral arches approach each other, the ligamenta flava are forced in both anterior and posterior directions; they then protrude into the cervical spinal canal and produce a corresponding deformation of the dura. In the presence of large space-occupying processes the ligaments—besides the vertebral arches—can accentuate any clamping or pincer action on the cervical cord in extension.

Nerve-fibres

Histological observations show that when the spinal cord shortens the axis-cylinders fold in irregular spirals (35). As the shortening due to the axial compression is most pronounced in the posterior part of the cervical cord, the increase in cross-sectional area is most marked in the region of the posterior columns (54). Because of the three-dimensional folding the cross-sectional area of the axis-cylinders is greater in extension than in flexion, when they are drawn out. The cross-section of the myelin sheaths also varies, but with a small range between the extreme spinal postures. For technical reasons it has been impossible to ascertain how the myelin sheaths and their sheaths of Schwann widen in axial compression (telescoping), and how this affects the intercellular spaces. The myelin sheath has been described as circular (20), and, more recently, as having a cog-wheel contour (19) (Fig. 14 A–C); the stained sections displayed no change in configuration of the sheath of Schwann (35). It is known that the myelin sheath both of the peripheral nerve and of the axis-cylinder in the spinal cord consists of spirally coiled lamellae composed of two contiguous membranes each consisting of a bimolecular lipoid layer with two affixed monomolecular protein and polysaccharide layers (97); the outermost end of the lamella of the myelin sheath is connected by the mesaxon to the surface membrane of the nucleated sheath of Schwann; the innermost lamella is adherent to the perimeter of the axis-cylinder at the edge of its investing membrane (20, 97, 174) (Fig. 14 D). As a consequence of the simultaneous growth of the axon and the Schwann cell, the concentric layers of the myelin sheath are, it would seem, adherent to the surface of the axis-cylinder (Fig. 14 F, G). It has been assumed that the coiled arrangement of the lamella is a device to protect the axis-cylinder process against damage through axial traction. However, we still do not know how the myelin sheath behaves during elongation and shortening of the cord. It is hardly likely that the membranes undergo dimensional change; there is, however, the possibility that the myelin sheath itself lengthens through axial extension of the coiled lamella (21). If the distance between the coils of such lamellae increases on axial compression, we may have an explanation of the increase in the cross-sectional area of the sheath in extension. It has been suggested that during the widening of the myelin sheath and the separation of the coils, cytoplasm of the Schwann cell enters the interspace between the coils (20, 96). From

the changes seen in transverse sections of the cord stained by Palmgren's method it would appear that the increase in the area of the myelin sheaths and Schwann cells is accompanied by a reduction in the intercellular spaces (Fig. 11).

Connective tissue and neuroglia

The stiff collagen fibres in the epipia surround the whole cord as a monolayer rhomboid network and they constitute the chief supporting element of the cord pulp (164, 192); they also invest the perivascular funnel-shaped layer and follow the vessels deep into the medulla (164) (Figs. 16–19). It is the rhomboid intersection of these collagen fibres with their concertina-like pattern that permits the shortening and lengthening of the cord (35). During this dimensional change there is a variation in the angle of intersection of the fibres forming the network; and in full elongation of the cord the fibres suddenly present a significant resistance to further deformation; axially disposed collagen fibres, too, such as those in the linea splendens—slightly telescoped in extension—suddenly present resistance as soon as they are fully drawn out (35, 192). A similar phenomenon has been recorded in maximum shortening of the cord; here, the collapse of the rhombi is arrested at a certain angle of intersection of the fibres (35). Any tendency for the cord to shorten further through the action of an abnormal force is resisted by the fibres and the cord will suddenly kink. The cross-sectional area of the cord, and hence that of the nerve-fibres themselves, are thus prevented from increasing beyond a certain limit (35).

The rigid collagen fibres that invest the cord converge at regular intervals to form the attachments of the dentate ligaments. These suspensory structures enter the dura, to which the cord is thus firmly anchored (192); when this network is drawn upon, either in the transverse or axial direction, it can broaden or lengthen to a limited degree through a change in the angle of intersection of the collagen fibres.

In both the grey and white matter the neuroglial fibres appear to form spirals or a rhomboid network. Through these structures, together with the presence of the intercellular fluid, a normal distance is maintained between the nerve-fibres. The arrangement of the neuroglial fibres suggests that they, too, are suddenly arrested in extreme functional positions, thereby preventing over-stretching of the nerve-fibres (p. 115).

Blood-vessels (54, 111, 254–6)

Under certain conditions the spinal cord tissue displays typical stratification, as is observed in histological sections. Transverse sections show numerous clefts—more prominent near the periphery of the cord—through which run vessels of both the extrinsic and intrinsic circulations; where they overlap they follow the same direction (Figs. 17, 24, 25). It was asserted in 1889 that the perivascular spaces in the brain and cord are artefacts, but it is evident from their arrangement and the characteristic biomechanical deformation of the surrounding tissue that these clefts are anatomical features; they can, however, apparently widen considerably through shrinkage during fixation (35). Moreover, these perivascular spaces are the lymph ducts of the cord (118, 146). From the architecture of the surrounding connective tissue and glial strata and the deformation that they undergo during the elongation and shortening of the cord it is evident that not only do these channels drain the cerebrospinal fluid but that their walls protect the blood-vessels against mechanical damage (Figs. 19, 20). Along the larger of these perivascular channels, at least, run collagen fibres which also are disposed in a rhomboid pattern (Figs. 21, 22). When they are drawn out and pressed together they, like the fibres in the epipia, presumably present sudden resistance. They thus behave similarly to the neuroglial fibres, which can be followed more readily in histological specimens because of their greater number.

When the cord *shortens* axially the transverse channels running between the intersecting glial fibres are kept patent by these fibres; they can be seen in both sagittal and coronal sections. At the same time the tendency for the tissue investing the channels to collapse is also counteracted by the resistance of the collagen fibres in the walls of the channels. The channels running axially are also kept open by the collagen fibres which, when compressed axially, bend away from these perivascular channels and displace the tissue towards the surface of the pia mater (Figs. 24 A, 25).

In *stretching* of the cord the protective function of the collagen fibres comes into play in the reverse sequence. The axially running nerve- and glial fibres are then pulled around the transverse perivascular channels (Figs. 24 B, 25). The tendency for constriction of these channels is then counteracted by the sudden resistance of those collagen fibres of the rhomboid network which run transversely and parallel to the channels. Narrowing of the axially coursing channels when stretched is presumably resisted by the stiffening collagen fibres running in the axial direction (192). The constrictive tendency of the stretched cord tissue is thus counteracted, and any lateral pressure on the blood-vessels is prevented.

These structural features and mechanisms may to some extent protect the blood supply of the cord also during pathodynamic pressure on, or slight transverse compression of, the cord tissue. The treatment of this question in the next chapter is anticipated here in its appropriate functional context.

The anterior spinal artery occupies a fairly protected position in the anterior median fissure. When the stretched cord is subjected to pressure—for instance, by an osteophyte located anterior to the cord—all arteries running anteroposteriorly in the cord are also protected from compression, so long as this is moderate (see below). On the other hand, the increase in transverse tension acting in the coronal plane of the cord and resulting from elongation of the spinal canal, tends to reduce the lumina of the arteries running transversely in this plane and thus to produce neurological damage (54, 148).

In true compression (pinching or clamping of the cord) it is chiefly those lateral branches of the central arteries running in the axial direction that are exposed to harmful over-stretching; the sagittal branches of the central arteries which have been telescoped in extension are at first elongated within the normal range, but when the local tension is great enough they rupture (Fig. 65). From experimental cord compression in the cadaver it would appear that tearing of vessels will start when compression has reduced the anteroposterior diameter of the cord by somewhat more than one-fifth.

Fig. 1. The cervical spine in full flexion and extension.

Diagram drawn from two superimposed radiographs with the base of the skull as the reference.

In flexion the cervical canal is elongated, in extension shortened. The change in length is greatest for the posterior aspect of the canal. In the illustrated case the difference measured in mid-canal is about 3 cm.

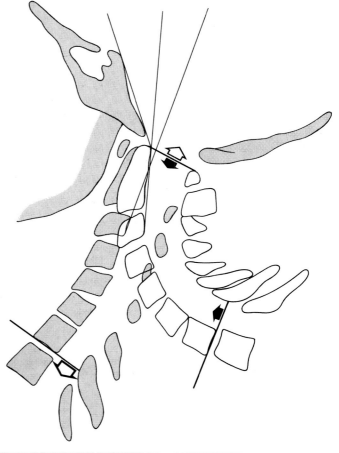

Fig. 2. Normal deformation of dura, cord and nerve-roots in the cervical canal in the cadaver due to full extension and flexion of the cervical spine.

A. *Extension*. The dura, cord and nerve-roots in the cervical canal are slack; the root-sleeves have lost contact with the pedicles (*lower arrows*), and the nerve-roots with the inner surfaces of the sleeves (*upper arrows*).

B. *Flexion*. The dura, cord and nerve-roots are drawn out, the root-sleeves come into contact with the pedicles, and the nerve-roots with the inner surfaces of the sleeves.

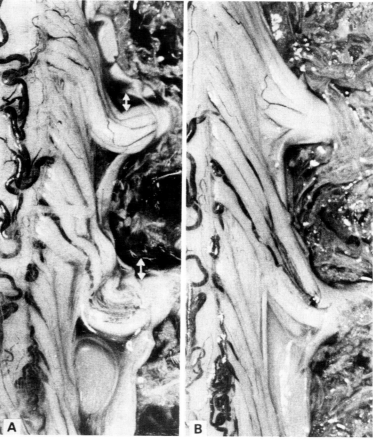

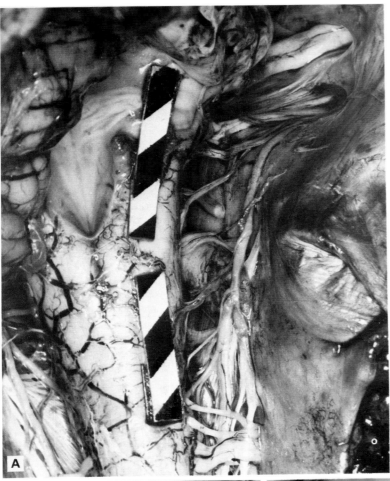

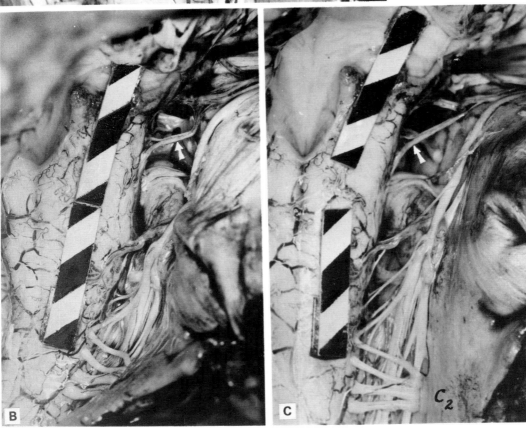

Fig. 3. Effects of flexion and extension of the head and cervical spine on the uppermost section of the pons–cord tissue tract and associated nerve-roots.

After removal of the occipital squama and the arches of the atlas and axis, the dura has been reflected and stitched to the bone; the right cerebellar hemisphere has been removed in order to expose the cranial nerves in the pontocerebellar angle. At the top of the photographs are seen the facial and acoustic nerves, and at the bottom the C_2 posterior nerve-roots. The junction between the posterior fossa and the upper cervical canal is located at the uppermost dentate ligament. Paper markers have been attached (at one end) rostrally, on the lateral aspect of the rhomboid fossa, and caudally, on the right lateral aspect of the medulla oblongata.

A. Survey of the area described; the cervical spine is in *slight flexion*.

B. With the spine fully *extended* the markers have been inserted so that their ends are just in contact. The section of the pons and oblongata seen in the photograph has shortened and slackened, as have the cerebral nerves in the posterior fossa and the nerve-roots in the upper cervical canal.

C. On full *flexion* the ends of the markers have moved apart. All the soft-tissue structures, including the nerves, running in the axial direction are elongated and stretched to their maximum physiological extent.

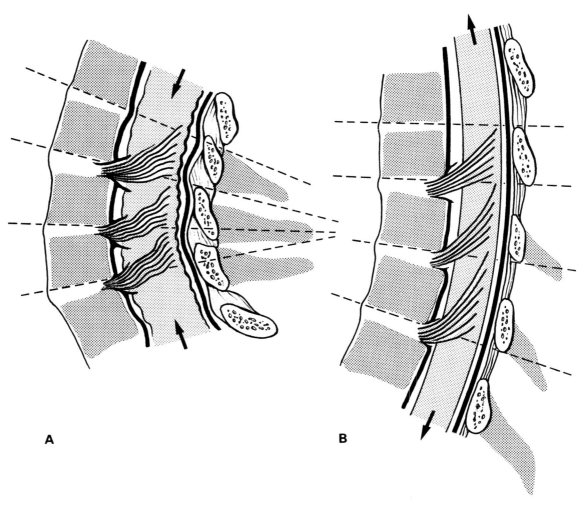

Fig. 4. The biomechanical effects of postural changes on the soft tissues in the cervical canal.

A. *Extension*. Slackened nerve-roots and protruding ligamenta flava.

B. On *flexion*, elongation of the cord and nerve-roots is permitted by the slackening of the cord tissue and the elasticity of the fibres.

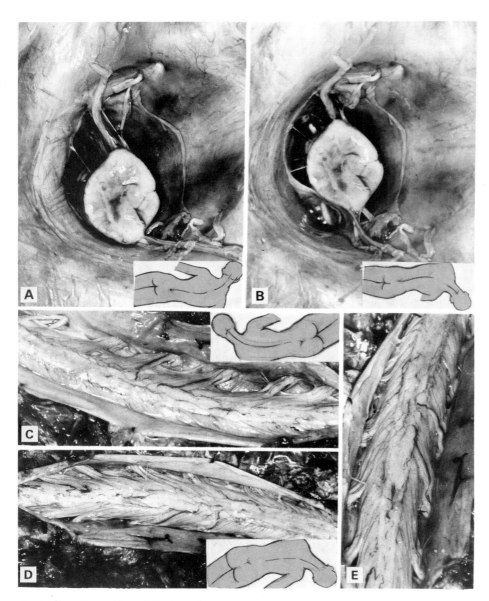

Fig. 5. The effect of lateral flexion of the cervical spine on the position of the cord in the canal.

Cord seen from the base of the skull.

A. With the body in the *right lateral position* and the cervical spine neutral but *flexed to the left* (away from the table), the left wall of the canal is shortened. This produces folding of the dura on this side, and hence relaxation of it and the dentate ligaments; as a result the cord drops on to the lower right surface of the (elongated) canal.

B. *Right lateral position* and cervical column *flexed to the right* (towards the table). The left side of the cervical canal is elongated, and the dura and dentate ligaments on this side are therefore stretched; this sets up unilateral tension in the dura and dentate ligaments and thus raises the cord to the middle of the canal. (Owing to an adhesion the arachnoid on the right side has been raised together with the cord.)

The cord seen from behind (same conditions as in A and B).

C. *Left lateral position* and cervical spine *flexed to the right*. The slack dentate ligaments and nerve-roots on the upper aspect of the canal are drawn out under the weight of the relaxed cord.

D. *Right lateral position* and cervical spine *flexed to the right*. As a result of the stretching of the dura on the upper surface of the canal the dentate ligaments and nerve-roots are stretched and the cord is raised to the middle of the canal.

E. *Erect position* and cervical spine *flexed to the right*. On the left side the dura, dentate ligaments, nerve-roots and half of the cord are stretched, and on the right side they are relaxed.

Fig. 6. The effect of extension and flexion of the cervical spine (and the resulting slackening and stretching of the dura) on the position of the cord in the cervical canal.

A. With the body in the left lateral position and the cervical spine *extended* the cord sags towards the left aspect of the canal.

B. In *flexion* of the cervical column, with the body in the same position, the cord is raised to the middle of the canal owing to the tension set up in the dura and the dentate ligaments.

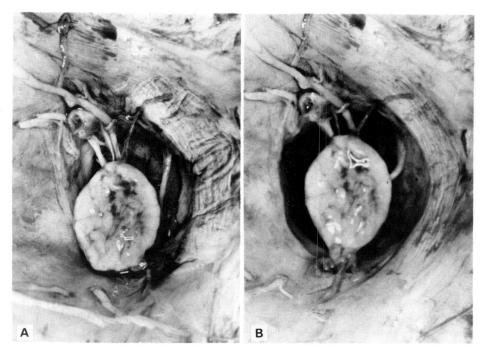

Fig. 7. The atlanto-epidural cavity.

A. Its posterior wall seen from the base of the skull. (The cavity has been exposed by removing the covering dura.)

B. The cavity filled with contrast medium in the cadaver.

C. A histological section showing the cavity walls.

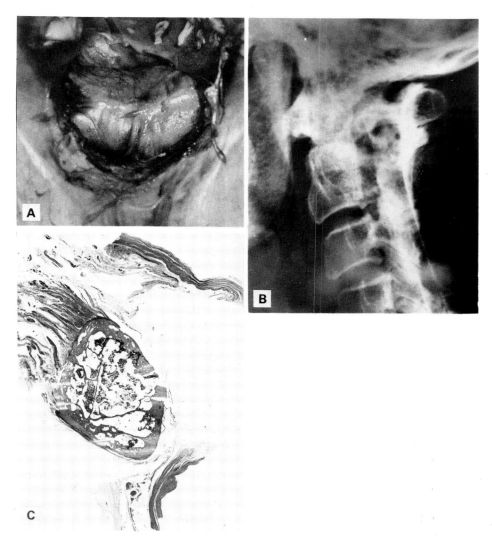

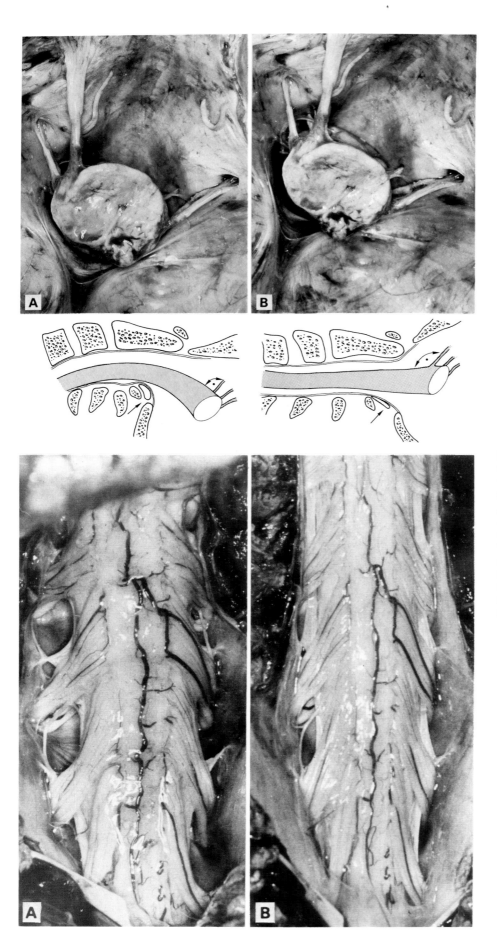

Fig. 8. The effect of extension and flexion of the cervical spine on the cranial nerves and cord. (The pons has been separated from the mesencephalon. V–XII on the left side and VI–XII on the right are preserved.)

A. *Extension*. Through the shortening of the cervical canal the dura mater together with the dentate ligaments and the cord has slackened and folded. This results in contact between the oblongata and the folds of the atlanto-occipital dura. The cranial nerves are stretched under the weight of the pons and oblongata (whose cerebellar support has been removed). The wall of the atlanto-occipital cavity, which bulges on extension, bears on the cord and thus prevents it making contact with the bone.

B. *Flexion*. Because the rostral anchorage of the mesencephalon has been severed there is no increase in tension in the pons–oblongata or the cranial nerves. On the other hand, the elongation of the cervical canal causes stretching of the dura, dentate ligaments and cord.

Fig. 9. Effect of slackening and stretching of the cord during postural changes of the cervical spine, with the body supine *(viewed from below)*.

A. *Extension*. Under the weight of the slackened cord the dura at the sites of attachment of the dentate ligaments has gone into folds, which bulge into the canal.

B. On *flexion* the dura is stretched, thus pulling the dentate ligaments taut and eliminating the folds in the dura. The nerve-roots now form a smaller angle with the axis of the cord, and the veins follow a straighter course.

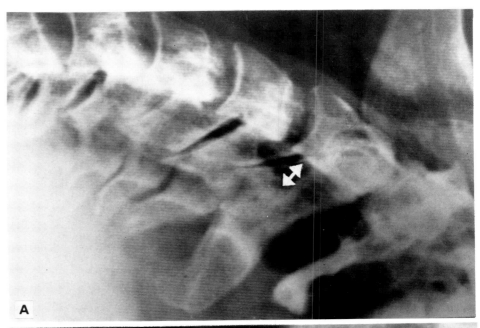

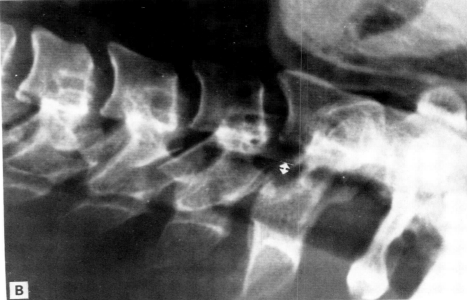

Fig. 10. Gas myelogram of the cervical cord in the supine cadaver.

A. *Extension* of the cervical spine. The cord has sagged on to the posterior surface of the canal. *Arrows* indicate the distance between the anterior surfaces of the canal and the cord.

B. *Flexion* of the cervical spine (slightly less than the maximum obtainable in the living subject). The cord has approached the soft-tissue structures on the anterior surface of the canal (*arrows*). The fact that they are now further from the bone (most clearly evident along the odontoid process) than in extension reflects the stretching of the dura. A wide radiolucent strip can now be seen along the posterior aspect of the cord, as far as the upper border of the fourth vertebra.

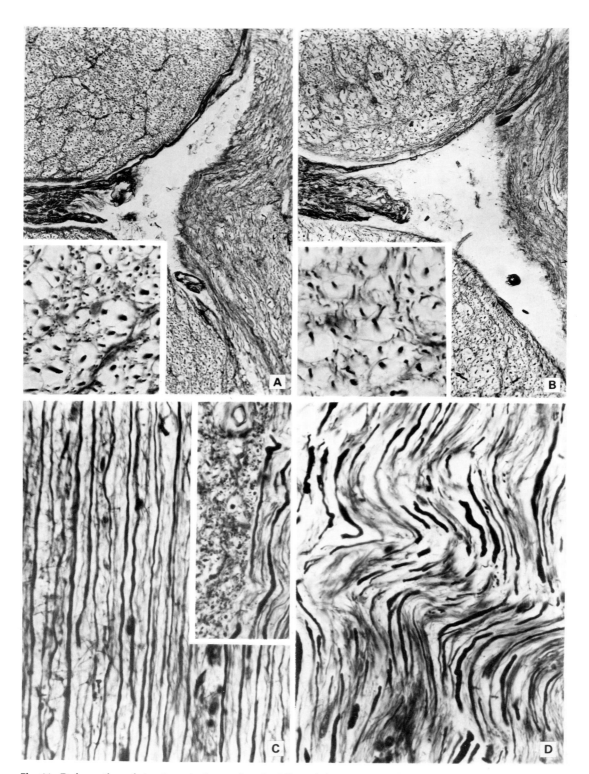

Fig. 11. Deformation of structures in the cord in changes of spinal posture.

A, B. Transverse section through the cord (×155).

A. Effect of *elongation of the cord*, produced by *flexion*, in the region of the anterior median fissure and the anterior white commissure. *Inset*. White matter of the sulco-marginal fasciculus (×525).

B. Effect of *shortening* produced by *extension*. The mechanical events are similar in principle to those observed in an elastic cylinder (Fig. 12); the fissures and the white matter increase in width. *Inset*. The widening is accompanied by evidence of an increase in cross-sectional area of the axis-cylinders and myelin sheaths, and a decrease in the intercellular distance.

C, D. Sagittal section through the cord (×525).

C. Effect of *elongation* on the nerve-fibres. *Inset*.—Boundary zone between grey and white matter (×490).

D. Effect of *shortening*. The fibres have separated, and, in some areas, increased in thickness. Because of the three-dimensional folding they cannot be followed throughout their length.

Fig. 12. Model of an elastic cylinder indicating the deformation of any cavity within the spinal cord tissue subjected to axial tension on flexion of the column.

Upper row, cross-sections. *Lower row*, longitudinal sections.

White arrows, applied force. *Black arrows*, direction of displacement of the material.

A. No force applied.

B, C. The cavity is elongated in the direction of the applied force and its cross-section reduced.

Fig. 13. The effect of axial compression *(left)* **and tension** *(right)* **of an elastic cylinder on any round hole containing a rigid cylindrical rod** *(darkly shaded area).*

(To simplify the presentation both the hole and the rod have been placed centrally in the cylinder.) This model represents the deformation of, and stresses produced in, the spinal cord containing an unyielding body when the cord is subjected physiologically to axial compression and tension.

On *compression* the cross-sections of cylinder and hole are widened and the rod becomes loose. On *stretching*, the cylinder's cross-section is reduced, and the rod is subjected to increasing pressure.

The circles (*upper left quadrant*) represent axis-cylinders with their myelin sheaths; the space around the rod represents any intracellular space in the tissue (Fig. 11) and the rod itself an unyielding pathological structure, such as a scar or circumscribed oedema.

The probable deformation of the myelin sheath during the shortening and lengthening of the axis-cylinders is illustrated by the rings adjoining each cylinder. When the membrane of the axoplasm is elongated the cross-sectional area diminishes, but as the surrounding myelin sheath is inelastic it tends to undergo compensatory folding. On experimental pinching of myelinated peripheral nerve-fibres, which results in their short-range over-stretching, the cross-sectional area of the axoplasm has, in fact, been observed to be accompanied by infolding of the myelin sheath.

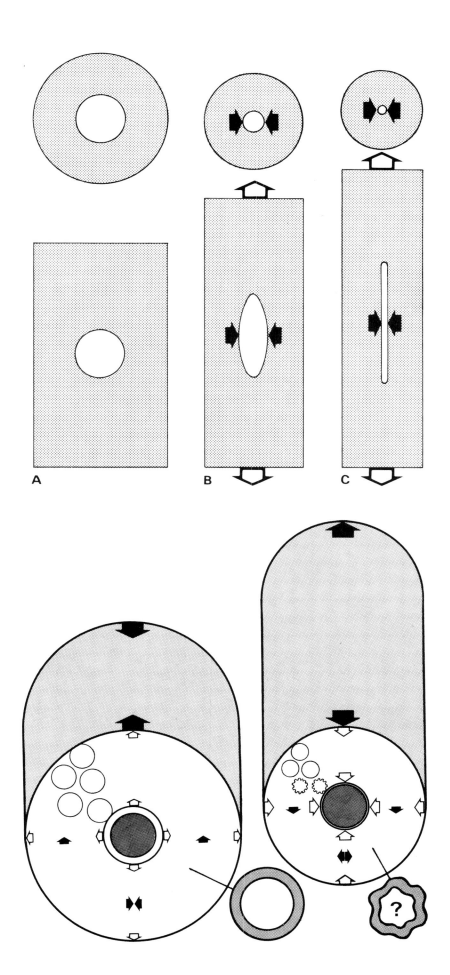

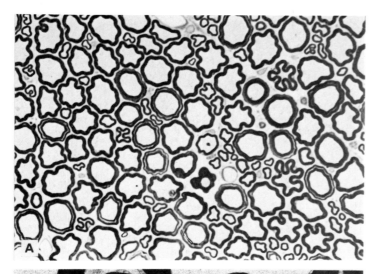

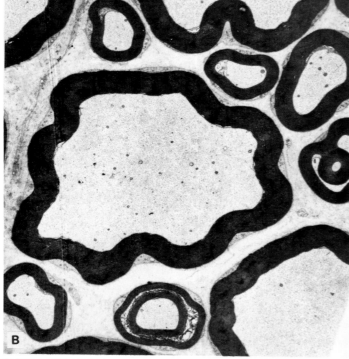

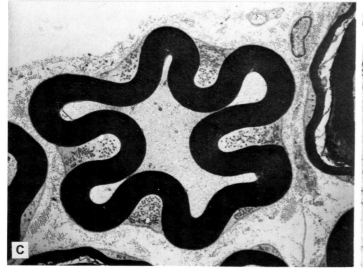

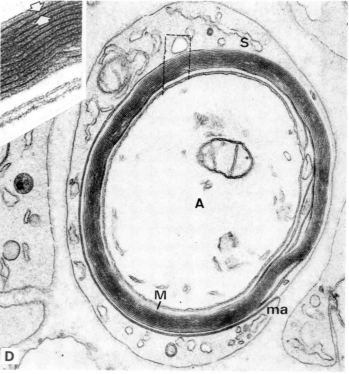

Fig. 14. Electron micrographs of myelinated fibres of nerve-roots and peripheral nerves.

A. Cross-section through L_7 anterior nerve-root (adult cat). Specimen fixed by perfusion with 5 per cent glutaraldehyde. Light micrograph, ×1140.

B. L_7 anterior nerve-root (adult cat); cross-section through internodal region. Fixation as in A. Electron micrograph, ×3800.

C. L_7 anterior nerve-root (adult cat); cross-section through paranodal region. Fixation as in A. ×2850.[1]

D. Cross-section through nerve-fibre of an 8-day-old mouse. *A*, axon; *ma*, mesaxon; *S*, Schwann cell, containing mitochondria and elements pertaining to the endoplasmic reticulum. Specimen fixed with $KMnO_4$; electron micrograph, ×21,000.
   Inset. Higher magnification of part of the myelin sheath showing its lamellar structure. *Arrows*, a lamella. Bottom, axon membrane. Electron micrograph, ×122,000.

E. Longitudinal section of a nerve-fibre (sciatic nerve) of a 15-day-old mouse. Circumferential structure of the segments of the myelin sheath: *A*, axon; *Nf*, neurofibrils; *Mi*, mitochondria; *V*, multivesicular bodies; *BM*, basement membrane.

F. The myelination process near a node of Ranvier.

G. A transverse and a longitudinal section through the node in F.[2]

[1] Courtesy of C.-H. Berthold, M.D., Karolinska Institute, Stockholm (19).
[2] Courtesy of A. Bischoff (21). (From A. Bischoff, Sandorama 8–9, 1958. With kind permission of the Editor.)

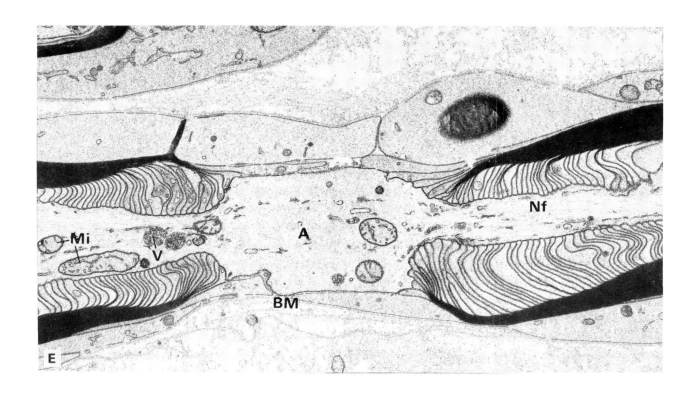

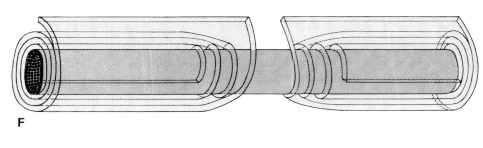

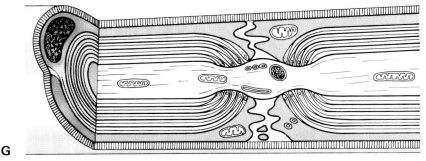

The most probable site of rupture of nerve-fibres in the spinal cord in over-stretching.

In some published histological sections the cross-section of the human myelinated nerve is seen to be roundish and contains a slight depression caused by the nucleus of the Schwann cell (20, 21). However, in the young mouse, cat and rabbit and reportedly also in the young human (19), a crenated myelin sheath has been observed.

The myelinated nerve-fibre adapts itself elastically to changes in length of the struc-tures to which it is anchored. A reduction of the cross-section of the nerve-fibre due to physiological stretching diminishes the cross-sectional area of the axoplasm and hence of the myelin sheath; this dimensional change seems to be accommodated by crenation. Conversely, on relaxation of the tension in the nerve-fibre the myelin sheath recovers its circular shape.

Micromanipulatory experiments in the frog have shown that—contrary to what one would expect—the weak point of the mye-linated nerve-fibre does not coincide with the node of Ranvier. The region that yields on pathological traction is instead located within one of the short myelinated sections of the fibre, where its (normally varying) calibre is narrowest (232). This seems to be true also in man. It has been observed under the operat-ing microscope that when a spinal cord speci-men is subjected to excessive tension the nervous substance diminishes in cross-sec-tional area before tearing occurs. Immedi-ately after the fibres are torn they retract and droplets form, which presumably consist of myelin (35).

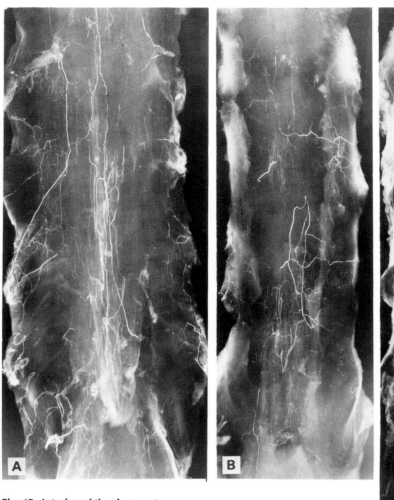

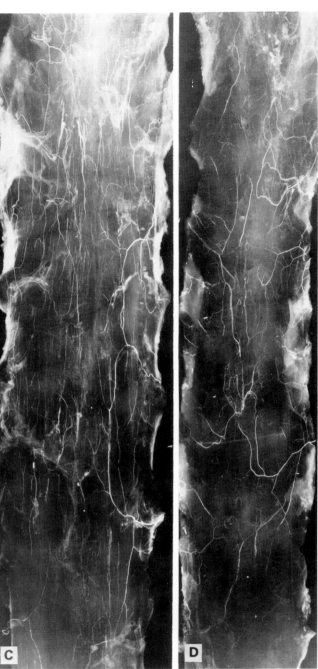

Fig. 15. Arteries of the dura mater.

A, B. Posterior walls. C, D. Anterior walls.

The arteries enter transversely at the level of the root-sheaths and soon assume an axial course—particularly on the posterior side. The posterior wall is thicker and slightly less elastic than the anterior one, and has a poorer arterial supply (186).

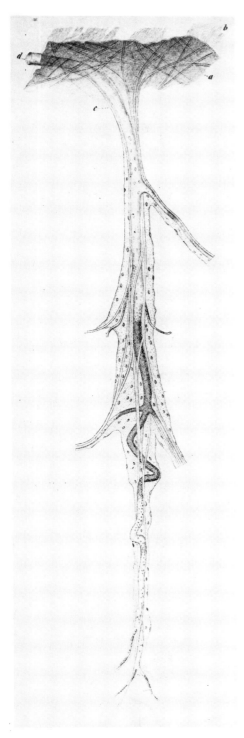

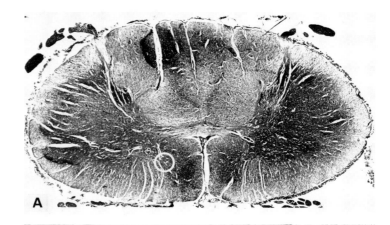

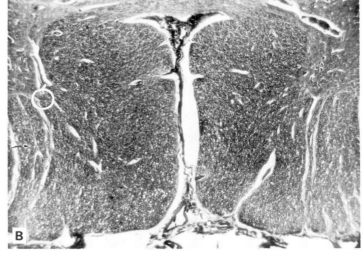

Fig. 16. The rhomboid pattern of the collagenous fibres in the pia.

They follow the arteries, and surround the wall of the perivascular space to form a funnel-shaped network (164).

Fig. 17. Transverse section through spinal cord at C_6 level, formaldehyde-fixed *in situ* **in neutral position of the spine.**

A, B. The most prominent clefts in the specimen are more or less parallel to the axons of the anterior and posterior nerve-roots.

C. Fibres from the ganglionic layer in the anterior horn follow an irregular course through the middle cleft. The neuroglial fibres in the clefts probably keep these open to accommodate minor blood-vessels. (Deformation of this region due to pressure exerted by osteophytes (Figs. 30, 31).)

Magnification, A, ×9; B, ×21; C, ×79.

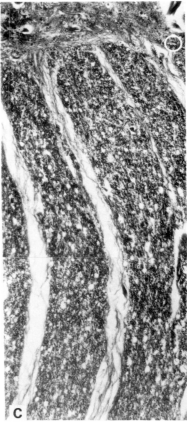

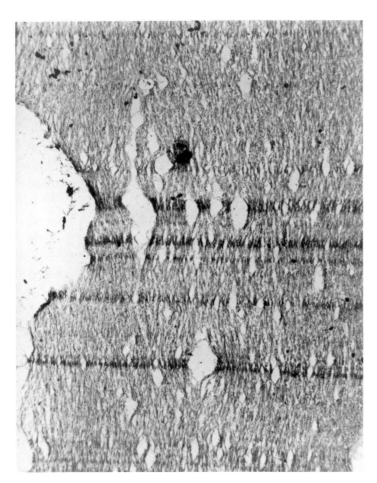

Fig. 18. The rhomboid pattern of the (three-dimensional) spinal cord network seen in a coronal histological section.

The pattern is fairly conspicuous in this specimen because nearly all the blood-vessels have been torn from their Virchow-Robin spaces.

(The dark transverse bands are obviously sectioning artefacts. The reason that they appear at levels where the transverse width of the spaces is greatest may lie with the greater resistance to sectioning of the more densely packed fibres at these levels.)

Fig. 19. Configuration of the fibres and the shape of perivascular spaces in the stretched and slackened state of the cord.

Coronal sections through the cervical cord fixed *in situ*. In, and on each side of, the mid-sagittal line (*centre of each picture*) are channels containing blood-vessels.

A, B. *Flexion*. When the cord is elongated the fibres approach each other so that the contours of the channels are denser (*darker*).

B. Two of the uppermost channels seen in A. Between the two channels there is evidence of a rhomboid fibre network (Fig. 22).

C, D. *Extension*. When the cord is telescoped the fibres in the network are folded.

D. In a greater magnification of the lowermost vessel in C a thin layer of tissue is seen to line the channel. The channels are kept patent by the deflection of the fibres that occurs when the cord shortens.

Van Gieson's stain. A, C, ×96; B, ×270; D, ×340.

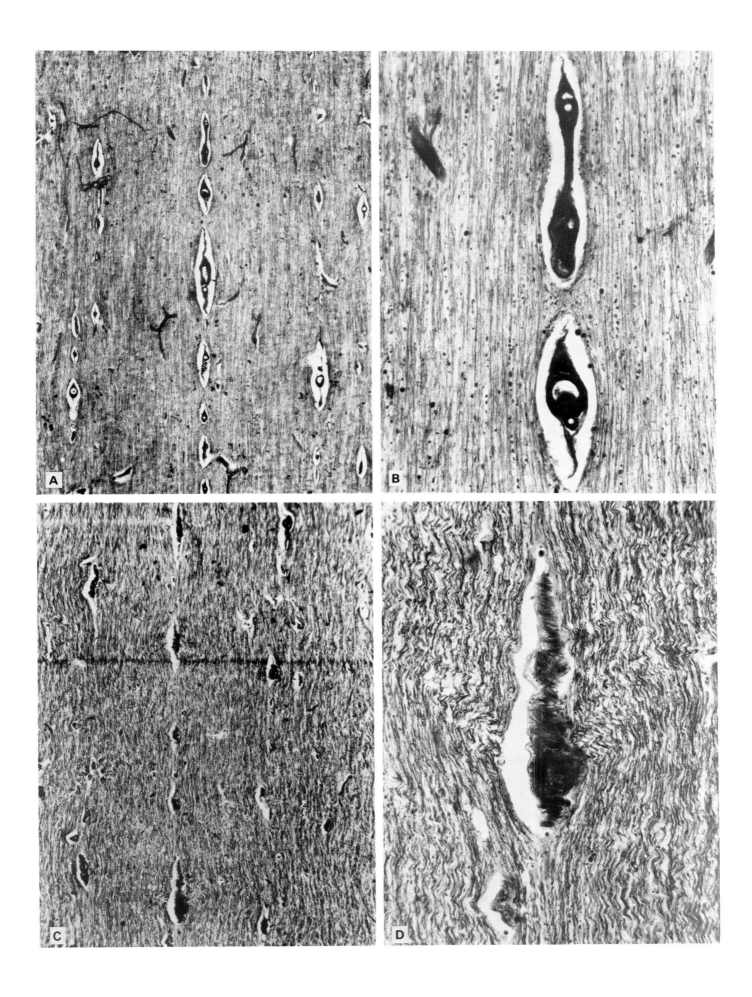

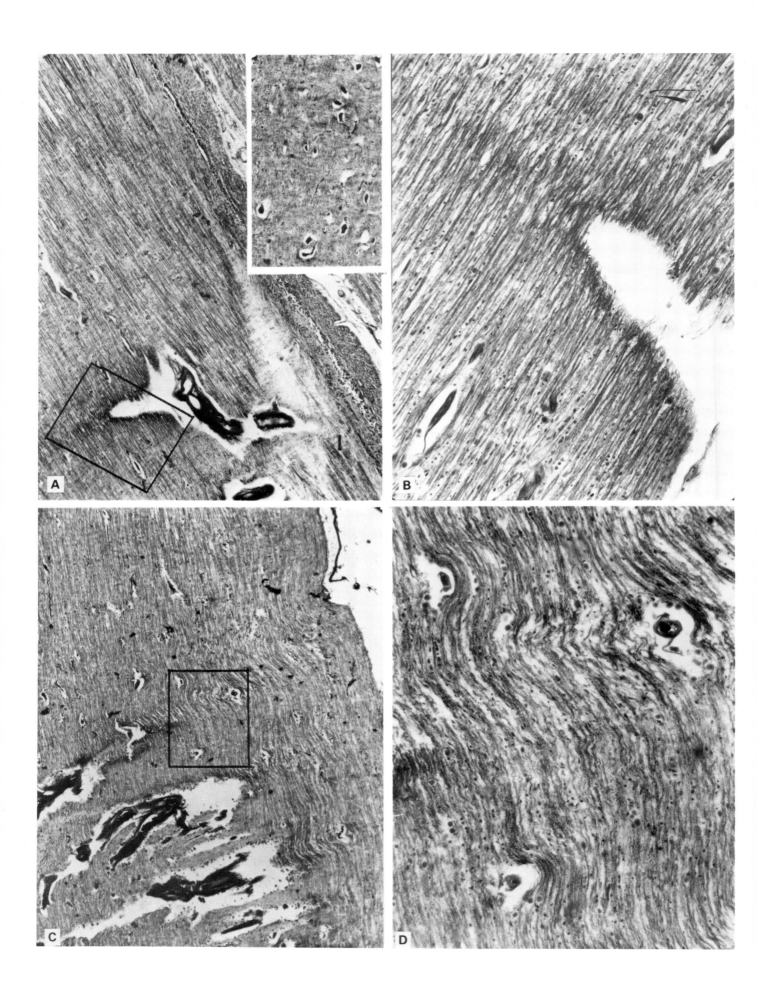

Fig. 20. Configuration of the fibres and the shape of the perivascular spaces in the stretched and slackened state of the cord.

A, B. *Flexion.* Mid-sagittal sections through the cervical cord fixed *in situ. Inset.* Area with channels running in the transverse plane of the anterior grey commissure.

B. (Framed area in A.) Bifurcated canal containing branches of the central artery. Around the canal the fibres are more compact, as in the coronal section in Fig. 19.

C, D. *Extension.* The fibres are curved around the channels, this resulting in denser packing.

Van Gieson's stain. Left pair, ×28; *right pair,* ×128.

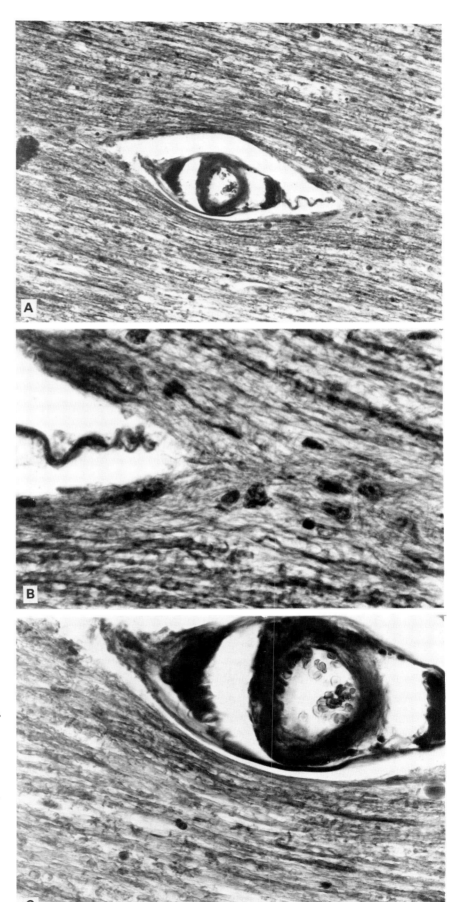

Fig. 21. Structural arrangement of the cervical cord tissue around a perivascular space.

Coronal sections through the cord, formaldehyde-fixed *in situ* with the spine flexed. The major axis of the space lies in the craniocaudal direction of the cord.

A. In flexion the axial nerve- and glial fibres bordering the perivascular space are approximated.

B. Between two spaces the fibres form a rhomboid network.

C. The fibres bounding the space are under particularly great tension. The artery (containing erythrocytes) is surrounded by an elastic sling (Fig. 23).

Palmgren's stain. A, ×330; B, C, ×900.

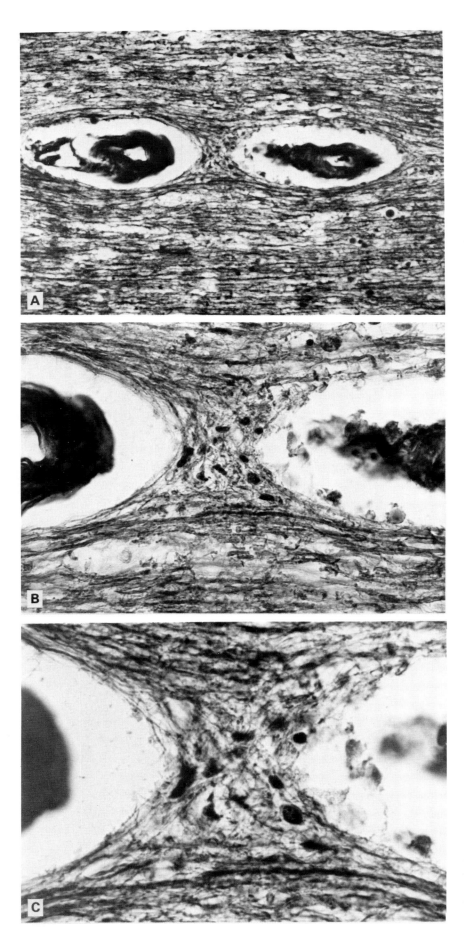

Fig. 22. Coronal histological section through the cervical cord showing the structure of the tissue between two perivascular canals.

The angle of intersection of the fibres forming the rhomboid network changes slightly when the cord is stretched and relaxed.

Palmgren's stain. A, ×250; B, ×500; C, ×900.

Fig. 23. Retinacula of the cord vessels; a structure preventing interference with the blood circulation during physiological deformation of the cord.

A, B. Coronal sections through the cervical spinal cord.

Arterioles suspended in their canals by retinacula. The vessels are surrounded by slings whose coiled ends are anchored in the cranial and caudal grooves of the perivascular spaces. If, as here, the retinacula are damaged on sectioning they retract and curl. Their elastic property is demonstrated by van Gieson staining. (A large number of retinacula are seen in Fig. 19.)

Palmgren's stain. ×350.

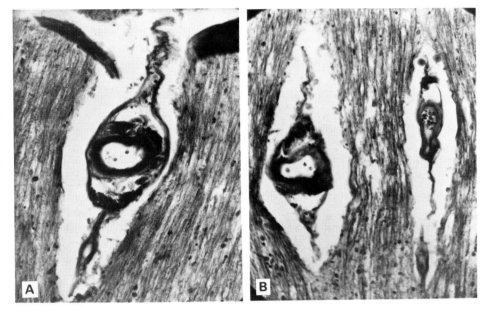

Fig. 24. The effect of extreme spinal postures on the blood-vessels of the cord.

Microangiograms of two transverse sections of the cervical cord at the C_6 level, formaldehyde-fixed *in situ*.

A. *Extension*. The area of the posterior columns has a U-shaped border, which is demarcated anteriorly by the anterior white commissure and laterally by the posterior horns. The posterior contour of the columns bulges outwards, and there is a definite impression between the medially located fasciculus gracilis and the adjacent fasciculus cuneatus (×12).

B. *Flexion*. The pia mater is drawn out axially, and at the same time stretched in the transverse direction by the dentate ligaments. The forces thus set up produce a slight, though perceptible, anteroposterior compression of the cord tissue. This has resulted in folding of the blood-vessels of the peripheral circulation, most clearly visible in the area of the posterior columns. There is also a marked local pathological tortuosity. The outward bulging of the contour of the posterior columns has been eliminated (×12,5).

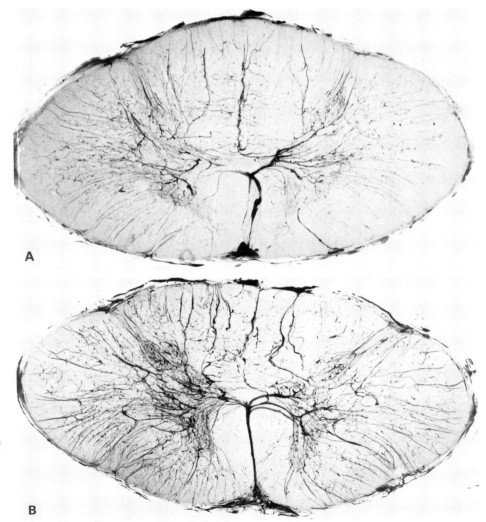

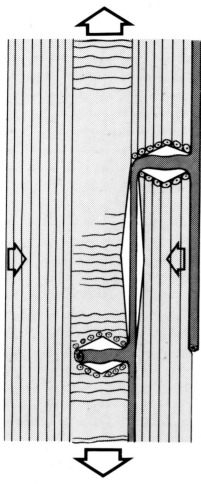

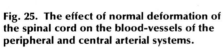

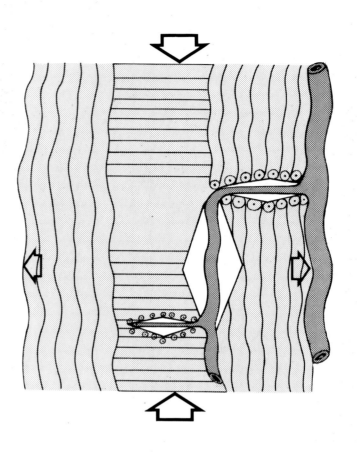

Fig. 25. The effect of normal deformation of the spinal cord on the blood-vessels of the peripheral and central arterial systems.

On elongation (*left*) the vessels running axially are straightened and those running transversely are folded; on shortening the cord (*right*) the effect on the respective vessels is reversed.

Pathodynamics of
the pons–cord tissue tract

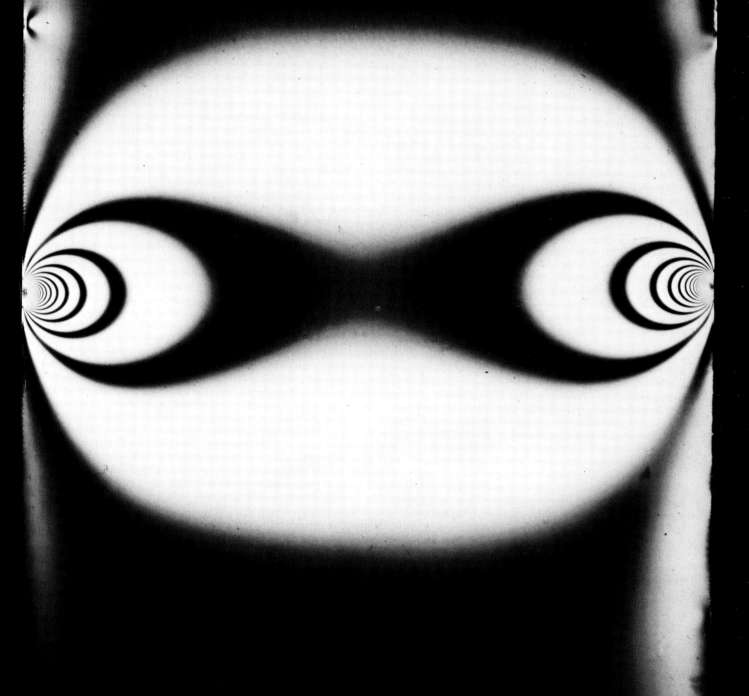

Compression

Pathodynamics of the pons–cord tissue tract

Transmission of tension by the soft tissues in the spinal canal

Physiological axial displacement

When the spinal canal is shortened by full extension of the column all the soft tissues within it slacken and go into folds. The tissue reserve so formed covers the requirements between full extension and the neutral position of the spinal canal, during which there is thus no axial displacement of the soft tissues in the canal. From the neutral position to full flexion the tension in the soft tissues steadily increases. During this phase there is an axial shift of the pons–cord tract within the dural theca (238) and also of the latter in the spinal canal, but this is quite small and difficult to discern (35). A better insight into the displacement of the dura in the spinal canal might be obtained by considering, instead, the displacement of the vertebrae along the dural theca.

The posterior aspect of each vertebral body, together with its arch, form a rigid skeletal tube. When the spinal canal is elongated during flexion these tubes move apart different distances according to their level, whereas the elongation of the elastic dural theca is uniform over its length. During this separation of the vertebrae there may be some axial shearing between them and the dura, even though the latter is anchored by fibrous attachments to the endosteum of the canal and the occipital bone around the foramen magnum. The tethering, slightly mobile, fibres in the anterior epidural space which form a network filled with lipoid tissue and veins, have been referred to as the 'displacement layer' (Verschiebungsschicht) (169). On separation of the vertebrae in forward and lateral flexion of the spine the vertebrae are displaced along this layer through the transmission of physiological and pathodynamic forces from one section of the dura to another (Fig. 28).

Pathological axial displacement

Stretching and displacement of the dura in the canal

If, in a cadaver, the cervical dura is gripped with Pean's forceps on its posterior border and pulled cephalad, a peculiar effect is noticed. At a distance of only 2 vertebrae caudal to the forceps the force of traction is transmitted round the entire dural theca so that the part of the dura diametrically opposite to the site of traction is stretched by about 2 mm in the cranial direction. Thus, the lateral and anterior aspects of the dura move the same distance in the cranial direction as the posterior aspect. This displacement is transmitted the length of the dural theca—to all the dentate ligaments, and hence to the thoracic and lumbar cord and the root-sheaths and nerve-roots, including those of the cauda equina. Conversely, traction applied caudally to the dura in the lumbar canal is transmitted to its cervical part. With the cervical spine flexed and the corresponding segment of the dura stretched, the tension is transmitted round the dura to its attachments at the foramen magnum. Unlike cephalad traction, which causes the root-sheaths to be drawn slightly closer to the pedicles of the vertebral bodies, caudad traction causes the sheaths and nerve-roots to move away from the pedicles. So long as the conditions in the regular displacement layer are normal these phenomena appear to be consistent.

The transmission of these tensile forces complies with a well-known physical principle, known as Saint-Venant's law, the precise explanation of which is still unknown. The application of axially directed traction at a point on the border of an elastic cylinder produces local stretching of the tube wall, the magnitude of which decreases parabolically on either side of the line of traction (Fig. 27 C). The force producing this local extension is thus distributed round the cylinder. At a distance below the rim of the cylinder not exceeding 2 times its diameter all points on the circumference will be displaced the same amount. The effect is the same irrespective of the magnitude of the elasticity of the material of which the cylinder is made.

Effect of displacing the dura in various postures of the spine

This study was performed on 9 cadavers. On applying traction cranially to the posterior part of the dura at the cervicothoracic level with the thoracolumbar spine extended, the dura could be moved an appreciable distance before a cranialward movement of the lumbosacral dura, conus medullaris and nerve-roots was seen. The resistance to traction was greater with the spine in the neutral position. When the thoracolumbar spine was flexed, resistance to cranial traction was immediate, and very little cranial movement of conus, lumbosacral dura or roots could be seen.

When cranialward traction was applied to the dura at C_1/C_2 with the neck extended the dura was initially slack and could be drawn up several centimetres before resistance was felt and the traction transmitted to caudally located structures. With the neck flexed the dura was taut and resistance to cranial traction was immediate. In the laterally flexed position, the cervical dura was taut on the convex side and slack on the concave, the differences when applying traction on the two sides being marked.

On lateral flexion of the thoracolumbar spine of the laterally recumbent cadaver, similar differences in tension of the dura on the two sides of the canal were seen. When cranialward traction was applied to the thoracic dura on the convex, stretched side, small diagonal folds were seen in the dura running infero-laterally from the point of traction to the concave side. This phenomenon visualizes the transmission of tension round the dural theca from the point of traction (Fig. 27 D). In the cadaver, of course, the only component of the cerebrospinal fluid pressure is hydrostatic; in the living subject the greater CSF pressure may inhibit the phenomenon of diagonal folding of the dura.

Pathological obstructions to transmission of the tension in the dura

In two 70-year-old cadavers the application of traction to the cervical dura with the cervical spine flexed produced no recordable effect on the dura or tract in the lumbar region. On the other hand, flexion and extension of the cervical spine produced the usual, though slightly less marked, stretching and slackening of the dentate ligaments, and hence of the tract, in the lower thoracic and lumbar regions. In these cases there was scarring of the dura and firm adhesion to the endosteum of the cervical and upper thoracic canal (222). It is evident from this observation that to obtain the described relative displacement between the dura and the endosteum in the spinal canal a certain relationship is required between the stiffness of the dura and the stiffness and mobility of the fibres in the epidural displacement layer. The stiffer the dura is, or becomes on applying traction, and the slacker the fibres in this layer, the further will the axial displacement be transmitted, though normally the local displacement at any level will hardly exceed about 3 mm.

Mechanical basis for physiologically and pathologically increased tension in the dura

On flexion of the spine the vertebrae are angulated and the posterior surfaces therefore separate. Between each pair of vertebrae the dura, which is otherwise anchored to the endosteum of the vertebrae, is stretched; the tension in the component sections is additive (37, 40, 41). (The presence of tension in the dura may be confirmed by making short transverse incisions at the levels of the intervertebral discs, when retraction results in oval gaps.) Local stretching of the cervical dura produces a high local tensile stress, while the resulting displacement of the dura in the lumbosacral region also gives rise to tension, though diminished because of transmission losses. If the normal cranialward displacement of the dura on flexion of the spine is prevented by a pathological structure in the lumbar region (osteophyte, herniated disc, tumour, etc.) the tension in the dura above the lesion will be increased by cervical flexion. If the cervical dura is already under abnormally high tension owing to a pathological alteration in the cervical region (and if the fibres in the displacement layer are intact) the resulting tension in the dura in the lumbosacral region will be still greater—if, for example, a herniated disc in this region interferes with the cranialward displacement of the dura. The root-sheaths and nerve-roots will then be exposed to a large increase in pressure. The greater the axial tension in the root-sheath the greater will be the pressure on the nerve-root; a bending tensile stress will then be set up in its tissue, and neurological symptoms, including pain, may be elicited.

Pathological tension in the dura and its sources

The most important of the numerous causes of tension in the dura is the presence of protrusions into the spinal canal, especially those from the anterior and antero-lateral direction. Another important source is epidural tumours; if these are large they can give rise to pathological tension even if they impinge on the posterior aspect of the dura.

From observations on the application of traction to the stretched dural theca it is evident that the pre-tension in it promotes immediate transmission of any additional tension over great distances. In the living subject the normal dilatation of the arachnoid membrane and dura by the CSF pressure produces a low uniform pre-tension in the dura, which is augmented by any abnormal tension; this accounts in some measure for the direct propagation of tension in it. Scarring in the epidural displacement layer can result in permanent fixation of the dura in a position of tension and thus limit the normal relaxation of the dura in extension (35, 222). It is important to bear in mind this possibility in neurosurgical operations undertaken to slacken the dura and pons–cord tract, for it might account for unsatisfactory results, especially as regards lumbosacral root symptoms.

If, in flexion of the cervical spine, two cervical vertebrae are abnormally angulated as a result of, for instance, osteochondritis or disc degeneration, the dura will be over-stretched along the posterior longitudinal ligament. Such an effect may also arise from a protrusion into the cervical canal from its anterior aspect, which raises the dura. In this case the conditions responsible for stretching of the dura are similar to those obtaining in experimental traction at a single site.

The local tension set up in various sections of the dura

by pathologically increased angulation between two or more vertebrae, or several large protrusions in the spinal canal is additive. Since the caudal end of the dura is firmly anchored in the sacral canal the aggregate tension in the cervical and, possibly also the thoracic, dura is transmitted to the lumbar region.

Mechanical effect of structures impinging on the spinal cord or a nerve-root

When a structure impinges upon biological tissue possessing elastic properties the mechanical consequences are dependent on the texture and other properties[1] of the tissues involved, the applied force, the area on which it acts and a variety of other factors. To determine the effect of the impinging structure is thus a complex problem. Nonetheless, a conception and a qualitative impression can be obtained from an analysis of the stress field in photoelastic models. In Fig. 136, an Araldite block[2] is subjected to bending alone and to bending combined with stretching; the isochrome pattern shows that the components of stress due to the axial and bending tension are additive.

Histodynamic effect of structures impinging on the dura and pons–cord tract from the anterior wall of the spinal canal

The term 'impinging structure' is used below to denote any pathological structure that protrudes into the spinal canal from its anterior or anterolateral wall and that exerts local pressure on the dura and pons–cord tract, thereby displacing them; the term is also used of pathological intradural structures exerting local pressure on the cord tissue. Such pressure on the dural theca with its root-sheaths, and on the pons–cord tract with its nerve-roots, occurs only in flexion of the spinal column; extra- and intradural impinging structures will then have much the same effect. Any analysis of neurological symptoms due to extradural structures must therefore take account of the effects of displacement and tension on the dura and root-sheaths.

Extra- and intradural impinging structures exert their maximum pathodynamic effect in full flexion of the spine, when the stretched dura and spinal cord are pulled against them. Because the path round the obstruction(s) is then lengthened, over-stretching of the whole pons–cord tract will result, and this will ultimately behave as an inelastic string. In theory, the full pathodynamic effect will then be transmitted uniformly from one end of it to the other; but in practice the pathodynamic tension acting in the whole pons–cord tract, and especially in the cervical cord, will be much greater when it is produced by an impinging structure in the *cervical* canal than by one located caudally. As the angles that the emergent thoracic and lumbar nerve-roots make with the cord are smaller than those made

by the cervical nerve-roots, there is a greater resistance to cord tension originating cranially than caudally (Fig. 93). For this reason a source of raised dural tension in the cervical region (for example, the deformation caused by osteophytes at, say, the C_5/C_6 level) is more likely to be a source of neurological symptoms than a comparable lumbar lesion. In the presence of both, the pathological tension set up by the cervical lesion may actually precipitate symptoms from the lumbar lesion, while the reverse effect is less likely (Figs. 29, 94).

Besides over-stretching of the tract, the impinging structures set up local bending tensile stress in the cord in both axial and transverse directions. This histodynamic stress will increase with the number of pathological structures protruding into the spinal canal. Depending on their prominence, the symptoms and neurological signs evoked by impinging structures may be widespread. Axial tension transmitted to the brain stem can affect the basal nuclei; transverse tension is transmitted direct to the cervical nerve-roots. If cervical flexion provokes radiating sciatic pain or a sensation of tension in the lumbar region, the over-stretching of the dural theca and the pons–cord tract will evidently have pulled and pressed one or more lumbar or sacral nerve-roots against one or more protrusions in the lumbosacral canal—that is, remote from the site of the movement responsible for the tension (Hyndman's sign). If there is a large impinging structure near a cervical intervertebral foramen that evokes symptoms on flexion of the cervical column, and a relatively small impinging structure near a lumbosacral intervertebral foramen that does not evoke symptoms on flexing the lumbar spine alone though it does on flexion of the cervical spine, the structure in the cervical section may be regarded as a 'generating protrusion' and the lumbar one as the 'precipitating protrusion'. It must be observed that the effect on the lumbosacral nerve-roots of a small protruding structure in the cervical region will be incomparably greater than will the effect of even a large lumbar protrusion on the cervical nerve-roots.

It is useful to observe a distinction between 'generating' and 'precipitating' protrusions if only to draw attention to the fact that, say, a thoracic kyphosis can produce over-stretching which, in the presence of a precipitating protrusion, in another region of the pons–cord tract may evoke neurological symptoms of even greater importance. This is illustrated by Maxwell and Kahn's case of a thoracic kyphosis (187), where there was probably a minor impinging structure in the cervical canal. (*Cf.* the conditions accompanying 'brachialgic sciatica' and 'sciatic brachialgia', p. 111.)

Remote symptoms may originate from over-stretching of nerve structures in regions where no precipitating (stimulating) factors would normally be expected. For instance, tic douloureux may conceivably be elicited at the same time as sciatic pain if the extended leg is

---

[1] E.g. plasticity, frictional resistance, compactness.
[2] Araldite, CIBA Products Company: Fair Lawn, N.J. USA; Duxford, Cambridge UK.

flexed at the hip-joint and there is a precipitating structure in the relevant region, namely, the trigeminal nerve-root. To understand the underlying mechanism it is necessary to recognize that in this movement (Lasègue's test) the lumbar spine is always flexed and that the sciatic nerve, the lumbosacral plexus and the whole pons–cord tract are thus stretched. If, in the case of a protrusion into the lumbar canal, there are pathological changes around the trigeminal root[3] then on performing Lasègue's test the trigeminal root will also be stretched[4] and thus stimulated to the point where a tic douloureux attack may be evoked (Figs. 94, 134) in addition to sciatic pain (author's observation in the case of a middle-aged male patient).

Experimental elimination of axial tension in the dura and the soft tissues of the spinal canal

If, after removal of, say, the C_7 vertebra, the bodies of the C_6 and T_1 are brought together until their facets articulate, the 'excess' of dura at the level of vertebra C_7 and the root-sheaths of segments C_7 and C_8 will be slack (Fig. 34). The upper thoracic dura will slip about 2 mm caudally (Fig. 35), but this effect may not be visible in the thoracic and lumbosacral canal. The dural theca will still be held by the fibres in the epidural displacement layer in much the same position as before the vertebra was removed. Therefore, so far as the relaxation of the dura at caudal levels is concerned, the effect of removing a whole cervical vertebra is no greater than that of lowering of a single intervertebral disc at a high level.

If the C_7 vertebra is removed with its articular processes the only connections between the cervical and the thoracolumbar spine are the skin, muscle, vessels, the dura and spinal cord. If the two parts of the spinal column are flexed or extended separately one will see the same biomechanical phenomena in the dura, root-sheaths, spinal cord and nerve-roots as before the separation. That is to say, the cervical and thoracolumbar cord with their nerve-roots will be drawn out in the same way and to the same extent as in the intact specimen when the two parts are flexed together, while in extension there will be the usual shortening and slackening.

Relaxation of the pons–cord tract

Of particular interest are the undetermined tensile forces in the nervous tissue in well-defined conditions of pathological stress. Since they are diminished by pons–cord relaxation an analysis not only of their magnitude but also of their range would be of value; but no method for such an analysis has been found. While it is recognized that relaxation of the pons–cord tract is due to slackening of its suspensory apparatus along the whole spinal canal, we still require to know the contribution of the component structures. One difficulty presented by a quantitative analysis is that their movements are too small to be seen with the unaided eye. Hence, it is difficult to compare the relaxation after resection of the C_7 vertebra with that obtained in extension of the cervical column.

An analysis of the magnitude and range of the tensile forces, rather than of the relaxation, may be more rewarding. The range of these forces by which histo-dynamic stresses are set up within the tissues can be found by a mechanical method. With the cervical and lumbar canal exposed, caudalward traction on the lumbar cord in the neutral position of the spinal column produces tautening of the cord along the cervical cord into the pons. This effect becomes increasingly marked the greater the flexion of the cervical spine, and can be observed for displacements of little more than one millimetre. On the other hand, when the cervical column is extended the effect of this traction extends only to the thoracocervical cord. Conversely, cranialward traction applied to the upper cervical cord with the cervical spine flexed and the thoracic spine in the neutral position is propagated only to the lower cervical cord; it exerts no visible effect on the thoracolumbar cord and cauda equina until the whole tract is brought under tension, as by raising the thoracic cord from the canal. The same effect results from full flexion of the thoracolumbar spine; there is then a small but visible cranial movement of the lumbar cord. On raising the lower cervical cord from the canal, or on pulling it caudally, the effect on its cranial end will decrease the more the cervical spine is extended, and increase with the degree of flexion. In other words, the greater the straightening of the pons–cord tract the greater the range of this tension in it and hence in its nerve-fibres; and the more marked the relaxation the shorter the range of displacement, until there is ultimately just a local effect. This means that the risk of histodynamic stress is eliminated.

To summarize, when the distance between two adjoining vertebrae is shortened the dura, nerve-roots, dentate ligaments and spinal cord in the associated section are relaxed; this is accompanied by a slight reduction in the tension in more remote structures (Figs. 34–39).

[3] For example, root-sleeve fibrosis, degenerative changes of the myelin sheaths of the nerve-fibres with consequent fragmentation or other pathological processes near the rim of the petrosal bone that can give rise to artificial synapsis (116).
[4] Bending tensile and notch stresses will also be set up in its tissue (Fig. 68).

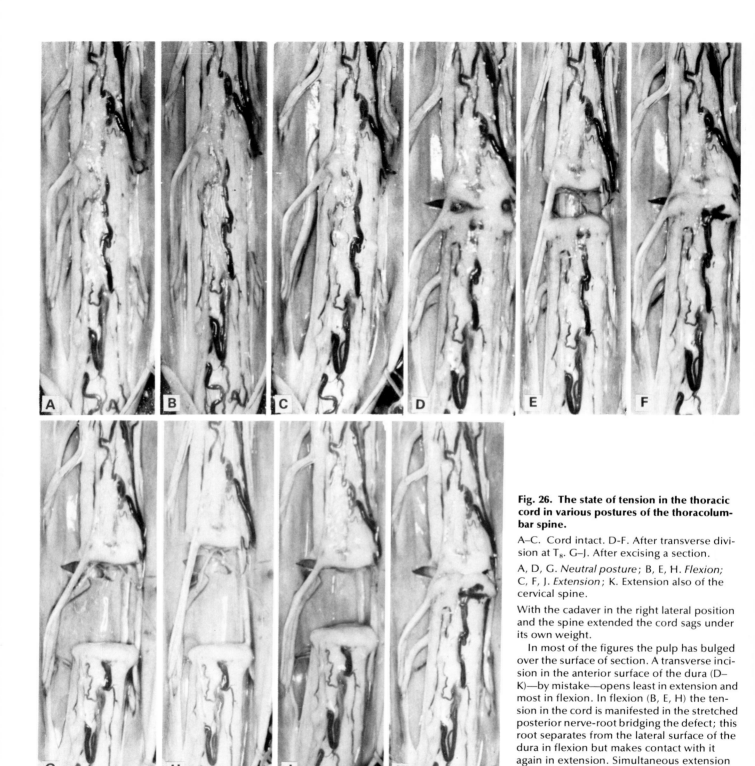

Fig. 26. The state of tension in the thoracic cord in various postures of the thoracolumbar spine.

A–C. Cord intact. D-F. After transverse division at T_8. G–J. After excising a section.

A, D, G. *Neutral posture*; B, E, H. *Flexion*; C, F, J. *Extension*; K. Extension also of the cervical spine.

With the cadaver in the right lateral position and the spine extended the cord sags under its own weight.

In most of the figures the pulp has bulged over the surface of section. A transverse incision in the anterior surface of the dura (D–K)—by mistake—opens least in extension and most in flexion. In flexion (B, E, H) the tension in the cord is manifested in the stretched posterior nerve-root bridging the defect; this root separates from the lateral surface of the dura in flexion but makes contact with it again in extension. Simultaneous extension of the cervical spine (K) has further relaxed the cord.

Fig. 27. Transmission of tension in the dura.

A. Exposed upper cervical and lower thoracolumbar canal.

B. *Cranialward* traction applied with a Pean's forceps to the posterior rim of the dura in the cervical region produces a small movement in the same direction around the whole circumference of the thoracic and lumbar dura. This movement is transmitted by the dentate ligaments to the spinal cord and the lumbosacral nerve-roots (*arrows in A*). The traction is mediated by the fine fibres composing the displacement layer of the dura.

C. Axial traction applied at a point on the rim of an elastic cylinder extends part of the cylinder wall (*upper shaded area*). Beyond a distance of about 2–3 times the diameter of the cylinder below the rim, the tensile force is distributed uniformly (*lower shaded area*) around the circumference (Saint-Venant's law).

D. The curved cylinder represents the dura in the cervical canal in lateral spinal flexion. On the convex side the dura is drawn out and stretched (*arrow*), while on the concave side it is slack. Any tensile force applied to the convex side will be immediately transmitted, whereas when such a force is applied to the concave side the slack must first be taken up.

The same effect is found in other elastic tissue cylinders—for instance, in the pia mater of the spinal cord and nerve-roots. It has implications in various pathodynamic contexts.

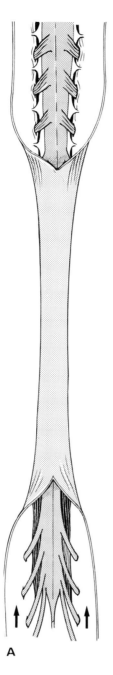

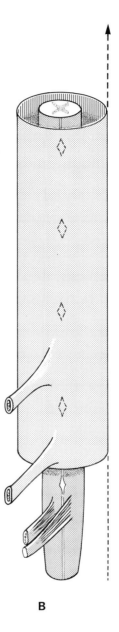

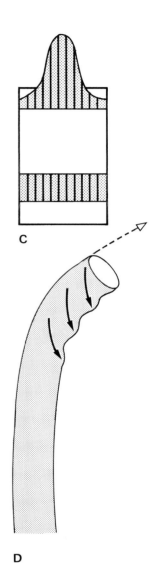

A   B   D

C

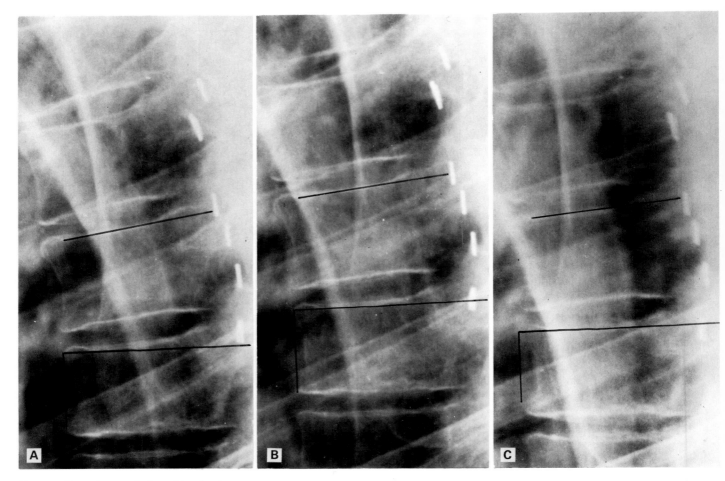

Fig. 28. Effect of transmission of tension in the dura of a living subject in postural changes of the spine.

Silver clips were attached to the thoracic dura at levels corresponding to two adjacent verte-brae in a patient operated on for rhizopathy.

The transmission is evident from the dis-placement of the silver clips in relation to the black reference lines.

A. *Flexion.* Cranialward displacement.

B. *Erect posture.* No displacement.

C. *Extension.* Caudalward displacement.

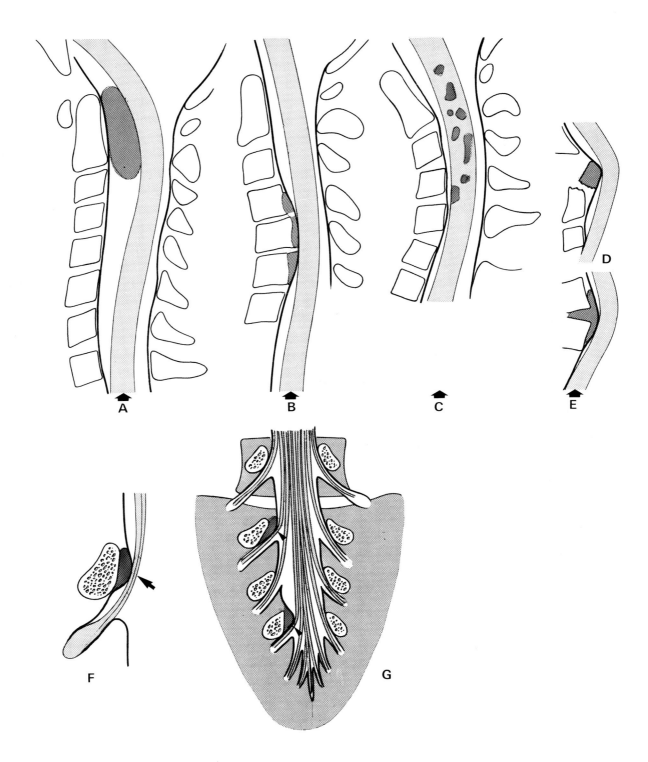

Fig. 29. Some common types of pathological changes outside and within the cervical cord causing over-stretching of the pons–cord tract, including the sacral nerve-roots.[1]

A. Anteriorly located foramen magnum tumour.

B. Spondylotic protrusions into the cervical canal.

C. Intramedullary glial tissue scar or circumscribed oedema, as in multiple sclerosis and spinal cord injury.

D. Fracture of the odontoid process.

E. Compression fracture of thoracic vertebra, with kyphotic angulation.

F, G. Pedicles deformed by osteophytic spurs.

[1] Because of pressure on, displacement of and consequently tension in the tract, produced on elongation of the spinal canal in flexion, the above sources of tension produce: (*i*) local stress fields, (*ii*) over-stretching of the whole tract, and (*iii*) secondary stress fields within remote sections of the tract—for instance, in the trigeminal or sacral nerve-roots.

Whatever their fundamental cause, these external (A, B, D, E) and internal (C) impinging structures alter the length of the path of the pons–cord tract or of the tract itself. The resulting increase in tension is transmitted caudalward from the impinging structures, along all the nerve-roots of the tract, and cranialward to the trigeminal nerve-roots. At the level of the impinging structures in the tissue passing over them, an axial and a transverse bending tension is set up. If this tension exceeds a certain magnitude, as is most likely to occur in flexion action potentials are elicited through development of

a discharging lesion (266) or the conductivity is blocked.

The increase in tension may result in over-stretching of the lumbosacral nerve-roots—which are drawn into contact with the pedicles (F, G)—especially if the pedicles are deformed or there are osteophytic spurs. Clinical experience shows that this situation also can result in neurological symptoms.

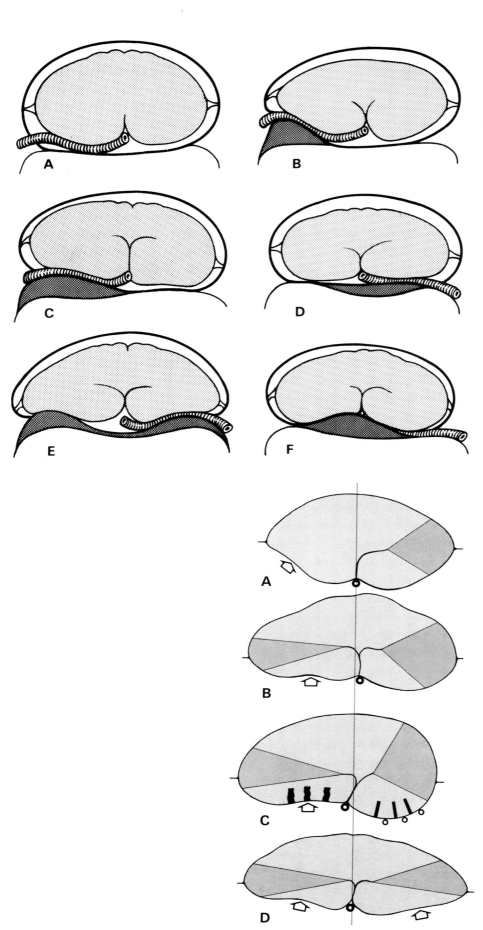

Fig. 30. Stress set up in the cervical cord by osteophytes, and constriction of the lumen of an anterior radicular artery on full flexion of the cervical spine.

Stippled area. Osteophytes.

A. Normal appearance of the cord and anterior radicular artery on flexion of the cervical spine.

B–G. If osteophytes occur at the level of an artery, the pressure they exert on the anterior aspect of the cord during flexion may result in narrowing or even complete occlusion of the lumen of the artery.

Note. On relaxation of the cord in extension of the spine the pressure of the osteophytes on the cord, and hence on the artery, is relieved.

Fig. 31. Areas of tensile stress *(stippled)* **set up in a spinal cord by pressure of osteophytes** *(arrows)* **during flexion.**

Pathologically increased transverse widening of right side (A–D) and left side (D) of cord. The resulting tension reduces the lumina of those arteries running in a transverse direction.

A–C, *left side of the cord.* Zones of physiological transverse widening of the cord tissue *(grey areas with relatively large angles)*.

C, *left side of the cord.* The vessels of the external circulation are normal *(small black lines)*.

C, *right side of the cord.* The vessels of the external circulation *(small black areas)* are folded and widened as a result of pressure exerted by the osteophyte on the anterior side of the cord.

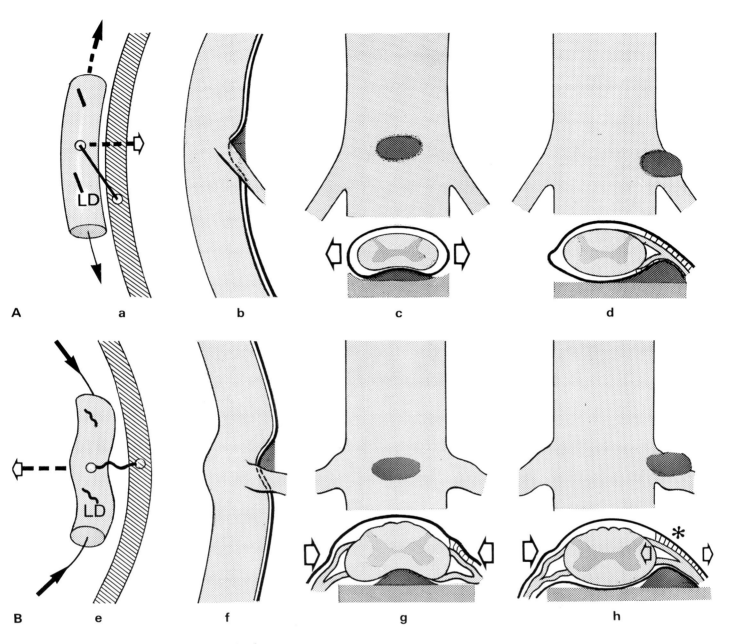

Fig. 32. Effect on a cervical cord section produced by a medial (c, g) and an anterolateral (d, h) protrusion during flexion and elimination of the effect on extension.

A. Model of the anterior wall of the spinal canal, cord and dentate ligament (LD) in flexion.

a–d. All soft tissues are stretched.
Owing to the tension set up in the cord, this is pulled towards the anterior wall of the canal.

b. The protrusion exerts local pressure on the cord and increases the axial and transverse bending tension.

c. The cord at the level of the protrusion is deformed by the transverse tension.

d. The anterior and posterior nerve-roots on the side of the protrusion are drawn into contact with it and stretched.

B. Model in extension.

e–h. All the soft tissues are slackened and (f, g) the potential pathodynamic effect of the protrusion is neutralized.

g. The deformation of the cord and nerve-roots by the protrusion is rendered innocuous by relaxation.

h. *Asterisk*. Clinically important exception. Acute anterolateral or intraforaminal discal herniation produces non-specific inflammation of the root-sheath and nerve-roots, and the swollen and thickened nerve-roots tend to shorten. This is counteracted by the fibres connecting the roots to the sheath, and the sheath to the periosteum of the intervertebral canal. The resulting bending tensile stress elicits neurological symptoms. Because of these attachments extension cannot give more than slight relief. Moreover, the resulting narrowing of the foramen may give rise to compression of the roots. The same situation applies in lumbar discal herniation.

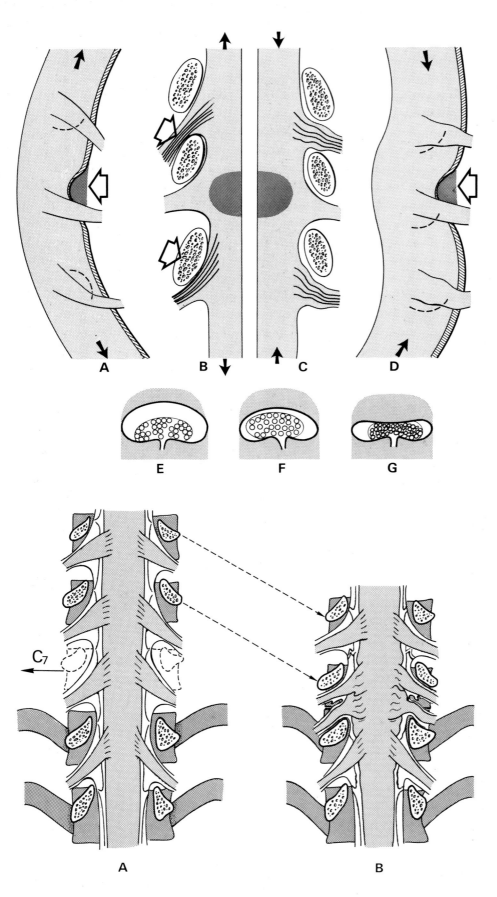

Fig. 33. Pathodynamic effects on the nerve-roots exerted during postural changes by a protrusion located on the anterior wall of the cervical canal.

Dark shading (A–D): Protrusion.

A, B. On *flexion* a pathological increase in axial and transverse tension is produced in the section of the cord that rides over the protrusion. This is reflected in flattening of the cord. Histodynamic tension is also produced in the nerve-roots at the level of and adjacent to the protrusion. As the roots are then drawn into contact with the pedicles (*white arrows*), quite small spurs—from, e.g., the uncovertebral joints—or other anterolateral pathological changes, will suffice to produce pressure and bending tension (E), and hence neurological symptoms. Protrusions located remote from the one responsible for the tension in the cord can also evoke symptoms.

C, D. In *extension* of the cervical canal, the cord and nerve-roots slacken—to a less degree near the protrusion. Although moderately large protrusions will bulge into the lumina of the intervertebral foramina (F), the relaxed roots will remain slack. The effectiveness of an operation—for instance, interbody fusion—may be ultimately determined by an unintended slight extension, which results in relaxation of the dura, cord, root-sheaths and nerve-roots. However, if the canal is narrow (G) the nerve-roots may be compressed.

Fig. 34. Effects of removing the vertebral body C_7.

A. Section of the spinal column (C_5–T_2). The appearance of the dura, dentate ligaments and cord with the body in the neutral position. The vertebral body C_7 is indicated with broken lines.

B. After removal of this vertebra the C_6 and T_1 vertebral bodies and intervertebral joints have been brought into contact. The head and cervical column are now unstable. The dura covering the vertebra C_7 has collapsed and folded. Below the vertebral body C_5 the dura and the pair of dentate ligaments have slackened slightly because the C_7 root-sheaths have lost their anchorage. Above C_5 the appearance of, and tension in, all the soft tissue structures remains unchanged. The dura along the whole of the spinal canal caudal to T_1 is also slackened to the extent permitted by the relaxation of the fibres in the epidural displacement layer and intervertebral canals. The cervical cord in the C_8 segment is telescoped to the fullest extent by axial compression. This and the resulting relaxation of the nerve-roots extend to the lower borders of the C_6 and T_1 root-sheaths. The relaxation of the root-sheaths and nerve-roots is greatest within the C_8 segment; caudal to this all the dentate ligaments, the whole of the cord, and the nerve-roots are as slack as in full extension of the cervical spine.

Fig. 35. The effect of resection of the vertebral body C$_7$ on the dura, dentate ligaments, nerve-roots and spinal cord in the lower cervical and upper thoracic canal (A, B) and in the lower thoracic and upper lumbar canal (C, D).

A. After bringing the vertebrae C$_6$ and T$_1$ together the dura at the level of resection is folded; the C$_8$ nerve-roots are quite slack and follow a serpentine course. While the nerve-roots of the C$_7$ (only the right one is visible) follow a normal course, those of the T$_1$ on the right side are clearly relaxed; the attachment of the dentate ligament passing between the anterior and posterior roots is under tension.

B. Through the extreme slackness of the tissue it is possible to raise the lowermost section of the cervical cord clear from the canal and displace it to the left. The level of resection is evident from the cleft in the anterior aspect of the dura below the now stretched C$_7$ root.

C, D. At the thoracolumbar level the soft tissues have been only slightly relaxed, as is evident when the cord has been drawn aside.

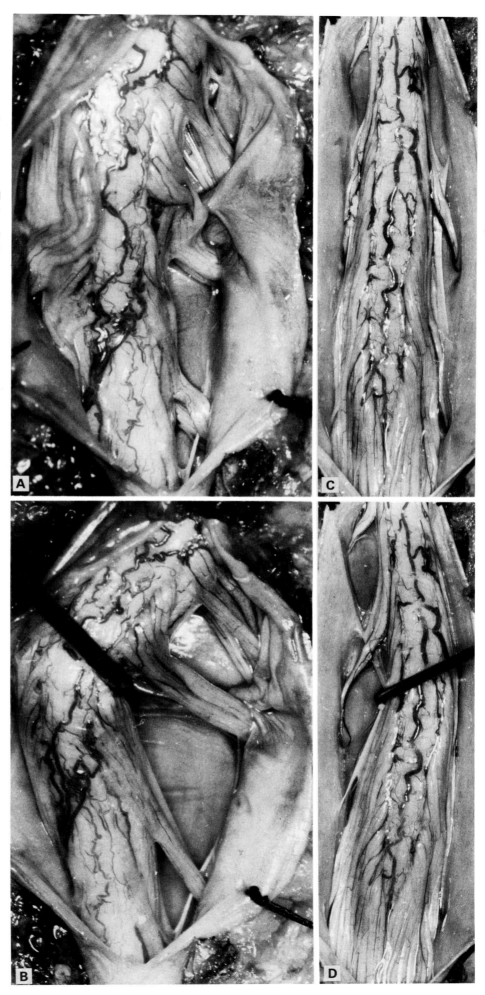

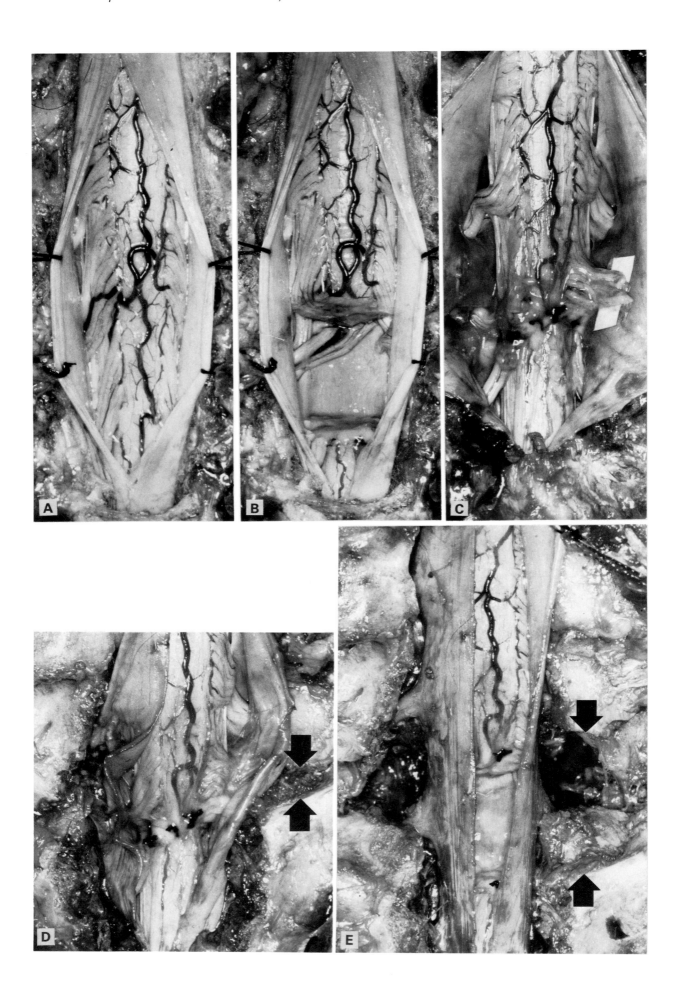

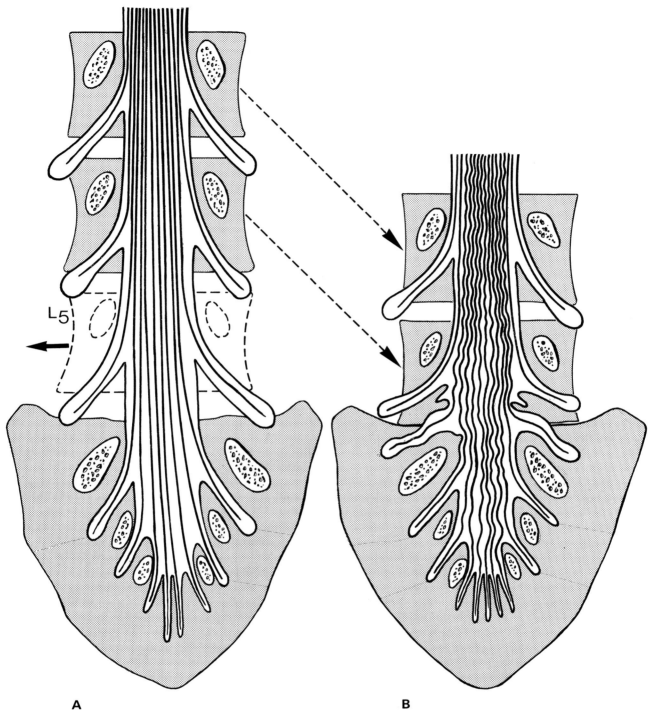

A

B

Fig. 37. Effects of resection of the vertebra L₅ on the nerve-roots; schematic representation.

A. L_3, L_4 and the sacrum; the vertebra L_5 is indicated by *broken lines*. The nerve-roots are still straight.

B. The L_4 body and the sacrum have been brought into contact. The dura at the L_5 level has collapsed and folded; its slackness can be followed to approximately the S_2 level.

Because the anchorages of the L_4 root-sheaths were not disturbed, the L_4 nerve-roots retain their tension, whereas all those caudal to the L_4 are slack, a state that can be followed to the tip of the conus medullaris. The tension in the pons–cord tract with the column fully flexed is reduced by the amount that would be contributed by the nerve-roots of the L_5–S_5 section if the column were intact.

Fig. 36. Approximation of the severed ends of the cervical cord after resection of the cord segment C_8 and the vertebral body C_7.

A, B. The posterior aspect of the lower cervical cord before and after the resection.

C. The severed cranial and caudal ends of the cord have been brought into contact and the pia has been sutured.

D, E. The borders of the lower articular facet of the C_6 and the upper facet of the T_1 after and before approximation of the vertebrae C_6 and T_1 (*black arrows*).

4–764371 *Breig*

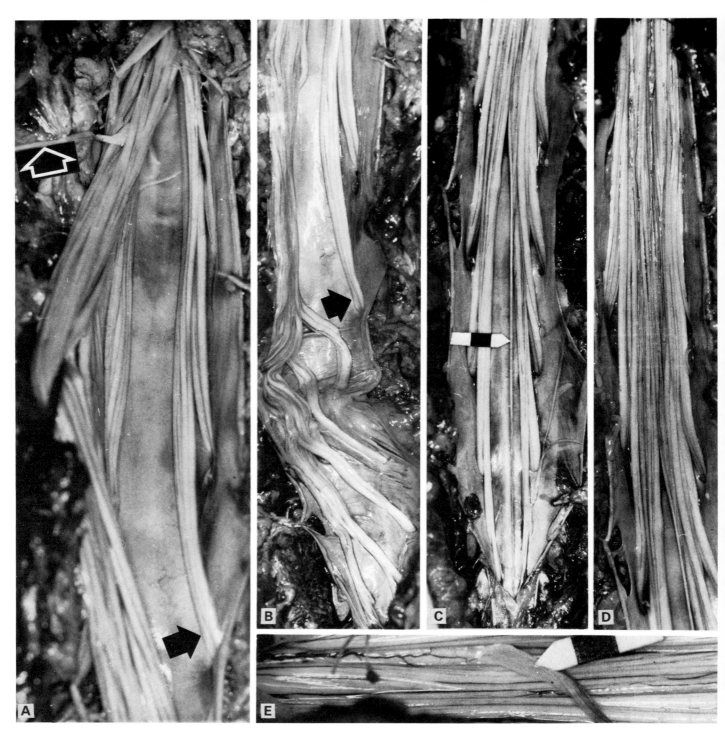

Fig. 38. Effects of resection of the vertebra L₅.

A. The completely relaxed L₅–S₅ nerve-roots, including the filum terminale, have been drawn to the side. The L₄ root (*black arrow*) is practically unaffected. The filum terminale (*white arrow*) has been severed and is deflected for clarity (higher magnification in E).

B. Completely relaxed dura below the vertebra L₄ with the slack nerve-roots. The transmission of the relaxation to the S₄ roots is seen in the sacral canal which has been exposed down to the S₄ body.

C, D. The division of the slender filum terminale (*black and white arrow*), does not contribute greatly to the relaxation of the pons—cord tract (for pathology *cf.* p. 183).

E. Higher magnification of the severed filum terminale.

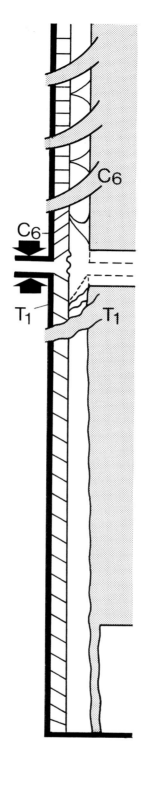
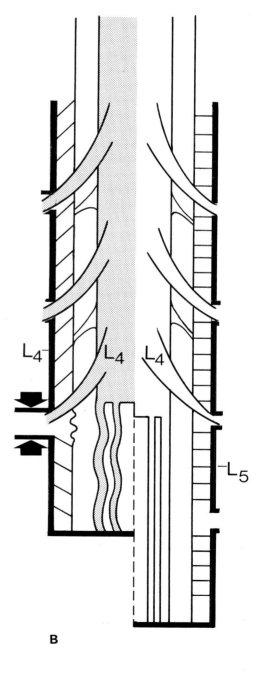

Fig. 39. Effects of resecting the vertebrae C$_7$ *(left)* and L$_5$ *(right)* on the suspensory fibres in the epidural displacement layer of the spinal canal.

(Vertebral column in neutral position.)

Opposed arrows. Section of the spinal canal as shortened by resection of the respective vertebrae.

Vertical bold lines. Limit of bone of the spinal canal.

Vertical fine lines. Dura; folded where the vertebra has been removed.

A. Along the vertebral body C$_6$ the fibres in the epidural displacement layer are drawn slightly cranialward, and below T$_1$, caudalward. As a result of the caudalward shift of the fibres the whole thoracolumbar cord and all the nerve-roots are slackened.

B. The course of the fibres in the displacement layer before *(light)* and after *(shaded)* resection of the vertebral body L$_5$.

A

B

Effects of pincer and clamping actions on the spinal cord

Both in over-stretching of the pons–cord tract on flexion of the spinal column and in compression of the tract on extension, it is in the first place the hard structures that exert pressure on the cord. In the former condition the pressure is exerted from one side on the *stretched* tract, with resulting pathological tension that is transmitted throughout the tract; in the latter condition the pressure is exerted from two opposite sides on the *slackened* tract, with resulting localized (short-range) axial tension in the cord. Factors governing the magnitude of the compressive force are the extent to which the canal lumen is reduced by protruding hard structures, the extent to which the tissues are folded and the resulting increase in diameter of the cord. The level of compression thus depends on the combined effects of the hard and soft tissues that pinch or clamp the cord. The same applies to compression of the nerve-roots in the intervertebral foramina.

For detecting compression of the cord tomographic gas myelography with the spine in *extension* has proved the most reliable method (see *Radiological diagnosis*, p. 127); but for demonstrating compression of nerve-roots in the intervertebral canal there is so far no radiographical method. The neurological indications of compression are deep muscle pain (accentuated by extension), paraesthesia and fibrillation, fasciculation and atrophy of muscles innervated by the affected nerve-roots (104). The resulting axial tension in the nerve-roots combined with the bending tension produced during *flexion* give rise to rapid, transient paraesthesia and possibly loss of power, but no specific muscular symptoms. In the case of protrusions into the intervertebral foramina the two types of symptoms not infrequently occur in the same patient on extending and flexing the spine, respectively.

As is evident from the literature, no distinction has been drawn between the two patterns of stress resulting from local compression and general over-stretching of the spinal cord and nerve-roots. Studies on the effects of compression of the cord in the dog (189) and experiments with foam rubber models (237) have thrown little light on the actual nature of the forces generated.

The forces due to pincer and clamping actions were accordingly investigated in two studies, one performed on a model and the other in the cadaver and on isolated cord and nerve specimens.

Stress field in a model

In order to visualize the state of stress that arises in a compressed material with elastic properties a transparent block of epoxy resin (Araldite) was subjected to a pincer action and the resulting stress field was observed through polarizing glass plates. The photoelastic pattern (Fig. 77 A) shows an intense axial tensile stress field at the level at which the pincer forces were applied. The axial tension is greatest in the central line and diminishes towards the surface of the compressed body (Fig. 77 B).

Cadaveric study

This study was performed to examine the effect of applying a compressive force to the spinal cord. The vessels were perfused with a radiopaque medium (18, 54) *via* a vertebral artery (Fig. 50). The cerebrospinal fluid was then replaced with 10 per cent formaldehyde injected by lumbar puncture. In 16 subjects a hole was drilled between two cervical vertebrae with the Cloward instrument, and through it a wooden dowel with a rounded tip (Fig. 42) was hammered different distances. With the cadaver prone, the neck was then extended and kept in this posture for 16 hours. The cervical dura and cord were then removed intact and preserved in 10 per cent formaldehyde for a week. The dura, dentate ligaments and nerve-roots were then dissected for microangiography.[1] In a further 6 subjects bilateral laminectomy at C_3–C_7 was performed and the cord was compressed by applying the index finger to the posterior dural surface.

Further experiments

Specimens of cord and peripheral nerves were removed for study; to the former finger pressure was briefly applied and removed, the latter were compressed by a screw-clamp (Fig. 86 A) and the specimens were fixed.

Artificial spinal cord oedema

On a fresh cadaver artificial spinal cord oedema was produced to study its probable effect on an intramedullary fissure. For this purpose a 3 mm deep and 10 mm long transverse incision was made in the exposed cervical cord at the C_5 level in the posterior columns. With the cadaver in the left lateral position and the carotid arteries and jugular veins ligated, distilled water was injected *via* a catheter in the right vertebral artery in portions of 20 ml every minute over a period of 10

---

[1] The absence of oedema and haemorrhage in the cadaver facilitates the observation of the relevant deformation and tearing of the nervous tissues.

minutes. The cord then stiffened and its mobility was reduced. It also increased in diameter and at the same time pulp was extruded from the incision, the margins of which now bulged roughly 1.5 mm over the surface of the cord. When about 200 ml of distilled water had been injected a circumscribed bulge appeared 11 mm cranial to the incision, which finally measured 7×3 mm. After about half an hour, when about 700 ml had been perfused from a suspended bottle at a pressure of about 40 cm H_2O, a similar bulge, 6×4 mm, had formed 32 mm caudal to the incision.

Skull traction with Crutchfield's forceps applied in the temporal plane and loaded with 5 kg increased the extrusion of the pulp. At the same time the actual incision, which had previously not been clearly visible, now formed a gap nearly 1 mm wide, from which distilled water oozed.

Experimental unilateral hydrocephalus

A thin rubber balloon was inserted into a lateral ventricle and inflated to produce an experimental unilateral hydrocephalus, which set up compressive stress within the brain tissue. The specimen was then fixed as above and examined, a comparison of the two halves of the brain being made (Fig. 87).

Results

The results of experimental compression of the cord *in situ* using a dowel and finger pressure are presented in Table 1 and the results of compression of isolated specimens (nos. 1–7) in Table 2.

When an isolated piece of cervical cord was compressed with the finger there was circumferential bulging above and below the site of compression. Following application and removal of light pressure the tissues retracted; but when a greater force was used the bulge was permanent. However, no appreciable deformation or displacement of the vessels could be discerned through the pia mater.

In most specimens where the anteroposterior diameter had been reduced by more than one fifth (Figs. 47, 57, 58) tears extending for three-quarters of the cord diameter were seen. In all instances of compression *in situ* the pia mater remained intact even when the spinal medulla was severely disrupted. In sagittal sections through the damaged cord transverse and diagonal tearing was found at the level of the compression. Moreover, there was a clear tendency for the ruptures to occur on the side of the cord opposite that to which the dowel was applied. Damage to the posterior grey commissure (189) and lateral displacement of the posterior columns by expressed grey matter behind the central canal (188) were rarely seen. There was evidence of tissue flow not only in the centre of the cord but also near the anterior and posterior parts of the pial sheath. Such flow below the anterior border of the pia

mater is discernible in Fig. 54, and in the centre of the cord with ensuing whirlpools in Fig. 60 Ac and C; in Fig. 82 the pons is seen stripped of the pia mater following expansion of an intracranially located balloon.

Discussion

Tissue rupture

From the transverse ruptures in the cord tissue, together with the high tensile stress demonstrated in the photoelastic model at the level at which the pincer force was applied, it is obvious that the rupture of nerve-fibres and blood-vessels is due to a pronounced local axial intramedullary tension. Comparable pincer or clamping actions *in vivo* would cause irreparable neural damage and haemorrhage. However, from clinical experience of adaptation to the pincer action exerted by hypertrophic spurs in the vertebral margins or by a slowly growing tumour it is evident that a time factor is involved: rupture due to an impinging structure will occur if the compression of the cord is too rapid to permit adequate adaptation to the tensile stress through growth of the axis-cylinders and blood-vessels. The constriction of the axis-cylinders will thus persist, with consequent impairment of conductivity.

Experimental compression of the cervical cord has been found to cause rupture of nerve-fibres identical with that observed following extension injuries of the neck (245). Transverse ruptures in the posterior zone of the cord were formerly ascribed to the forward protruding ligamenta flava; though not stated explicitly, it was presumably considered that the cord substance was torn as a result of its depression by the bulging ligament. The presence of ruptures opposite the anterior site of depression of the cord by the experimental dowel is not necessarily evidence of an impinging structure producing elevated local tensile stress, for there is another, more likely, mechanism. Because of friction between the protruding dowel and the cord the local axial tension will not be fully developed in its anterior border zone. Besides the frictional resistance between the dowel and the dura and pia mater, there is the resistance presented by the radially disposed septa and blood-vessels just below the surface of the cord, and this will also prevent superficial damage by stiffening the tissues. If it were not for the resistance due to these factors the deformed anterior border zone of the cord would also rupture. In the posterior border zone of the cord, however, a distinctly different set of mechanical conditions obtains. Even if the posterior aspect of the dura were pushed further than normally towards the centre of the cervical canal by a thickened layer of ligamenta flava, this arachnoid—dura surface is rendered so smooth and slippery by the CSF that the result of the local axial over-stretching of the cord tissue close to the pial sheath is unmodified by friction.

In the experiments there was no evidence that the

TABLE 1. Compression of the cervical spinal cord *in situ* on the fresh cadaver.

Speci-men no.	Method	Direction	Duration	Estimated (a) & actual (b) extent of constriction	Main type of damage to cervical cord at level of pincer action	Figures illustrating deformation		
						Gross	Histolo-gical	Micro-angio-graphical
1	Intercor-poral drill hole, level C_5/C_6	From anterior	Ca. 16 h	(a) 2/3, (b) complete	Total compression	50	51, 52	50, 53, 54
2	As no. 1	From anterior	Ca. 16 h	(a) relatively slight	2/3 transverse rupture in posterior zone just cranial to max. compression (>1/3)[a]		47, 60, 61	
3	Intercor-poral drill hole, level C_6/C_7	From anterior	Ca. 16 h	(a), (b) 1/3–1/2	Transverse & diagonal rupture in posterior zone of subject[a]	57		57
4	Intercor-poral drill hole, level C_4/C_5	From anterior	Ca. 16 h	(a), (b) >1/3	No rupture visible externally[a]			56
5	As no. 1	From anterior	Sudden trauma	?	Perforation of half of cervical cord. Evidence of damage in anterior zone of left half[b]			66
6	As no. 1	From anterior	Ca. 16 h	(a), (b) extremely small	No rupture visible externally[a]	43		
7	As no. 1	From anterior	Ca. 16 h	(a), (b) <1/3	Transverse rupture visible externally[a]	43		
8	As no. 4	From anterior	Ca. 16 h	(a)?, (b) <2/3	Transverse rupture visible externally[a]	43	61	58
9	As no. 1	From anterior	Ca. 16 h	(b) <1/2	Transverse rupture visible externally[a]	43	63	58, 59, 64
10	As no. 1	From anterior	Ca. 16 h	(b) <1/2	Transverse rupture visible externally[a]	43	63	58, 59, 64
11	As no. 1	From anterior	Ca. 16 h	(b) 1/2	Transverse rupture visible externally[a]	43		
12	As no. 1	From anterior	Ca. 16 h	(b) 1/2	Transverse rupture visible externally[a]	43		
13	As no. 1	From anterior	Ca. 16 h	(b) 1/2	Transverse rupture visible externally[a]	43		
14	Lamin-ectomy C_3–C_7	From posterior	Fraction of a s	(a) 1/2	Transverse rupture in anterior zone[c]	48		
15	As no. 14	From posterior	Ca. 16 h	(a) 1/2	Transverse rupture in anterior zone[c]	48		
16	As no. 14	From posterior	Ca. 16 h	(a) 1/2	No rupture visible externally[c]	48		
17	As no. 14	From posterior	Ca. 16 h	(a) 1/2	No rupture visible externally[c]	48		
18	As no. 14	From posterior	Ca. 16 h	(a) 1/2	Transverse rupture in anterior zone[c]	48		
19	As no. 14	From posterior	Ca. 16 h	(a) 1/2	Transverse rupture in anterior zone[c]			
20	As no. 1	From anterior	Ca. 16 h	(b) 1/2	Almost total compression[a]			
21	As no. 4	From anterior	Ca. 16 h	(b) 1/2	Transverse rupture in posterior zone[a]			
22	As no. 4	From anterior	Ca. 16 h	(b) 1/2	No rupture visible externally[a]			

Notes. *Functional position of cervical spine.*—Extended, except for specimens 5, 16 and 17 when spine was *straight*, and specimens 15, 18 and 19 when it was *flexed*.

Extradural compressing body.—Round wooden dowel, diam. 1.5 cm, except for specimens 14–18 (index finger) and specimen 19 (metal punch).

Mode of fixation.—Filled subarachnoid space with 10% formaldehyde just after compression, except for specimens 5 and 14–19, which were fixed outside the body.

Duration of formaldehyde fixation.—Sixteen hours, except for specimens 5 and 14–19, when it was several days.

[a] In all the experiments the cord had been fixed *in situ* with the cervical spine extended and the dowel in place in the intercorporal drill hole. The intramedullary fissure had presumably been kept open by the local tension produced by the compressing dowel; had the dowel been removed immediately after the compression, the surfaces of the intramedullary fissure would have approached each other, thus rendering the fissure less prominent.

[b] Drill hole (C_5/C_6) made—exceptionally—only after filling cord vessels with medium on mistakenly piercing dura with drill. Total derangement of tissue and vessels in traumatized zone; no appreciable histodynamic effect outside it. Type of damage similar to brain laceration in open skull trauma.

[c] The annotations concerning the position of the cervical spine at the time the cervical cord was compressed from behind with the tip of the index finger are missing. However, since the laminectomy had been performed with the cervical spine in the flexed position, the pressure on the closed dura was most probably exerted in this position. The tension produced in the cord was thus probably a maximum; for the high local axial tension in the medullary tissue due to the compression of the cord, and its normal tension associated with spinal flexion are additive.

TABLE 2. Types of deformation set up in isolated specimens of the spinal cord, nerve-roots and peripheral nerves.[a]

Specimen no.	Fig. no.	Type of deformation	Specimen embedded so that section passes through
1	73	Compression of *cervical nerve-root* specimens.	Cross-sectional constriction
2	75	Compression of *sciatic nerve* specimens.	Cross-sectional constriction
3	89	Tissue deformation produced in an artificially *stretched* cord specimen by *cone* inserted in anteroposterior direction.	Hole in sagittal direction
4	92 A	Distention of a cervical cord specimen by a *cylindrical body* of relatively large cross-section inserted in the sagittal direction; the specimen is stretched as much as in the *neutral* posture of the spine.	Hole in transverse direction
5	92 B	As 92 A but specimen *stretched* as much as in *flexed posture*.	Hole in transverse direction
6	92 C	As 92 A but specimen *folded* as much as in the *extended posture*.	Hole in transverse direction
7	89	Distention of a cord specimen by a *spherical body* inserted in its substance.	Hole in coronal direction

[a] The experiments were performed to obtain an impression of the deformation of nervous tissue produced in a patient by the corresponding type of histodynamic stress.

rupture in the posterior border zone of the cord at the level of the dowel was due to the ligamenta flava, nor that the posterior aspect of the cord was deformed by a single protruding ligament (52). It would thus seem that the type of damage ascribed to these ligaments can occur even in the absence of any appreciable bulging; of course, the existence of a prominent ligament might well mean that compression occurs earlier than would otherwise have been the case. At all events it is against the upper rim of the vertebral arch (*crista arci*) that the pressure is ultimately exerted; furthermore, the experiments indicate that the moving component of the pincer is a fairly firm body protruding into the cervical canal from the anterior direction; clinical observations suggest that this structure is most likely to be the lower rim of a vertebral body that has slipped posteriorly or, less often, another smaller or larger part of a fractured vertebra that has been displaced in the posterior direction (Fig. 45 A).

In most of the cord specimens where the anteroposterior diameter had been reduced to somewhat more than one-fifth tearing could usually be followed for about three-quarters of the cord diameter (Figs. 57, 60). This phenomenon was observed at all levels of the cervical cord subjected to compression *in situ*. The experimental material is too small to determine accurately

the minimum constriction for which tearing will occur, but it would seem to be relatively small. In a more detailed analysis account should be taken of the shape of the impinging structure; the effects of constriction would presumably diminish in severity the greater the area of the pincer surface. For a given force, pinching would thus be potentially more deleterious than clamping.

Tissue displacement

In compression of the cord the tissue displacement at the axis of the medulla is mainly cranial in direction (189) owing to the convergence caudal to the cervical enlargement of the cord, and because of its greater diameter cranially.

In the case of deep depression of the cord medullary tissue can be displaced from the site of rupture as discrete masses; the damage is then no longer confined to the level of compression (Fig. 60 A–C) (123, 124). If a reconstructive neurosurgical operation is contemplated in the future, the consequences of pulp displacement (heterotopia) (188) through previous depression must be recognized and taken into account.

The preferential site of rupture of nerve-fibres

In some published histological sections the cross-section of the human myelinated nerve is seen to be roundish and to contain a slight depression corresponding to the nucleus of the Schwann cell (20, 174). However, in the young mouse, cat and rabbit and, reportedly, also in the young human subject (19), a crenated myelin sheath has been observed.

The myelinated nerve-fibre undergoes elastic adaptation to changes in length of the structures to which it is anchored. A reduction in the cross-sectional area of the fibre due to stretching is accompanied by a decrease in the cross-sectional area of the axoplasm; this dimensional change seems to be accommodated by crenation of the myelin sheath. Conversely, on relaxation of the tension in the nerve-fibre the myelin sheath recovers its circular section (Fig. 11 B, *Inset*).

Micromanipulatory experiments in the frog have shown that the weakest point of the myelinated nerve-fibre does not, as might be expected, coincide with the node of Ranvier. Yielding due to pathodynamic traction occurs instead within one of the short myelinated sections of the fibre, where its (normally varying) calibre is smallest (232). This seems to be true also in man. It has been observed under the operating microscope that when a spinal cord specimen is subjected to excessive tension the nervous substance diminishes in cross-sectional area before rupture occurs. Immediately after the fibres are torn they retract and form isolated flocks, which presumably consist of protoplasm and myelin (35).

In patients with partial cross-sectional lesions of the cord due to compressive trauma (to judge from the neurological deficit), damage to pain fibres often seems to exceed that to other types of fibres. Sensitivity of pain fibres has been demonstrated in peripheral nerve-fibres of small diameter in the cat (179) (though not in man). It would thus seem probable that also in man the smaller calibre of non-myelinated 'pain fibres' renders them more vulnerable than, for example, the medium calibred myelinated 'touch fibres'.

Hypothetical and verified pincer and clamping mechanisms

In some cases of tetraplegia due to extension injury—for instance, young persons diving into shallow water—no external cord injury or ligamentous damage of the spine was observed at autopsy (247). Normally, in full extension of the cervical spine the space in the canal required to accommodate the widened cord and the bulging ligaments is provided by the cranialward flow of CSF and by epidural venous drainage; but in sudden trauma there may not be time for this displacement of fluid. A pressure wave and ensuing trough would then presumably be created in the subarachnoid space and spinal cord tissue, analogous to those produced by an underwater explosion (46), and neural conductivity would be impaired. Similar conditions are probably set up by the pressure wave and cavitation effect of a bullet passing near the spinal cord; again, the ensuing cord lesion, which has been ascribed to 'cord concussion', is not visible externally. Recently, in experimental high-speed impact in the canine cadaver a pressure wave followed by a trough in the fluid of the spinal subarachnoid space has been registered (266).

In hyperextension injuries, the fracture or dislocation of a vertebra and lesion of the intervertebral disc is often accompanied by tearing of the anterior longitudinal ligament and other ligaments; separation of the posterior longitudinal ligament from the back of a vertebra has been found (22), and it has been considered that buckling of this ligament may have squeezed the cervical spinal cord back against the subjacent vertebra (123) and damaged it above and below the fractured vertebra (123).

In the light of the experimental findings reported here, it would seem that for compressive spinal cord injury to occur there must be a rapid backward slipping of a fractured or dislocated vertebra.

Aim and measures of surgical intervention

With the recognition of the destructive nature of the tension set up in the nervous tissue when the cord is pinched or clamped, the importance of eliminating the causes of spinal cord compression without delay (9) has become increasingly evident. But removal of the compressing body by one of the measures of protective neurosurgery, however promptly, cannot undo the damage, namely the over-stretching or rupture of nerve-fibres and blood-vessels. There is still, however, an ur-gent need to relax the cord, for the surfaces of the rup-tured cord tissue must be approximated as early as pos-sible to improve the blood supply to the damaged area and to prevent growth of glial and/or connective tissue into the intramedullary fissure. We are now in a posi-tion, moreover, to choose the appropriate surgical measures according to the cause of the compression and the resulting pathodynamic situation in the in-dividual case. This may sometimes be assessed on the basis of symptoms and signs, radiographs and other ob-jective criteria, which, under favourable conditions, en-able the critical and subcritical grade of compression to be differentiated.

Effect of experimental intramedullary oedema on a fissure in the cervical spinal cord

The experimental findings of the effect of artificial oedema and traction on the medullary tissue—visual-ized by an incision in the cervical cord—presumably illustrate the effects of oedema and skull traction on an intramedullary fissure produced by trauma in a com-pressive spinal cord injury. Potentially deleterious ef-fects of such oedema are probably the following:

(i) because of the increase in the intra- and the inter-cellular pressure, squashed pulp is pressed into the widening fissure; serum or blood leaks from the blood-vessels.

(ii) skull traction accentuates this phenomenon and hence its other harmful effects on blood-vessels and nerve-fibres.

(iii) the bulges of the tissue of the posterior columns cranial and caudal to the incision evidently show hither-to unrecognized effects of post-traumatic oedema; the neurological symptoms and signs that may be ascribed to circulatory disturbances in the spinal cord may be due, wholly or in part, to a remote rheological effect within the plasm of the axis-cylinders.

Thus, in the treatment of patients with fresh spinal cord injury effective therapeutic measures to prevent the development of oedema should be taken as early as possible after the trauma (17).

Critical compression

From the above observations it is evident that even momentary compression of the cord beyond the critical limit will inevitably result in irreversible damage.[2] It is nonetheless important to take immediate steps to elim-inate the possibility of extending any rupture through adoption of unsuitable spinal positions, or movements of a fractured or dislocated vertebra. This applies also when the compressing structure is a disc or loose pieces of bone that may easily change its position and exert a greater pressure on the cord. Finally, it is necessary

---

[2] Just as a complicated cord trauma due to piercing, uncom-plicated critical compression is invariably followed by either upward or downward Wallerian degeneration, since here, too, the nerve-fibres are ruptured.

to bear in mind the untoward effect of developing oedema, namely, the retraction of the swollen nerve-fibres; the resulting tension will be superimposed on the local axial tension within the cord tissue due to the pincer or clamping action of the offending body (Fig. 70).

For these reasons protective arco-cristectomy or protective bilateral laminectomy, followed by cervico-lordodesis and—where it is needed—some form of stabilization of the spine, may be regarded as the most logical and potentially rewarding surgical procedure. It should preferably be performed as an emergency operation.

Subcritical compression

If the spinal canal is shallow and there are large osteophytes, calcified ligaments or other firm structures that, in extension, might be expected to produce compression of the cord, the tension set up in the cord tissue on slight extension of the neck is as a rule subcritical. Since full extension of the cervical spine is seldom assumed, any neurological symptoms provoked under the above predisposing conditions are probably ascribable to relatively moderate and intermittent compression of the cord. (The sudden paraparesis that has been experienced in the dental chair by the patient who forces his head backwards is, of course, a typical result of critical compression.) The consequent, chronic local, subcritical over-stretching of the axis-cylinders can then result in a reversible interruption of their conductivity. As in cervical myelopathies, in which histologically demonstrable damage to the lateral pyramidal tracts can result from hypoxia through over-stretching and consequent constriction of transverse branches of the central arteries supplying this area of the cord (54, 148), damage to the central cord may well develop if there is prolonged over-stretching of the descending and ascending central branches of these arteries. For this reason it is also important to eliminate without delay any subcritical short-range tension in the cord.

From the above analysis it would seem that the nature and location of the neurological manifestations of subcritical compression of the cervical cord are dependent on where in the cord tissue the compressive forces are acting; their severity is determined largely by the magnitude of the tensile stress, which is, in turn, dependent on the magnitude of the compressive forces.

Even in moderate, subcritical compression of the cord occurring in extension the nerve-fibres are stretched in a wide zone around the centre of the cord. So long as the magnitude of this short-range tension is not excessive it may produce functional deficit unaccompanied by substantial damage; if there is no oedema the conductivity will start to recover as soon as the pincer action on the cord has been eliminated.

Because the histodynamic tensile stress field is concentrated centrally in the cord a neurological picture resembling that of central cervical cord injury (233) may be expected, with impairment of the motor power and tendon reflexes of the arms (the fibres to the arms in the lateral pyramidal tracts pass nearer the centre of the cord than do those to the legs). From the fact that in spondylotic myelopathies due to chronic intermittent forces the neurological manifestations are often reversible, it would seem that the compression is mostly subcritical.

Difficulties in distinguishing between subcritical and critical compression

In many compressive conditions over-stretching of the nerve-fibres even to just below the limit of rupture is hardly to be expected. Even in the case of relatively slight compression some nerve-fibres will almost invariably tear and tension will be set up in blood-vessels, with consequent intramedullary oedema and, possibly, extravasation with neurological manifestations. When the pincer action has been eliminated and the oedema has dispersed, many symptoms may prove to be only temporary (50); the persistent ones will probably be due to rupture of the nerve-fibres and damage produced by hypoxia or anoxia.

Without an insight into the fundamental bio-mechanical conditions the neurological manifestations of a complete cross-sectional lesion would hardly be attributed to the same type of stress as that producing central spinal cord injury (233); in fact, the difference is only one of degree. For safety's sake both should be treated as emergency situations. Even subcritical compression may have serious sequelae, if prolonged.

Comparison of effects of unilateral thrust and pincer action

Whether over-stretching of the spinal cord is due to unilateral thrust or to compression by a pincer or clamping mechanism, the stress set up in the medullary tissues is tensile and differs only in its location, direction and intensity. In *compression* the axial tension is localized to an area around the site of application of the force(s); it is a maximum beneath the centre of the cord, where it may lead to tearing. On the other hand, the over-stretching produced by structures impinging on the anterior surface of the cord during *flexion* ultimately involves the whole pons–cord tract; besides the local bending tensile stress in the transverse and sagittal planes, there is a general axial tension throughout the tract. Because of this distribution the over-stretching during flexion will seldom, if ever, result in tearing.[3]

[3] However, at autopsy of persons dying after high-speed frontal car collision, haemorrhages have been found at various sites throughout the brain, pons and spinal cord (114). These suggest that the forcible stretching of the nervous tissues, resulting mainly from the ultra-rapid acceleration of the mass of the brain on forward bending of the head and the cervical spine, can lead to rupture of their fibres. (When the brain is decelerated just as rapidly on encountering the rigid vault of the skull, the impact—and possibly a consequent cavitation effect—might well account for the superficial lacerations.)

The differences between these two types of tension are manifested in the type and severity of the neurological symptoms.

When, in traumatic hyperflexion of the cervical column, the already over-stretched cord is compressed—for example, by a fractured, anteriorly displaced vertebral arch (an injury that has been recorded in pole-vaulters and persons using the trampoline (209)), the resulting local over-stretching at the level of compression is presumably superimposed on the general stretching due to the pathological lengthening of the canal. This may result in total rupture of the cervical spinal cord and hence irreversible tetraplegia (Fig. 49).

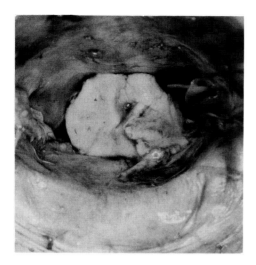

Fig. 40. View into the cervical canal from the base of the skull, showing structures potentially involved in a pincer action on the cord during extension.

With the cervical spine fully extended the spinal cord makes contact with the anterior and posterior surfaces of the canal. The anterior aspect of the cord is in contact with the dura-covered odontoid process, and its posterior aspect with a fold of the dura (raised by the ligamentum flavum between the vertebral arches C_1 and C_2).

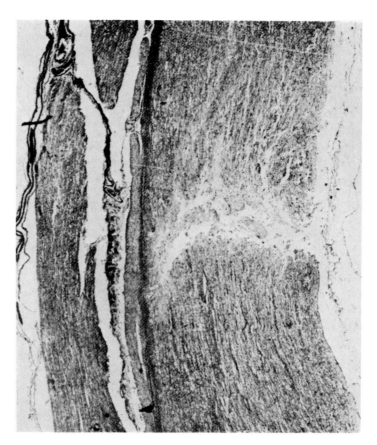

Fig. 41. Trauma of the cervical spinal cord giving rise to tetraplegia.

In tetraplegia resulting from forced extension (so-called hyperextension) of the neck it has generally been considered that the neurological deficit is due to compression of the cord by the forward-bulging ligamentum flavum. Proof for this explanation was seen in this histological section through the cord in the area of the lesion at the C_4/C_5 level; the subject was a man aged 67 years, who had fallen and sustained a large bruise on the forehead; he died 9 weeks later. Interruption and fragmentation of the nerve-fibres, mainly in the transverse plane, extends from the posterior aspect of the cord almost to the central canal. At the boundaries of the fissure there is marked gliosis. The damage extends into the anterior columns, where compound granular corpuscles are also seen, but where the gliosis is less severe and there is no gross rupture of the nerve-fibres.

Courtesy of A. Taylor, M.D. (245). With kind permission of the Editor of The Journal of Bone & Joint Surgery.

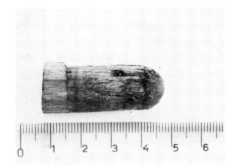

Fig. 42. Device for artificial compression of the spinal cord.

The device used for extradural compression of the cervical spinal cord from the anterior aspect was a wooden dowel. It was inserted in a hole drilled with a Cloward's instrument in the C_5/C_6 or C_6/C_7 vertebral bodies. So that it would slide better on the dura, the rounded tip was rendered smooth by rubbing with wax. The thickness of the vertebral body was marked with pencil on the side of the dowel. When the spinal cord had been filled with opaque medium *via* a vertebral artery (256), and formaldehyde had been injected into the subarachnoid space after draining the CSF, the dowel was tapped different distances into the hole so that graded compression of the cervical spinal cord was obtained. The cadaver was then stored in a refrigerator for about 16 hours in the prone position, the cervical spine in full extension. In some cases compression was performed as rapidly as possible and in others slowly.

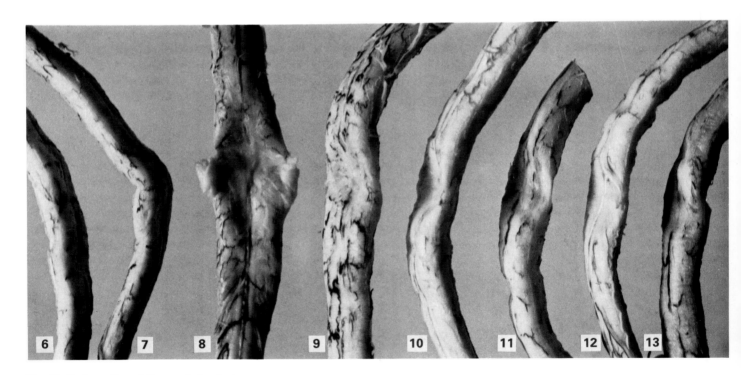

Fig. 43. Deformation of the cervical spinal cord due to different degrees of compression *in situ* with the spine extended.

(Specimens nos. 6–13, Table 1.) Compression technique, see Fig. 42. Technique for filling the vessels (18). Fixation technique, see p. 54.

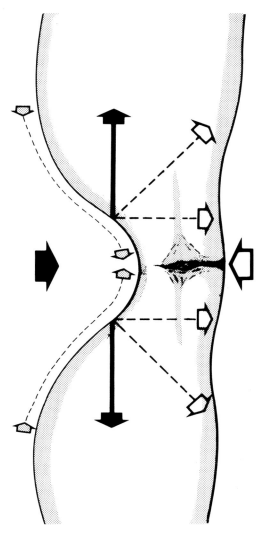

Fig. 44. Forces acting in the cervical cord tissue produced by a pincer mechanism.

Large black arrow. Direction of pressure exerted by the impinging body.

Large white arrow. Reaction at the posterior wall of the canal.

Small black arrows. Axial component of the tensile force resulting from the pincer action.

Small white arrows. Oblique and transverse components of the resulting tensile force.

Grey arrows. Direction of the resulting traction in the pia mater.

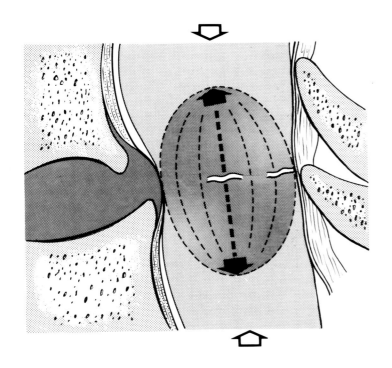

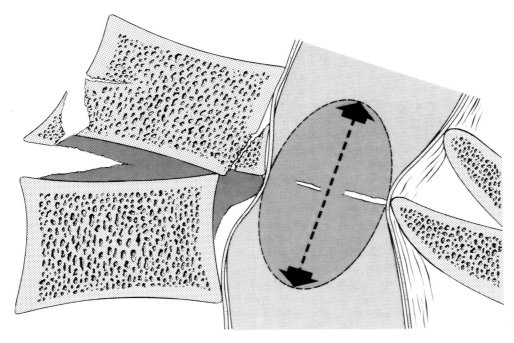

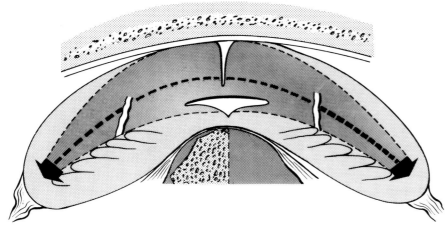

A

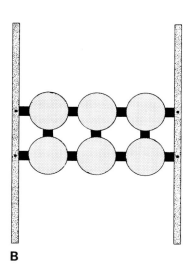

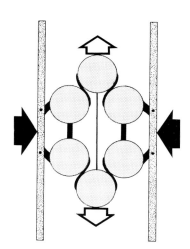

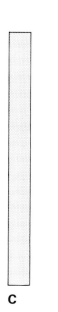
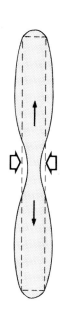

B

C

Fig. 45.

A. Intramedullary tensile stress field (*shaded*) **produced by a pincer action on the cord during extension of the cervical spine** (Fig. 77).

Upper and *Middle*. Extent of the histologically visible three-dimensional field in sagittal sections through the cord. *Black arrows*. Direction of the resultant forces acting in the tissue and stretching it in all directions. As the distance between the opposing pincer surfaces is decreased the tensile forces, and hence the intensity of the stress field, increase.

The cord fibres, which normally are folded in extension, are immediately drawn out straight when the pincer action starts. When the anteroposterior diameter of the cord has been reduced by about 20–30 per cent the axial tension is so great that some of the axial fibres tear. Maximum tearing occurs in the transverse plane, approximately at the level of the line connecting the pincer surfaces. If the movement of the dowel is arrested just as tearing has begun, the rupture can remain as a transverse fissure (Fig. 41); but if the dowel continues to move there will be further displacement of tissue, promoted by the forces of elastic retraction.

Lower. The approximate extent of the histologically visible stress field in the transverse section through the cord, on a level with the site of the pincer action. As a result of transverse tension (*black arrows*) set up by the pincer action, fibres running in the transverse direction have been torn. As has been shown experimentally, the tearing can be manifested as gaps on each side of the anterior median fissure (Fig. 63). If the dowel continues to move in the posterior direction the tearing will be followed by internal mass displacement.

The palisade structures along the anterior aspect of the cord, which in the unloaded state run in an anteroposterior direction, may to a certain extent account for the arcuate form of the transverse tensile field (Figs. 17, 85).

B. Model demonstrating the origin of tension set up in a compressed body perpendicular to the direction of the applied force.

The forces set up in an incompressible body when it is subjected to compression (clamping) may be visualized in a simple model consisting of two parallel rows of three smooth spheres, initially equidistant from each other and connected by short elastic strings of equal length and thickness. The spheres are located between two plane surfaces to which the outer pairs are attached with identical elastic strings.

Approximation of the two plane surfaces causes the spheres to be pressed against one another. Between the two plane surfaces and each of the middle spheres there are a total of two laterally attached elastic strings; as the total elongation of the strings on stretching is greater for the middle spheres they have a greater freedom of motion than the others. Since the spheres are smooth and not exactly in line, slipping can occur between them. The two middle spheres will tend to be pressed out of line with the neighbouring spheres, either in the same or opposite directions. When the middle spheres are displaced in opposite directions the strings connecting them will be under much greater tension than any of the strings attaching the spheres to the plane surfaces.

The model shows that the application of bilateral pressure to a body results in a rearrangement of its incompressible components; it also illustrates that the tension thus set up in the body acts perpendicularly to the plane of compression. By adding more layers of spheres a three-dimensional stress field can be simulated.

C. Model illustrating the internal stress set up in an axis-cylinder subjected to a pincer action.

Left. Axis-cylinder in normal state.

Right. Axis-cylinder subjected to a pincer force (*large open arrows*). The visco-elastic plasm reacts to this load in two ways. Its fluid component tends to flow towards the free ends of the cylinder, where it causes increasing bulging of the axon membranes. The cohesive elements of the plasm take up the tension (*small arrows*) produced by the pressure that displaces them towards the axis of the cylinder.

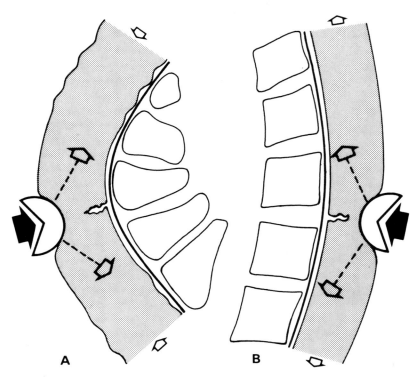

Fig. 46. Sites of tearing in the cervical cord resulting from its compression by a body impinging on it from the anterior (A) and posterior (B) directions.

A. Transverse tear in the posterior side of the cervical cord produced by a dowel applied on its anterior aspect with the cervical spine extended. The resulting lesion appears identical to that regularly observed after an extension trauma, hitherto ascribed to penetration of the cord by a protruding ligamentum flavum.

(For a given degree of impression of the cord the injury produced by the dowel would presumably be less severe in extension than flexion, where the cord is already under tension.)

B. When the dowel enters the cervical canal from the posterior side the lesion is located on the *anterior* aspect of the cord irrespective of whether the cord is extended or (as here) flexed. An example of this traumatic situation is when a fractured vertebral arch enters the cervical canal from the posterior side while the cervical spine is flexed.

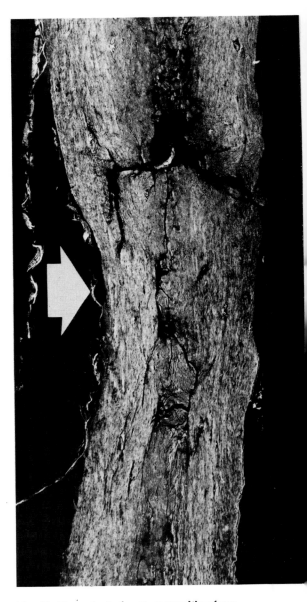

Fig. 47. The extent of rupture resulting from moderate compression. (Specimen no. 2, Table 1)

A mid-sagittal section through the cervical cord that has been exposed to transverse compression *in situ* with the cervical column extended (p. 54). The site where the rounded wooden dowel impinged on the anterior aspect of the cervical cord is marked with an *arrow*. Although the anteroposterior diameter of the cord has been reduced by less than one-third, there is a practically complete rupture. On each side of the site of compression there is a clear compensatory increase in the diameter of the cord.

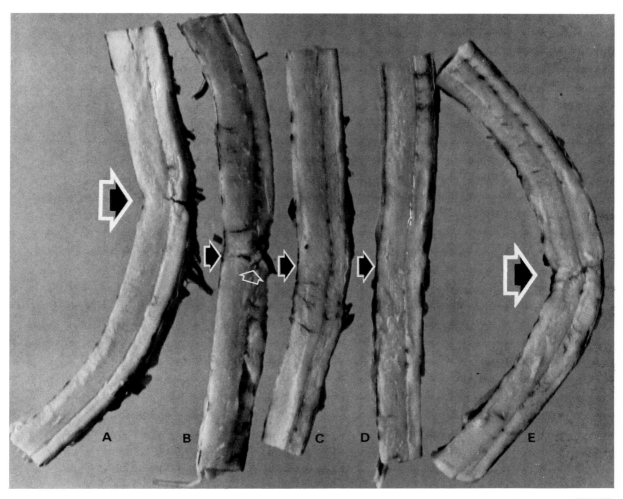

Fig. 48. Transverse fissures in the anterior aspect of the left half of the cervical cord in a control series of subjects in whom the posterior surface of the cord was compressed with the finger in various postures. (Specimens nos. 14–18, Table 1)

A. Prone, cervical spine extended.

B. Prone, cervical spine flexed.

C, D. Erect, cervical spine in neutral position.

E. Prone, cervical spine extended.

(So as to check visually that the impression was the same in each subject the dura was opened for a few centimetres in the midline, but without draining the CSF.) Immediately after the compression the cord was removed and preserved in 10 per cent formaldehyde. The specimens compressed with the spine extended retained their extended (backward flexed) shape even though they were not fixed *in situ*. The specimens compressed in the neutral body posture contained no gross fissures in the plane of section.

The results confirm (*i*) that the compression trauma occurs instantaneously; (*ii*) that (despite some shrinkage on fixation) the fissuring is not an artificial product of fixation *in situ* over a long period; and (*iii*) that the fissuring is greatest on the side of the cord remote from the finger. Evidently it is not the ligamentum flavum that is responsible for the compressive trauma in sudden extension of the cervical spine, but rather the pressure exerted by the lower margin of a posteriorly slipped vertebra, bone fragment, disc, encapsulated fluid or the like, on the cord from the anterior side of the canal (see Fig. 47).

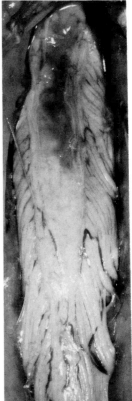

Fig. 49. The squashed portion of the cervical cord of a young patient who died from a trampoline accident. (See p. 60.)

Courtesy of K. Rietz, M.D., Karolinska Hospital.

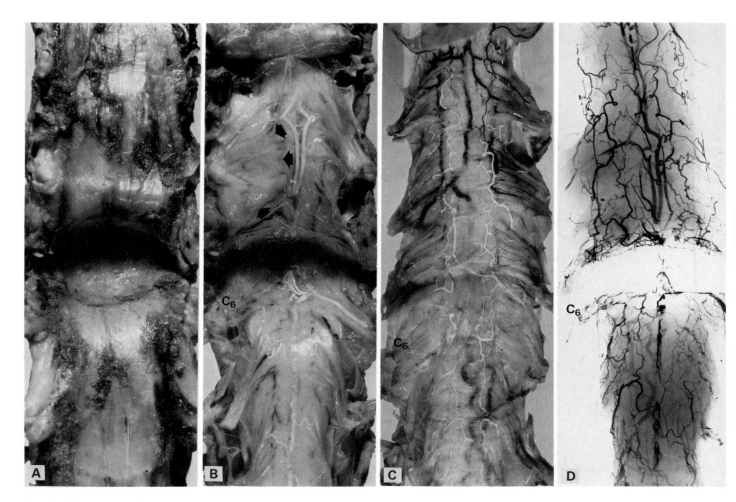

Fig. 50. Effects of complete compression of the cord with the wooden dowel at the C$_6$ level, cervical column extended. (Specimen no. 1, Table 1)

A. The impression in the anterior side of the dura.

B. Anterior aspect. Dura removed. The cord pulp has been completely displaced, so that the anterior and posterior surfaces of the pial sheath have come into contact; at the bottom of the impression the pia has been widened; contrast medium remains in the C$_6$ radicular artery and the superficial pial vessels (Fig. 53); the expressed pulp bulges anteriorly below the C$_6$ root.

Arrows. Sub-pial herniation of the pulp.

C. Posterior aspect. Pia and vessels are intact.

D. Microangiograms showing the increase in volume above and below the site of compression.

Fig. 51. Coronal histological section through the herniated pulp, just cranial to the site of complete compression. (Specimen no. 1, cranial part)

Part of the pulp expressed from the pia has not separated from the rest but bulges outwards (70).

Palmgren's stain. ×6.4.

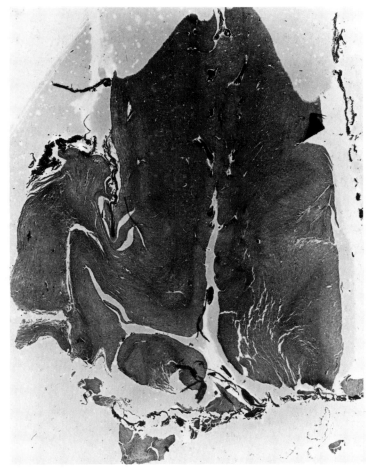

Fig. 52. Sagittal histological sections through the caudal part of the cervical cord just below the site of complete compression showing tissue deformation. (Specimen no. 1, caudal part)

Along its posterior aspect (*right*) the folding of the tissue network produced by extension appears to have been largely retained, though with some distortion. In the physiological axial shortening accompanying extension the network becomes more rigid, and tearing and fissures are therefore more likely to occur. The whorls reflecting the displacement extend caudalward over at least 3 segments, below which level the cord regains its normal diameter. The displacement of the tissue by the dowel approaching from the anterior direction is greatest on the anterior half (*left*).

Palmgren's stain. ×5.2.

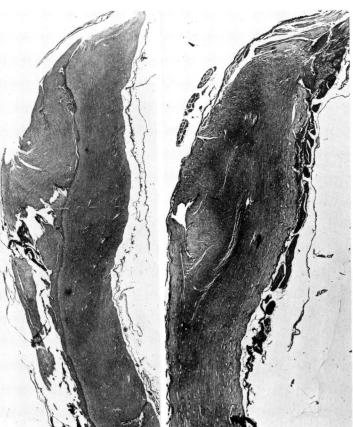

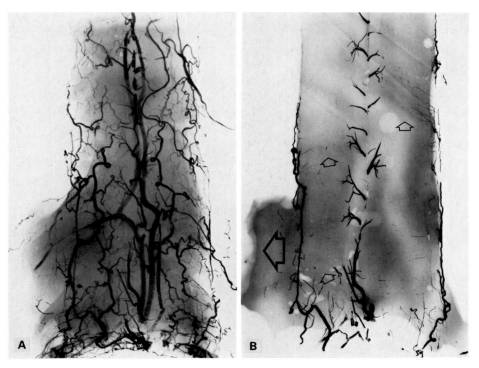

Fig. 53. Microangiogram of the area above the site of complete compression. (Specimen no. 1, cranial part)

A. Anteroposterior projection before sectioning.

B. Anteroposterior projection of a 4 mm coronal section. The cranialward deflection of the lateral branches of the central arteries, which is most pronounced in the immediate vicinity of the impression, decreases greatly at a distance of about 2 segments. The displacement of the pulp (Fig. 51) is most clearly manifested by the course of the finest branches of the arteries entering from the external circulation *(small arrows). Large arrow.* Direction of herniation.

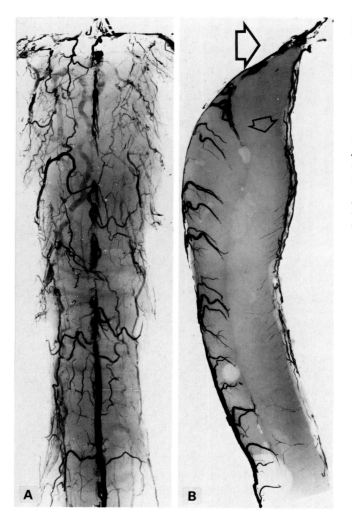

Fig. 54. Microangiogram of the area below the site of complete compression. (Specimen no. 1, caudal part)

A. Anteroposterior projection before sectioning.

B. Lateral projection of a 3 mm sagittal section. The displacement of the pulp is reflected in the increase in diameter over a distance of nearly 4 segments. Immediately below the site of total compression *(white arrow)* the main branches of the central arteries are deflected caudalward and pressed against the anterior aspect of the pia mater *(small arrow)*. Below the level at which the deflection of the vessels and the bulging of the cord ceases there is presumably no further structural damage.

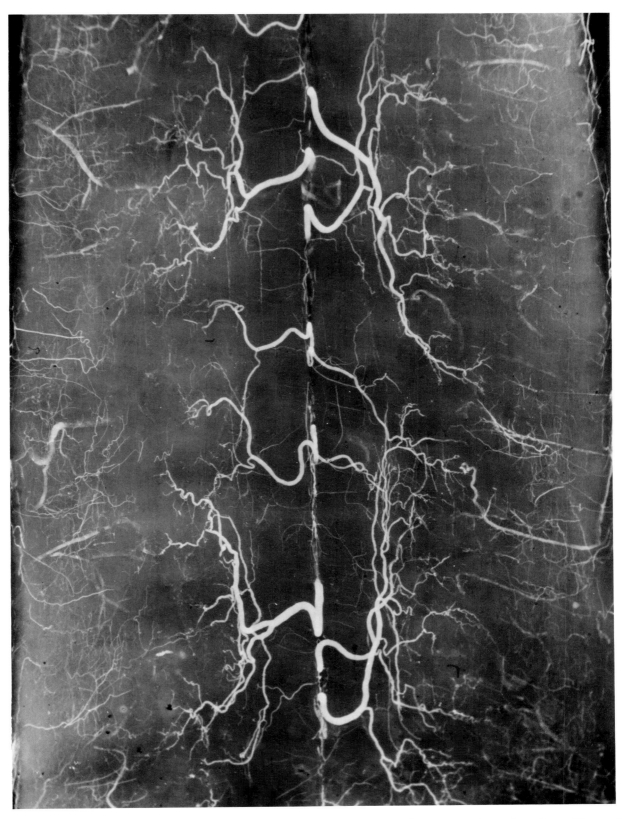

Fig. 55. Normal vascular pattern of the cord
—a valuable basis for assessment of deformation produced by a unilateral thrust or a pincer action.

Microangiogram of a 2 mm mid-coronal section of a cervical cord specimen, not under tension.

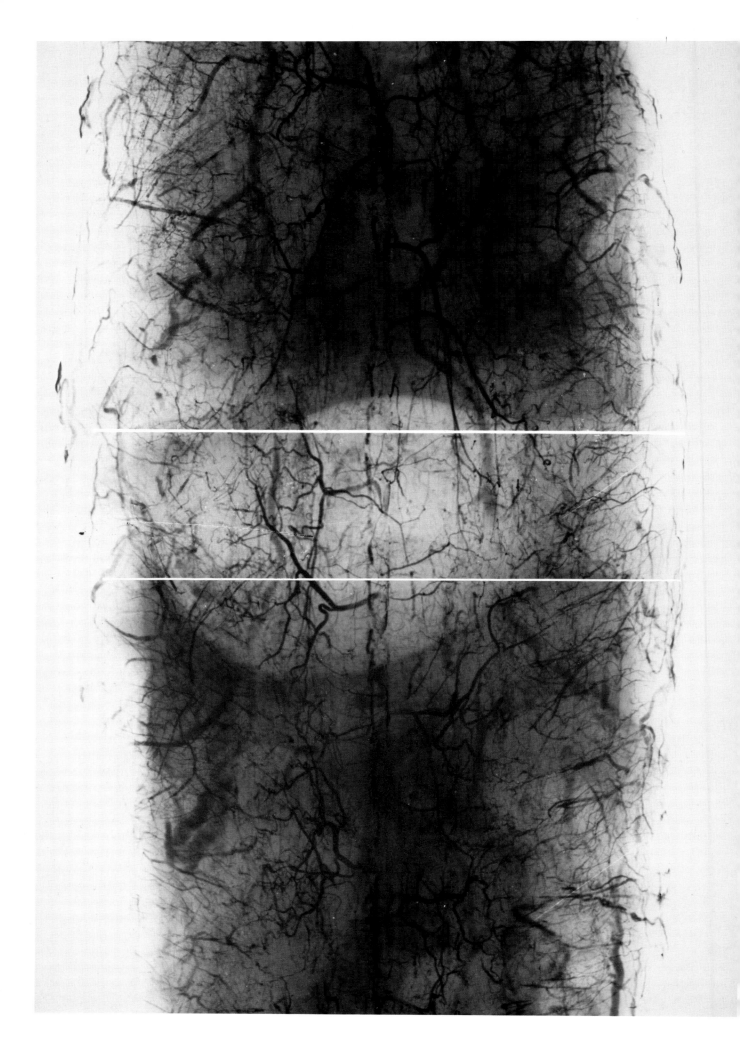

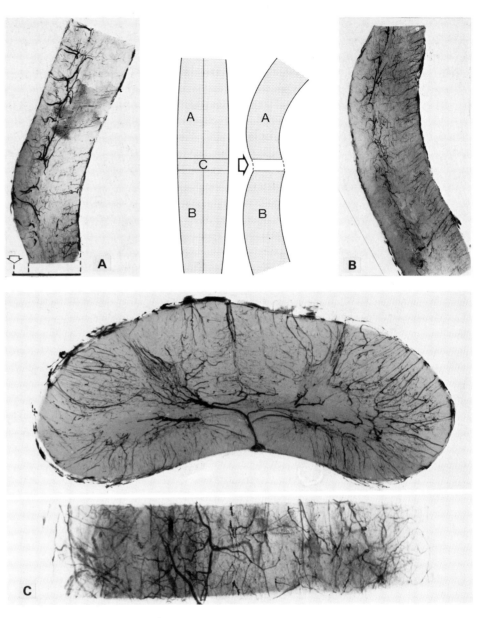

Fig. 56. Non-deleterious (subliminary) compression of the extended cervical cord at the C$_6$ level causing a reduction of about one sixth in its anteroposterior diameter. (Specimen no. 4, Table 1)

Left. Anteroposterior microangiogram, general view. The light zone indicates the region of compression of the cord ($\times$10.6).

Right. A. Microangiogram of a mid-sagittal section of the cord, cranial to the cross-section C in the diagram. Slight but definite cranial deflection of the central arteries in the extreme caudal part of the section.

B. The caudal mid-sagittal region (corresponding to A in the diagram). A slight caudalward deflection of the central arteries, though less distinct, is discernible in the extreme cranial part of the section ($\times$2.1).

C (*upper*). Microangiogram of a 3 mm cross-section at the level of the maximum antero-posterior compression. The impression of the anterior aspect of the cord by the dowel has resulted in flattening and widening of the cord, shortening of the anteroposteriorly running vessels of the peripheral arterial system, and, at the same time, stretching of the transverse branches of the central arteries and a branch of a (*right*) central artery supplying the basal part of the posterior columns. The stretching of the vessels transversing the posterior columns has greatly reduced their lumina. The interpretation is facilitated by reference to the anteroposterior projection of the subjacent transverse section.

C (*lower*). Anteroposterior view of the same transverse section ($\times$7.1).

In all the sections the presence of a tensile stress field near the site of the pincer action is clearly reflected in the transverse, axial and diagonal stretching of the centrally located vessels.

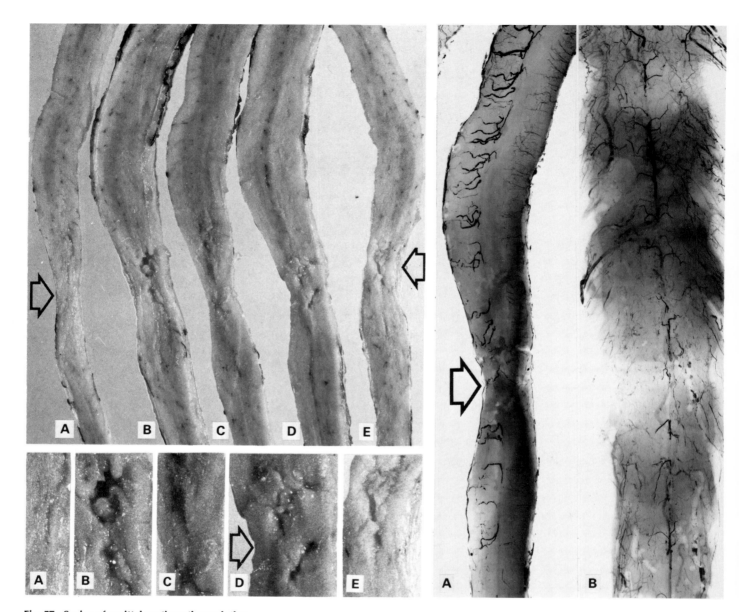

Fig. 57. Series of sagittal sections through the cord showing artificial compression injury produced in extension of the cervical column. (*Left*, A–E.) Same procedure as in Fig. 46 A. (Specimen no. 3, Table 1)

Arrows. The direction of the wooden dowel. The specimen on the right (section E) has been rotated 180°.

Insets. Zone of rupture of specimens A–E under higher magnification.

Right. A. Microangiogram (×2.5), showing the deflection of the central arteries above and below the site of compression.

B. Frontal view.

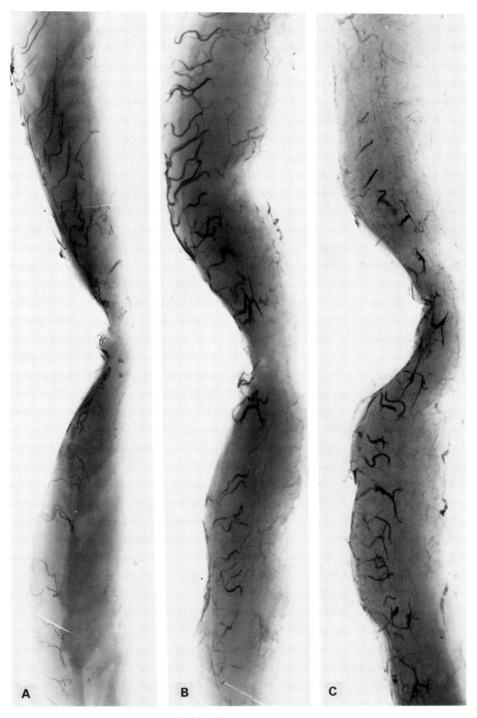

Fig. 58. Lateral microangiograms showing the range of the effect of compression of the cord (×3.3). (Specimens nos. 8–10 in Fig. 43)

At the level of compression the anteroposterior diameter of the cord has been reduced by about 80 per cent (A), 50 per cent (B) and 60 per cent (C). The displacement of the arteries due to tension—cranially in the upper and caudally in the lower part of the specimen—clearly increases with the degree of compression. The range of the increase in diameter caudally and, especially, cranially of the level of compression (B, C), confirms that the cord substance has been squeezed out more in the latter direction (189).

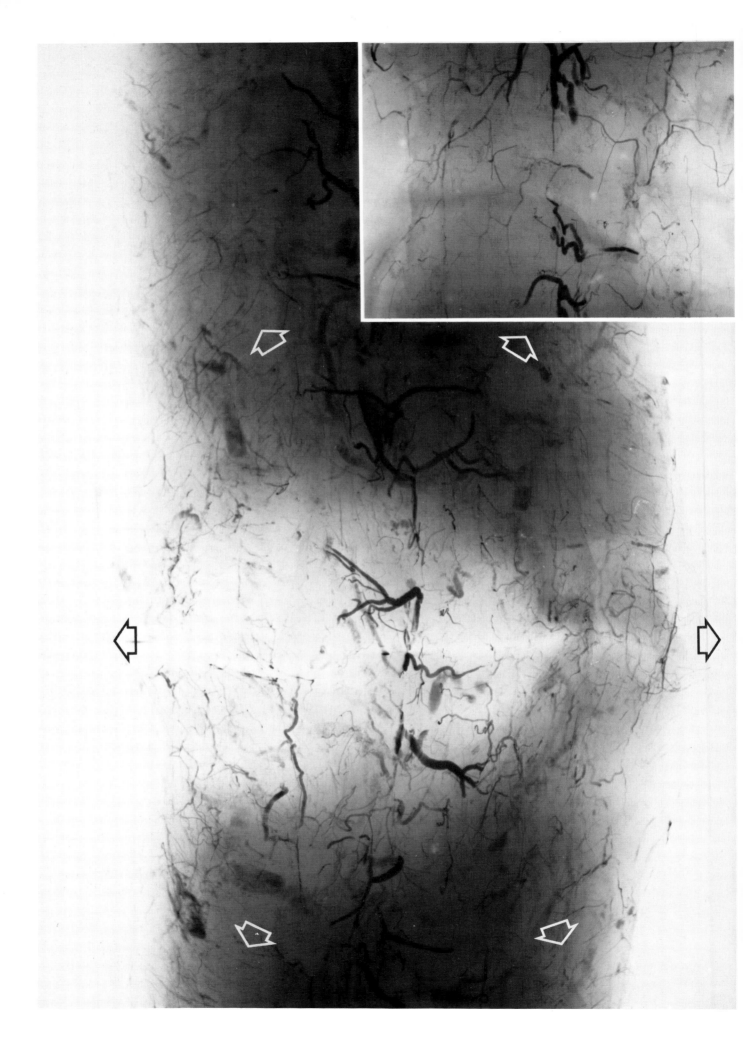

Fig. 59. Anteroposterior microangiogram of a cervical cord specimen (no. 10 in Fig. 43) illustrating deflection of blood-vessels due to a (anteroposterior) pincer action. The narrow radiolucent strip is the site of rupture, and the radiopaque areas above and below indicate the displaced tissue. *Arrows.* Direction of the stress field produced by the dowel (applied from the anterior direction). On close inspection numerous small torn vessels are seen to have retracted and coiled up.

Inset. Zone of rupture in Specimen no. 9, Fig. 43 (×10.0).

Fig. 60.

A. Effects of compression of the cervical cord by a punch applied to the anterior surface with the cervical spine extended (3 specimens, a and d identical, no. 2). (a, ×3.4; b, ×1.8; c, ×2.6; d, ×3.8).

a, d. At the level of compression, which reduced the thickness of the cord substance by about one-third, a transverse tear and various other fissures are seen. Running in both axial and oblique directions, they confirm the multi-directional nature of the stress field produced by a pincer action. Like the tears, the shearing in the tissue is a secondary phenomenon, localized chiefly at the level of the pincer action.

b, c. The same phenomenon as in a and d but with total rupture; the pia mater is undamaged. In c a tendency for a vortex formation in the tissue is evident about 2 or 3 segments above and below the level of compression.

B. Formation of vortices in the cord pulp as it flows in the cranial and caudal directions after rupture and persistent compression.

The extrusion of cord substance by the fractured or displaced bone usually continues for a time after this has produced a transverse intramedullary fissure. The viscous tissue elements, with their high fluid content, are thus forced into the pial sheath, and flow in the cranial and caudal directions. This flow is augmented by the elastic retraction of the membranes of the severed nerve fibres, the cytoplasm of which has already been displaced in the same directions. As in other fluids, resistance to flow can set up vortices in the intramedullary tissue.

(From the microangiograms in Figs. 53, 54 and 58 it would appear that the cranially and caudally directed intramedullary shearing forces act chiefly in the anterior part of the cord rather than in its posterior border zone, as indicated in this figure. Cranialward and caudalward extrusion of the tissue would therefore occur at first in the anterior border zone, and flow would take place in the reverse directions.)

When tissue—turn loss by the actual forces—is undergoing malacia, intramedullary cysts may form (*cf.* "Trauma and Syringomyelia" in: Barnett, H. J. M., Foster, J. B., Hudgson, P.: Syringomyelia. Saunders, London, 1973).

C. Cross-section through a vortex in the cervical cord below the level of pinching (*Upper,* Fig. 62 in: (188); *Lower,* Fig. 68 in: (188).[1] (Surrounding structures retouched.)

[1] Courtesy of E. Th. Mayer, M.D. (188).
With kind permission of the Editor of Hdb Neurotraumatologie, Urban & Schwarzenberg, München–Berlin–Vienna.

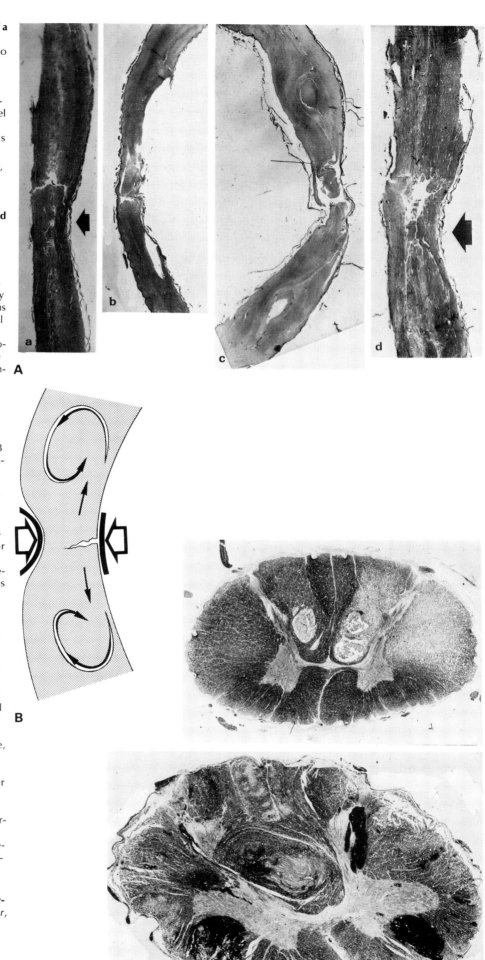

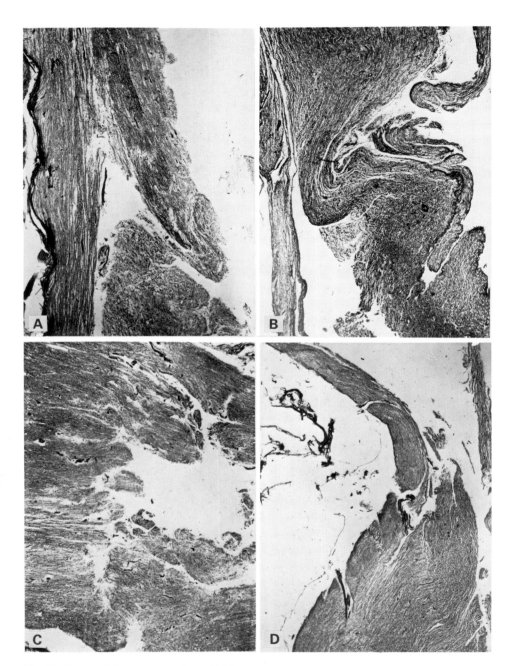

Fig. 61. Zones of tissue rupture in artificial spinal cord injury showing various types of deformation; higher magnification (×1100).

A. Shear zone (in Specimen b in Fig. 60) resulting from cranialward displacement of tissue after tearing, with the largest ruptures running in axial and oblique directions.

B. The fibres near the shear zone are amply folded (Specimen c in Fig. 60).

C. Zone of tearing, mainly transverse, with numerous isolated remnants in the form of flakes floating inside the pial membrane, as sometimes seen in acute spinal cord injury (Specimen d in Fig. 60).

D. Tissue deformation between the zones of stretching and telescoping (Specimen no. 8 in Fig. 43).

Fig. 62. Zones of rupture in the cord tissue.

A. Zone of fissuring. Folding of fibres after retraction (×550). (Specimen B in Fig. 61.)

B. The zone of tearing, with fibres running more or less at right angles to the plane of section (×550).

C, D. The zone of tearing with fibres running largely parallel to the plane of section. In C, in the immediate vicinity of the zone of rupture, there is a transparent substance (myelin droplets?). In D a number of nerve-fibres in the border of the zone of tearing have curled up into balls, probably owing to elastic retraction of the axoplasm after rupture (×550).

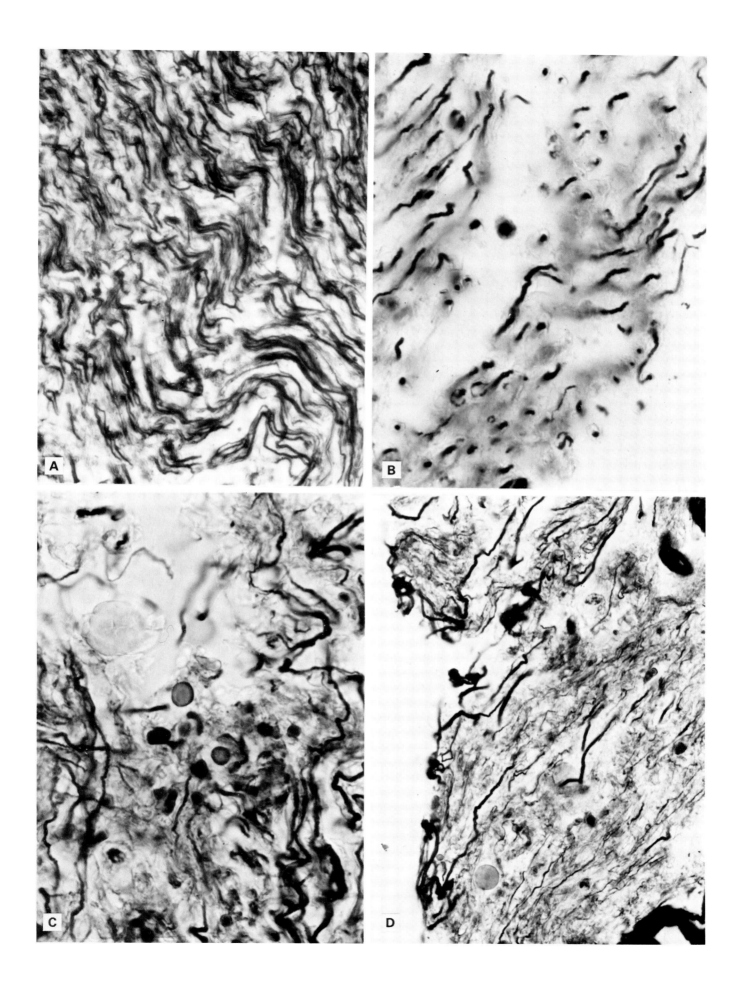

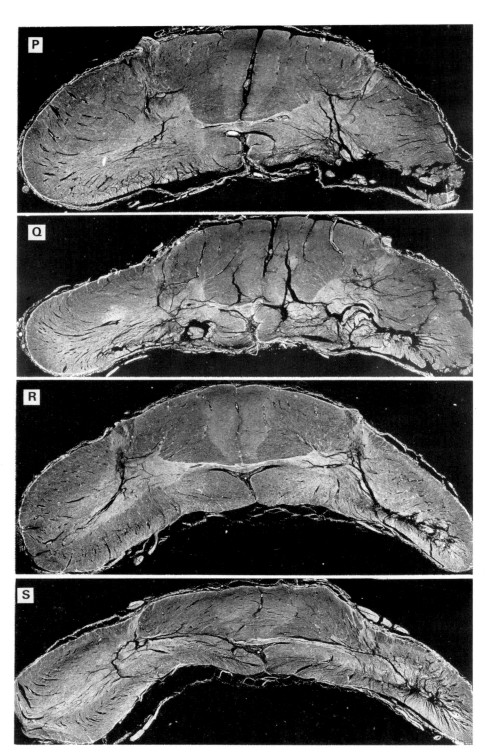

Fig. 63. Pairs of adjacent histological transverse sections at the level of maximal compression (C_5/C_6) in two cervical cord specimens compressed from the anterior direction *in situ*.[1]

P, Q. (Specimen no. 10 in Fig. 64, *left*.) Compression has resulted in powerful transverse tension, reflected in the marked bilateral displacement of the tissues (funnel-shaped depression towards the lateral aspects of the cord). The numerous fissures and clefts run chiefly in the anteroposterior direction, as would be expected from the results obtained in the photoelastic experiments.

R, S. (Specimen no. 9 in Fig. 64, *right*.) The same basic histodynamic features in the specimens from another subject.

[1] The usual histological cross-sections in articles on the effects of spinal cord compression depict fissures in the tissue similar to those shown in this figure. Although in most such cases the cord will not have been fixed *in situ* the direction of these fissures is invariably that of the compressive force. This rules out the possibility of them being artefacts (47), even though the slight shrinkage due to formalin fixation (35) renders them easier to see. (*Intra vitam* they are masked by oedema.) On compression of the cord from the anterior or posterior direction fissures appear which follow an anteroposterior or posteroanterior direction, respectively, in the cord section. When, more rarely, the spinal cord is compressed in the transverse direction the fissures (and their sequelae in the form of intramedullary scars) follow a transverse course (Fig. 65 (188)). Cross-sections through the cord above or below the compressed area may show symmetrical 'contusion sequestra' or 'heterotopia'. Severe deformations in the form of heterotopia have been presumed to be artefacts caused during removal of the spinal cord from the canal (188). In the sagittal section in c, Fig. 60 A, where the cord was fixed *in situ* after compression, the tissue is seen to be displaced in a cranial direction. If only one cross-section had been taken at the level of the displaced tissue, it could not have demonstrated that this heterotopia is actually due to flow of, and vortex formation in, the medullary tissue caused by the compression.

The anteroposterior fissures in the spinal cord cut only transverse (horizontal) neuronal transmissions. Of much greater importance for the occurrence of neurological symptoms are the rarely demonstrated *transverse* fissures which interrupt the long pathways.

Fissures form only when the limit of extensibility of all elements composing the nervous tissue has been exceeded. At low compressive deformation of the spinal cord, fissuring occurs only sporadically, but reversible over-stretching of the axis-cylinders is frequent. As the deformation is increased there is further rupturing of axis-cylinders and the fissures extend in various directions; areas containing over-stretched axis-cylinders are now fewer, as is reflected in the duration of the absence of responses (evoked cortical potentials 72, 75) and by the constancy of the neurological symptoms.

Fig. 64. Microangiograms of 5 mm serial sections from two specimens *left* **and** *right* **of artificially compressed cervical cord.** The sections are shown cranially to caudally from top to bottom (×3.0).

Left. Cervical cord specimen 4 cm long[1] (no. 9 in Fig. 43).

Right. Cervical cord specimen 3.5 cm long[1] (no. 10 in Fig. 43).

The transverse width of the cord increases through the series as far as the level of the dowel (*P* and *Q* left; *R* and *S* right) and then decreases. The trunk of the anterior central artery and its lateral branches increase and decrease in length, correspondingly (Figs. 56, 58 and 59).

[1] *P*, *Q*, *R* and *S* are the same sections as those so labelled in Fig. 63.

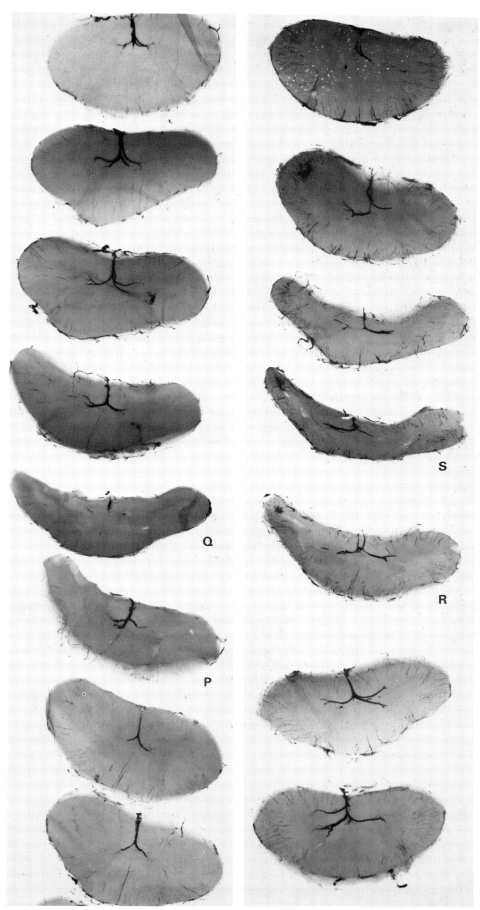

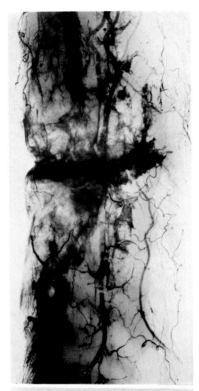

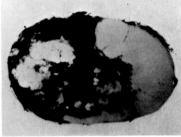

A

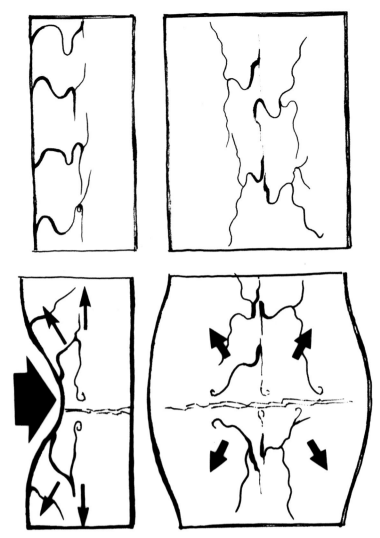

B

Fig. 65.

A. Pooling of contrast medium indicating rupture of blood-vessels at the level of a transverse fissure in the tissue produced by compression.

Upper. Microradiograph of a length of cervical spinal cord injected *in situ* with Micropaque after compression by approximately 40 per cent of its anteroposterior diameter. The pressure was applied by means of a dowel inserted through a borehole from the anterior side at the C$_6$/C$_7$ level.[1]

Extravasated contrast medium collected in a zone along the transverse tear. This rupture was produced by the axial component of the tensile stress set up by the compression. The leakage of medium suggests that if the tensile stress attains a certain level there will be rupture not only of the axis-cylinders but also of microvascular branches.

Apart from the slight depression in the right surface of the cord there was no damage visible from outside even in the tear zone.[2] However, a transverse incision through the cervical cord at the level of the depression disclosed total destruction of the right half— except for a relatively narrow band of apparently intact white substance near the pia mater.

Lower. A microradiograph of a transverse section at this level disclosed ruptured vessels also in this band. In the left half the lesion was situated lateral to the central

canal of myelon, where it involved a large area (white in the radiograph because the medium had escaped from this pool), and also to a lesser degree the left posterior horn of grey matter and the dorsal funiculus. While this feature suggests that the deleterious stress (due to the pincer action) is greatest in the centre of the field, its site and effect are apparently much dependent on the direction of the force and the volume of tissue compressed. The haemorrhage due to the tissue lesion in this specimen essentially resembles that associated with spinal cord injury in man (124, 140, 147, 188, 257, 272) and experimental lesions in animals as visualized in the microangiograms (84, 95, 101)[1] and fluorescence photomicrographs (84). On the side of the cross-section opposite that containing the extravasation in the white matter, the microvasculature in the white mattter is hardly discernible. Here, the bleeding centrally in the cord is distinctly ramified, indicating spread along the perivascular spaces of the lateral branches of the central arteries.[3]

[1] The dowel was removed after the epidural compression of the cervical cord since in experimental compression in the cadaver no contrast medium leaks out from the severed vessels so long as the compressing body remains in place; the contrast medium was then injected into the cord *via* a vertebral artery in order to examine whether the vessels had also been damaged.

[2] In specimens where the dowel remained in place the tear zone is usually transparent on translumina-

tion because no contrast medium has leaked out.

[3] The fact that compression haemorrhage is located mainly in the central grey matter of the spinal cord (zone 1 of the microvasculature) (82, 84, 88, 95, 254, 262) is thus due to (*i*) the concentration of the maximum tension at the central axis of the stress field in the spinal cord tissue, (*ii*) the axial course of the lateral branches of the central arteries in this region, and (*iii*) the technique widely adopted in experimental spinal cord injury in animals, whereby tapered weights are dropped on the cord (5, 6, 84, 95, 262); this produces a conical depression in the tissue and thus increases the tendency for the damage to be located mainly at the centre of the cord. When the weight and the distance that it falls are increased, the tensile stress field within the cord is intensified and widened. The distortion of the cord and the simultaneous internal distortion of the tissue might well lead ultimately to over-stretching also of the transversely coursing vessels of the extrinsic circulation; bleeding in the white matter might then result (84, 142).

In the above specimen the small blood-vessels that, for this reason, were torn from the surrounding tissue and coiled up after retraction are seen only occasionally in the microangiograms despite high magnification (Figs. 56, 59).

B. Diagrammatic representation of the retraction of axial branches of the intramedullary blood-vessels after tearing of the cord.

Upper row. Normal conditions.

Lower row. Ruptured small vessels that have retracted and coiled up.

Black arrows. Direction of tension.

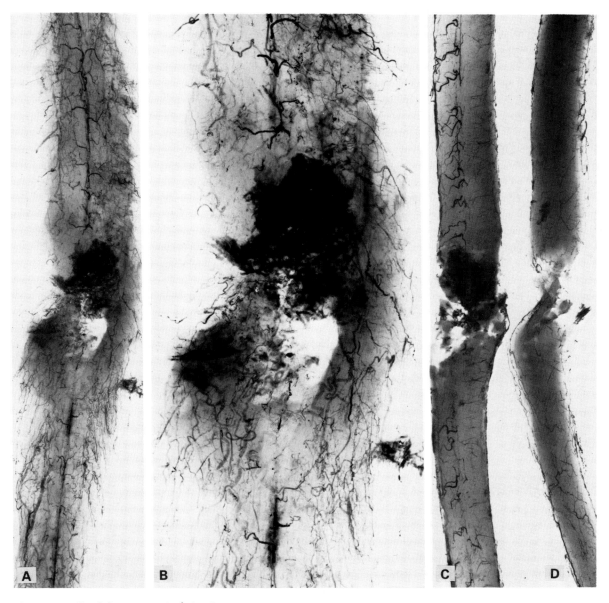

Fig. 66. Localized derangement of structures in cord laceration. Cervical spinal cord damaged with a Cloward drill *in situ* after filling with contrast medium (Specimen no. 5, Table 1).

A, B. Anteroposterior microangiograms; lower and higher magnification, respectively. The specimen was removed and fixed in formaldehyde.

C. Mid-sagittal section about 3 mm thick.

D. Section lateral to C.

Outside the lacerated region the tissue and blood-vessels are entirely unaffected—as in the case of an open brain laceration. (If even a rather small rupture, with haemorrhage and oedema, is located within the hind-brain or spinal cord, the lesion will inevitably lead to distension of the surrounding tissue. This might well be a cause of the signs and symptoms in cerebral palsy (251).)

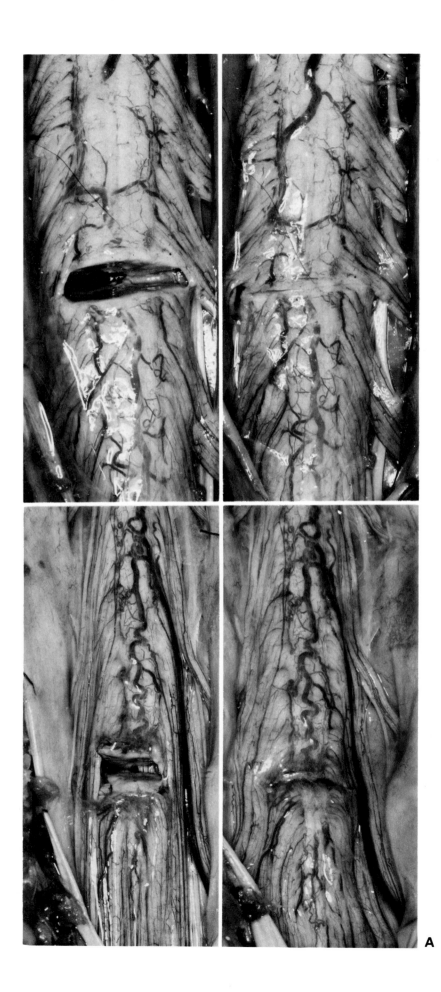

Fig. 67.

A. Effects of the normal tension and relaxation of the pons–cord tract on a transverse incision in the spinal cord at cervical and lumbar levels.

Left, upper and lower. In full flexion of the head and cervical spine there is retraction of the wound surfaces at the cervical and lumbar levels, respectively.

Right, upper. In the neutral position of the cervical spine (moving from flexion) the wound surfaces at the *cervical level* come together.

Right, lower. At the *lumbar level* the wound surfaces meet only when the cervical spine is fully extended.

A

B. Effects of normal tension and relaxation of the pons–cord tract on the transected half of the cervical spinal cord *in situ.*

Left. In full flexion of the head and the cervical spine the wound surfaces in the transected half of the cord have been drawn apart. (The dentate ligament that had not been severed is fully stretched.)

Right. On assuming the neutral position of the cervical spine from flexion the wound surfaces are brought into almost complete contact. (It is incomplete at the lower margin of the sagging cord—the body is in the right lateral position.)[1]

C. Effects of normal tension in the canine pons–cord tract on the transected half of its cervical section *in situ.*
(Control experiment on the fresh cadaver of a 50 cm long beagle.)[2]

Left. Hemitransection of the right half of the cord at the C_1/C_2 level. Cadaver in the prone neutral position. While making the sagittal incision in the dura the pia mater was inadvertently severed at two places a few millimetres to the left of the midline.)

Middle. On bending the dog's head forward the edges of the incision opened to form a cleft. Pulp was extruded from both the cleft and the rifts in the pia.

Right. On full forward bending of the head and the whole spine the cleft in the right half of the cord widened considerably and a large amount of pulp was squeezed out from both the cleft and the rifts. (The obvious disintegration of the medullary tissue was probably caused by the drug used in sacrificing the dog.)

D. The cervical spine of a dog in full flexion (*right*) **and extension** (*left*)**.** Drawn from radiographs of the cadaver.

The difference in the length of the central axis of the cervical canal in the two positions was 2.7 cm. (Length of the dog and breed not known.)

[1] This study was performed to obtain an impression of whether, in prospective animal experiments, hemitransection of the cord might be a useful technique for investigating regeneration of the nerve-fibres. Hemitransection would obviously result in a less severe neurological deficit than total transection, thus facilitating the postoperative care of the experimental animal and increasing its chances of survival.

The observed tendency for the edges of the incision to dehisce due to sagging of the cord indicated the need for microsurgical repair of the pial sheath (Fig. 36).

The main inference to be drawn from the above observations is that after the hemitransection has been performed the cervical column of the experimental animal must be held in extended (upright) position to keep the cord relaxed and its wound surfaces in contact.

The advocated canine experiments are at present being carried out by the author at The Erasmus University, Rotterdam, The Netherlands.

[2] With permission of Birger Schantz, M.V.D., School of Veterinary Medicine, University of Stockholm. Photo: Matts Johansson, Veterinary College, Stockholm.

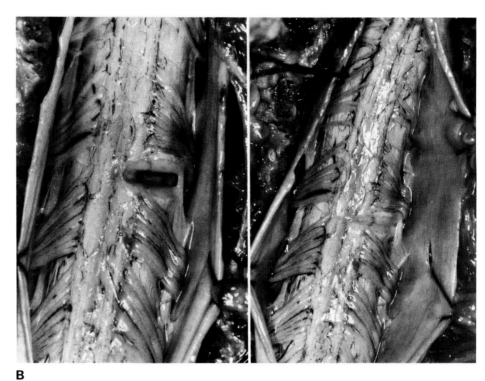

B

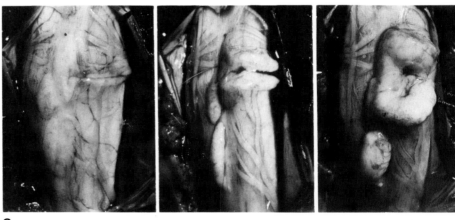

C

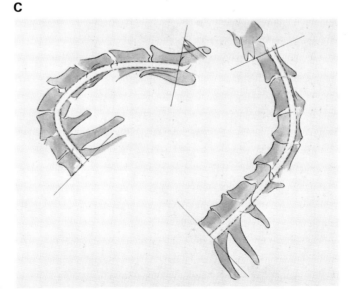

D

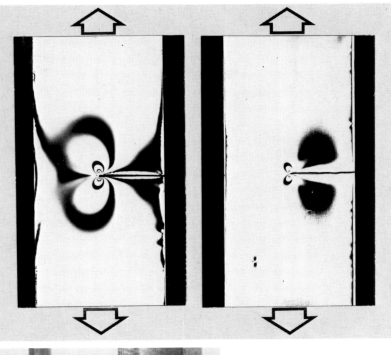

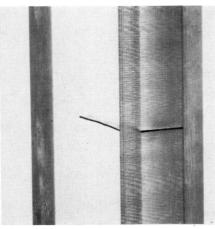

Fig. 68. The stress concentration around a tear in the cord tissue subjected to axial traction (notch stress), visualized by means of a photoelastic model.[1,2]

Upper, left. A rectangular Araldite block has been cut half way through from one edge to the midline. On applying traction to the ends of the block the cut opens to form a notch; the stress field set up around the end of the cut is indicated by isochromes.

Upper, right. Another Araldite block with an identical cut has been cemented between two intact Araldite blocks. This sandwich plate was similarly subjected to traction. The isochromes show that despite the presence of the stabilizing intact block on each side, the stress concentration at the end of the notch persists.

Lower. The structure of the sandwich block.

[1] In the nervous system this type of stress can interfere with the conductivity of the nerve-fibres. It occurs, for instance, around an intramedullary tissue rupture in spinal cord injury (Fig. 41) and fragmentation of disorganized myelin sheaths in a pathologically altered Gasserian ganglion and trigeminal nerve-root (15, 163).

[2] These phenomena suggest that the application of skull traction in the former condition increases the tension acting in the damaged spinal cord. Not only is the conductivity of the cord interrupted by the primary rupture, but it is impaired by the increased tension in the intact nerve-fibres around the rupture. It would thus seem that, besides flexion of the cervical spine, skull traction can aggravate a neurological deficit (Case 2, p. 233).

Fig. 69.

A. The effect of skull traction on a transverse incision in the cervical cord with the cervical spine in neutral position.

Left. The wound surfaces of the transverse incision in the cord are approximated.

Right. During skull traction the wound surfaces separate. (Forceps attached to the parietal bone in a coronal plane through the auditory meatus; load 5 kg.)

Photo: Stellan Linzander, M.D., Stockholm.

B. Representation of the elongation of the normal cervical spinal canal during skull traction.

Diagram of superimposed radiographs of the cervical spine of a patient who had sustained a compressive fracture of the C_5 vertebral body (Case 2, p. 233). *Blank.* Cervical spine unloaded. *Shaded.* Spine subjected to skull traction some hours after the injury, the forceps loaded with a weight of 5 kg. As indicated by the cranial displacement of the odontoid process, the length of the cervical spinal canal had been increased by 10 mm (the enlargement factor subtracted), as measured between a line tangential to the lower surface of the C_7 vertebral body and the tip of the odontoid process of the axis. From the diagram it is seen that the elongation of the canal is due to the increase in length of *all* the intervertebral spaces; in addition the C_5/C_6 space, where the intervertebral disc had been damaged, is enlarged by practically the same amount as the undamaged neighbouring intervertebral spaces. Note also the separation of the articular surfaces of the intervertebral joints.

C. Diagrammatic survey of the harmful effects on the cervical cord of its compression *(left),* **of a fracture reduction and/or dislocation of the cervical spine by skull traction** *(right).*

Left. Transverse fissure in the cord at the level where it has been pinched (clamped).

Right. The intramedullary (subpial) wound surfaces have been drawn apart by skull traction.

D. Device for measuring the interdependent shift of spinal structures in the cadaver *in situ* **due to changes in position of the spine and application of external forces to it.**[1]

The pointers can be moved in both lateral and vertical directions, so that structures deep in the spinal canal can easily be reached. A long distance is measured as the sum of a series of short distances of convenient length. By turning the crank, one of the pointers, which is attached to a wheel rolling in a track, can be moved to the next point. This procedure gives a value to an acceptable degree of accuracy.

The instrument was applied to a score of biomechanical analyses.

[1] Constructed by The National Defence Research Institute, Sweden, to author's design. Courtesy of Pehr Clements, Civ. Eng., Stockholm.

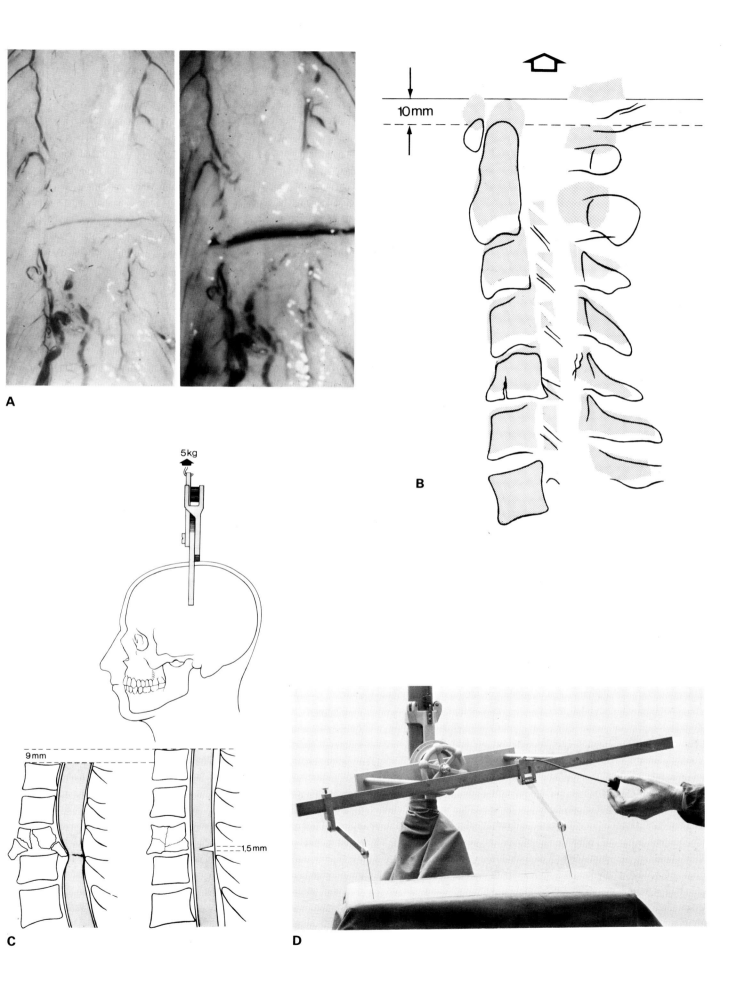

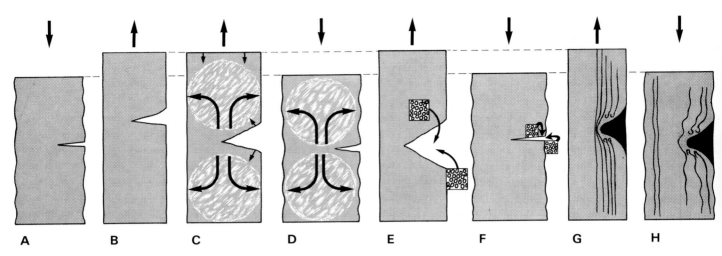

Fig. 70. The local effect of normal tension in the cord containing a partial transverse rupture.

A. A transverse tear, a typical result of compressive trauma inflicted with the cervical spine extended.

B. When the spinal cord is stretched during flexion the wound surfaces separate and the remaining intact fibres are exposed to over-stretching.

C. Owing to the appearance of reactive oedema (*stippled*) there is an increase in the cross-section (p. 55) of the involved length of the cord (*arrows pointing laterally*) and the wound surfaces retract further (*oblique arrows*).

D. The relaxation of the cord tissue on extension leads to a reduction in the axial tension and hence narrowing of the gap.

E. *Flexion.* If the cord is kept *stretched* during the repair stage, glia and connective tissue grow into the wound gap (*large squares*).

F. *Extension.* If the cord is kept *slack* during the repair stage and the wound surfaces are approximated, the gap is narrower and less repair with glia and connective tissue is required (*small squares*).

G. Unless widening of the fissure is prevented by relaxation of the spinal cord, the scar will be wider and the residual intact fibres in its vicinity will be subjected to pathological bending tensile stress even during normal stretching of the cord.

H. The bending tensile stress produced by the scar in G is eliminated by relaxation.

(In the figure the tearing of the cord tissue has been emphasized by exaggerating the separation of the wound surfaces; the pia mater cylinder has been omitted at the level of the rupture.)

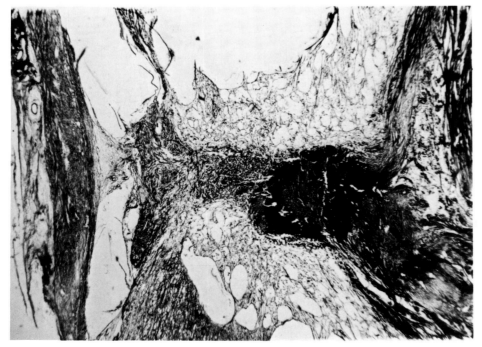

Fig. 71. An experimentally modified collagenous scar (*dark*) **in the sectioned spinal cord** (*light*) **of a dog, showing an attempt at promoting spinal cord regeneration, by inserting a piece of cerebellar tissue.**

"Two types of barrier to axonal regeneration in the spinal cord were found in experimental spinal cord transection in dogs. One was an astroglial scar formed within the spinal cord, and the other a collagenous scar in the gap between proximal and distal stumps (141)."

(This situation is essentially equivalent to that in E and G in Fig. 70)

"Three weeks after the transplantation in some of the above experiments axon collected in bundles, penetrated the scar and travelled a few millimetres to meet the transplant in the former gap that was converted into a spongy structure."

Courtesy of Chun C. Kao, Department of Surgery (Neurological Surgery), Indiana University Medical Center, USA.

Fig. 72. Histodynamic background to nerve-root damage in spinal cord injury.

Analysis of the traumatic and post-traumatic tissue deformation in the C_8 right posterior root and the posterior horn after acute compression of the cervical spinal cord in a 20-year-old victim of a road accident; he had received a blow on the upper part of the forehead, resulting in (unspecified) dislocation of the C_6 vertebra (on hyperextension of the cervical spine?) followed by immediate tetraplegia; survived 7 days (188).

Part of a cross-section through the cervical cord and a longitudinal section through the posterior root.[1] Extensive vacuolization in the posterior horn; ruptures between pia and pulp; at *F*, evidence of an anteroposterior fissure. Fibres in the distal stump of the nerve-root clearly folded; of the proximal stump only a marginal zone is preserved; centrally in the root, fragmented tissue. Likewise in border zone of posterior horn, possibly root tissue retracted into the cord; just anterior to this the section passes through vacuoles in the posterior horn, which follows an axial direction. These injuries to the root and posterior horn have previously been ascribed to tearing of the root from the posterior horn.[2]

The post-traumatic alterations of the C_8 root indicate that, together with the cervical spinal cord, the root had been clamped against the bone wall of the cervical canal, and that one of the affected areas was at the place where the root enters the posterior horn. To judge from the damage the resulting stress field in the root tissue extended fairly far distally. As a result of the summation of the stresses maximum tearing has occurred just at the point where the nerve-root joins the posterior horn. The fissures parallel to the axial direction of the root may have arisen because the erected filaments had been forcibly compressed in their axial direction.[3]

Courtesy of E. Th. Mayer (188). With kind permission of the Editor of Hdb Neurotraumatologie, Urban & Schwarzenberg, München–Berlin–Vienna.

[1] On the cord cross-section the left pyramidal lateral tract is impaired more than the right. Together with the damage to the root on the right side this points to compression from the left front towards the back right, or vice versa. The cord was not fixed *in situ*.

[2] The longitudinal and cross-sections through a cervical spinal cord subjected to compression portray the histodynamic effects of the axial and transverse components of the intramedullary stress field, respectively. In general, only a few hours after the trauma its immediate histodynamic consequences are more difficult to discern owing to oedema and vacuolization (stretching of the axoplasm (59, 77, 79, 207)), periaxonal oedema (33), myelin-sheath oedema (83, 102, 262), tearing and retraction of myelin sheaths (83, 262), interstitial oedema in the supporting framework of neuroglia (83, 262) and secondary degeneration of axis-cylinders (83, 103). On extension of the cervical spinal column the tissue of the nerve-roots is also telescoped (35). The stems of the filaments of the posterior roots are erected at their sites of entry into the spinal cord.

[3] The biological and histodynamic alterations, the effect on the damaged tissue exerted by movements of the spinal cord and nerve-roots in the living

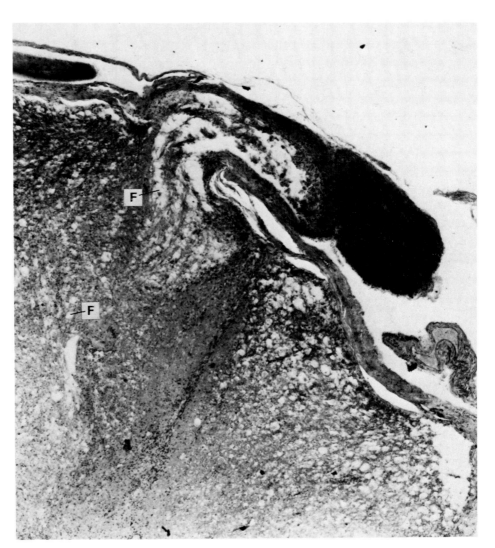

patient and the inevitable fixation and sectioning artefacts have complicated the histological picture to the point where a more detailed analysis would be meaningless.

The severe injuries to the nerve-root might perhaps excite doubt as to whether the relatively minor changes observed in artificial compression of isolated nerve-roots are consistent with reality (Fig. 73). Suturing of the extensive tears in the nerve-fibres such as those seen in the present picture is ruled out even with the Millipore technique (13, 249). The only treatment method that can offer the patient a chance of at least partial restoration of function is relaxation of the nerve-roots by spinal extension. Moreover, this method should be applied also when the tubulization technique employing Millipore is used (58, 249).

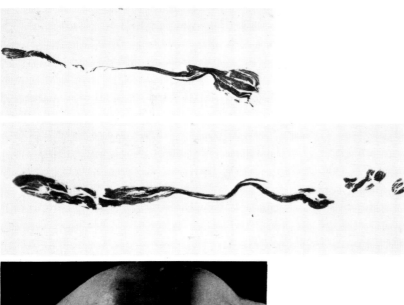

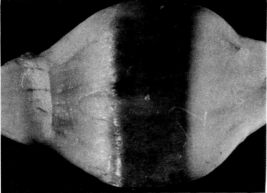

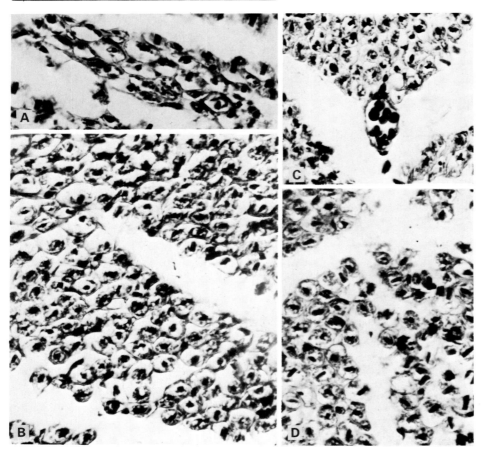

Fig. 73. Effect of a pincer action on isolated cervical nerve-roots. (Specimen no. 1, Table 2)

Longitudinal sections through an artificially compressed posterior (*top*) and anterior (*middle*) cervical nerve-root. (The breaks anterior and posterior to the clamped zone may be sectioning artefacts.) (×12.5). *Formaldehyde fixation, Palmgren's stain,* ×6.4.

In spite of extensive squashing of fibres in the clamped nerve-root, which has resulted in local stretching, there is no definite rupture in the region of maximum compression. *Bottom.*—Fresh specimen of nerve-root.

The nerve-roots are obviously more resistant to compressive stress than the spinal cord. This is consistent with earlier observations (264, 265). *Cf.* recent view in Fig. 75.

Fig. 74. Transverse section through a C$_6$ nerve-root subjected to pinching *in situ.*

The contours of the transversely cut axis-cylinders near the surface of the nerve-root (A) and just below (B, upper half) are oval (flattened), presumably because of their attachment to the pia, and the transverse tension caused by the high contact pressure. The irregular (crenated ?) contour of the more centrally located cylinders is evidently due to axial tension in the root (B, *lower half,* C *and* D). The endoneurial spaces remain patent.

Osmium tetroxide, ×280.

Fig. 75. Effect of pincer action on an isolated length of sciatic nerve. (Specimen no. 2, Table 2)

A. Clamped sciatic nerve fixed in formaldehyde (×ca. 2.0).

B. Translumination of the nerve and the impressed zone. The compressed fibres have only slightly increased in width.

C. Longitudinal section. The fibres are clearly stretched both within and just outside the actual zone of clamping, and there are signs of tearing. There is folding of the fibres, which increases with distance from the clamped zone, and evidence of a compensatory increase in the circumference of the nerve-root (60, 207). (Some of the fibres have been sectioned obliquely (×ca. 5.6).)

The sciatic nerve, just as the nerve-roots, thus presents a fairly great resistance to damage by compressive forces.

Recent view. When a section of a spinal cord, nerve-root or peripheral nerve is pinched between two firm structures *in situ*, the nerve-fibres take up the tension resulting from their inward deflection. When such a section is resected and subjected to the same degree of pinching, the cut ends of the nerve-fibres are able to retract more readily and the tension in them is lowered. Thus, a realistic picture of the biomechanical events *in vivo* can be obtained only when the pathological load is applied to the intact nervous tissue *in situ*.

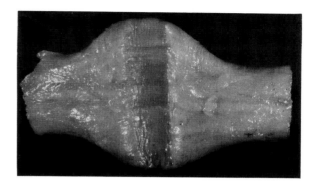

A

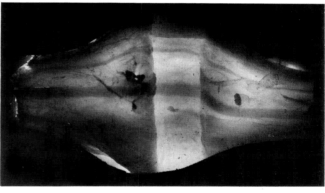

B

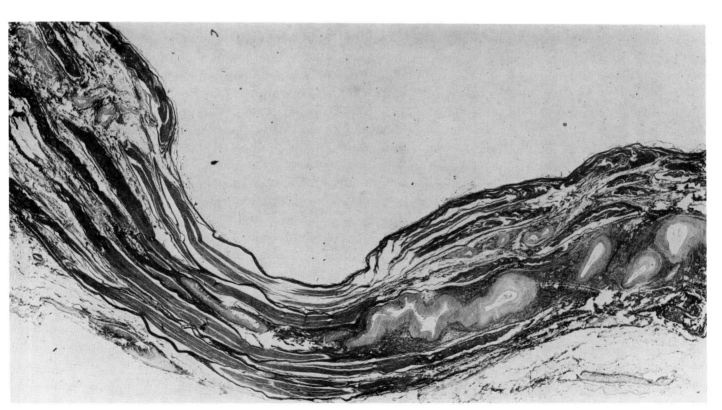

C

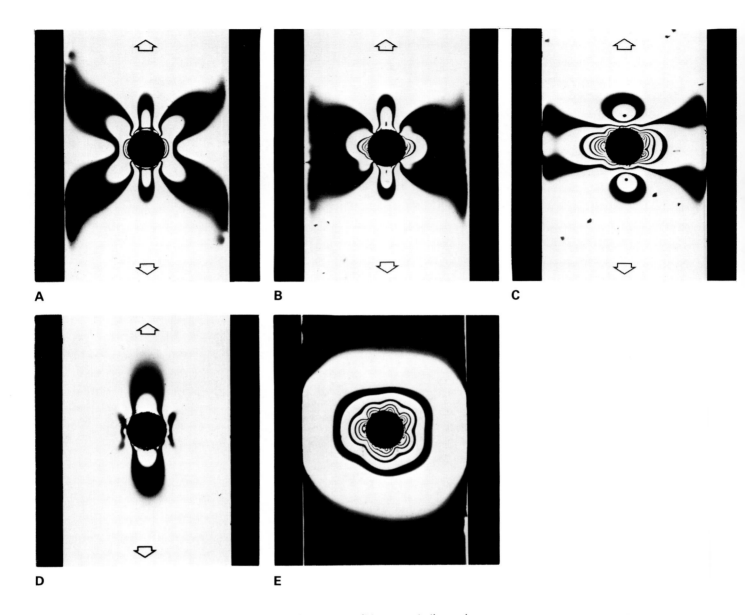

Fig. 76. Photoelastic models simulating stress fields set up by various types of pathological changes in the spinal cord.[1]

The isochromes (lines joining points of equal stress) show the differences in stress concentration in a homogeneous elastic rectangular Araldite block subjected to traction (A–E).

A. The block with a round hole, under tension. *Clinical analogy:* Representation of the stress set up by, for example, an intramedullary malacic cyst on stretching of the spinal cord; the isochrome pattern suggests that in flexion of the spine there is an increase in the tension in the cord tangential to the cyst (*black circle*).

B. The block, likewise under tension, with a rigid rod inserted loosely in the hole. *Clinical analogy:* Representation of the stress set up by a circumscribed deformable haematomyelia or cyst (hydromyelia, syringomyelia, etc.), assuming that there is a membrane that prevents escape of the liquid into the tissue. The

histodynamic conditions are similar to those under A, with the exception that the cyst is subjected to a radial pressure. If the conducting nerve-fibres that previously passed through the site of the cyst have been destroyed (as illustrated in A, and in some cases also in B) the stress perpendicular to the axis of the cavity is of no practical significance.

C. The rod forced into the hole while the block is kept under tension. *Clinical analogy:* According to the model, expanding lesions, such as intramedullary tumours, central gliosis, vascular fibrosis, invading scar tissue after spinal cord injuries and circumscribed oedema, exert a powerful pressure on the surrounding tissue, thereby setting up high tensile bending stress in the nerve-fibres (C'). This stress increases in flexion and decreases, or even disappears, in extension.

D. The rod cemented in the hole while the block is kept under tension. *Clinical analogy:* Glial scarring in, for instance, multiple sclerosis without constriction of the axis-cylinders around the rigid structures. The most promi-

nent of the stress phenomena is the elevated axial tension in the cylinders passing through the actual scar and in those cylinders displaced around the lesions.

E. The block *not* under tension, with the rod forced into the hole. *Clinical analogy:* The high local stress that may be exerted on the surrounding tissue by an *expanding* lesion even in the neutral position of the column.

A'–E'. Graphical representation of the corresponding stress distributions for Figs. A to E.

[1] The deformation of the elastic fibres of the spinal cord, which are arranged in a fairly loose network, differs considerably from the deformation of a homogeneous elastic body. The effects in the spinal cord tissue therefore do not correspond exactly to those in the above model. Nonetheless, as shown in Fig. 78, there would appear to be similarities in the mechanical effect in the two materials.

The author recognizes that this analysis is inexact—qualitative rather than quantitative.

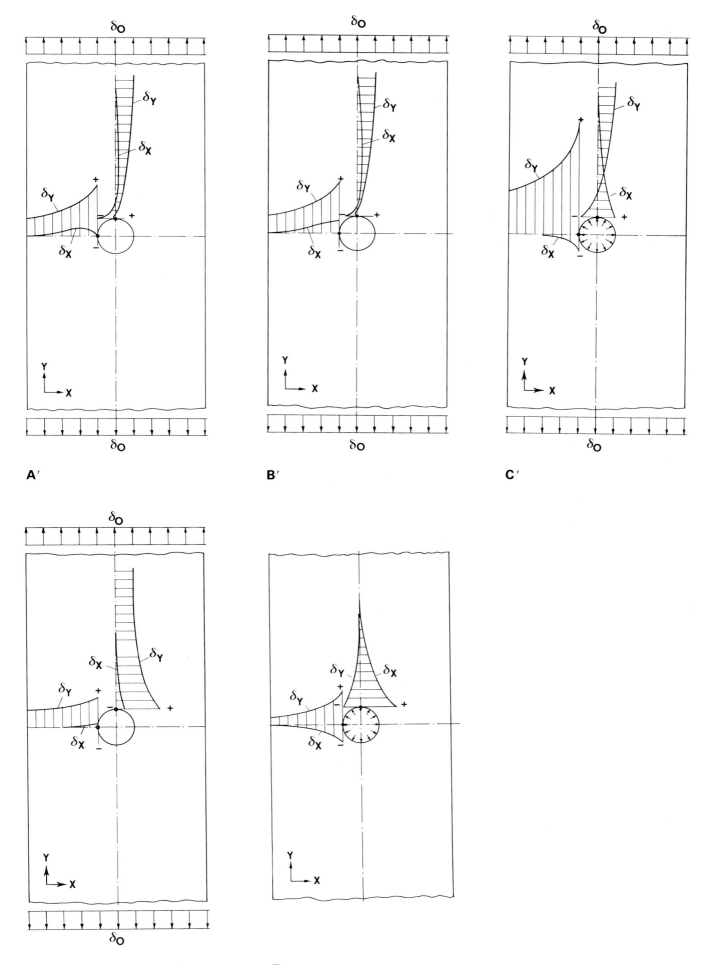

A'

B'

C'

D'

E'

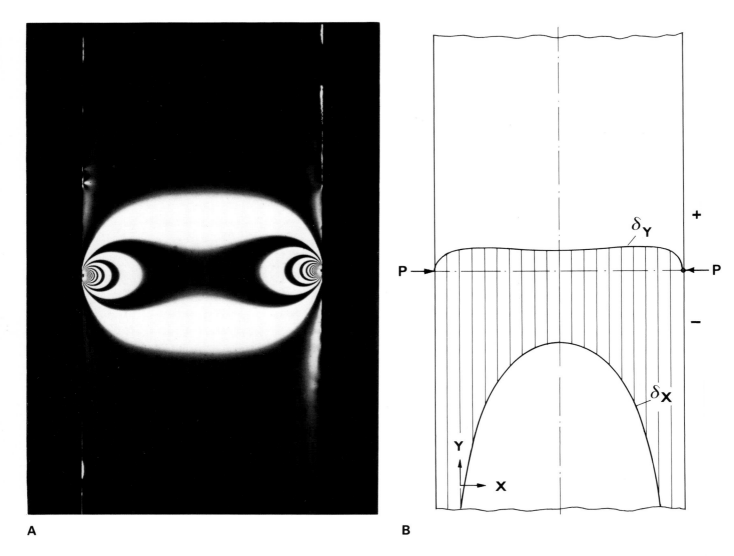

A   **B**

Fig. 77. Analysis of the physical effects of compressive stress.

A. The stress field produced by a pincer action on the Araldite block.

B. Graphical representation of the isochromes. P, point of load. δy, variation in axial tensile stress (upper, positive, part of the curve), δx, variation in transverse compressive stress (lower, negative, part of the curve). The axial stress is zero at P and then increases rapidly to a maximum in a zone about one-tenth the thickness of the block; towards the middle of the block there is a slight dip. The compressive stress is infinitely high at the margins and falls rapidly to a minimum at the middle of the block.

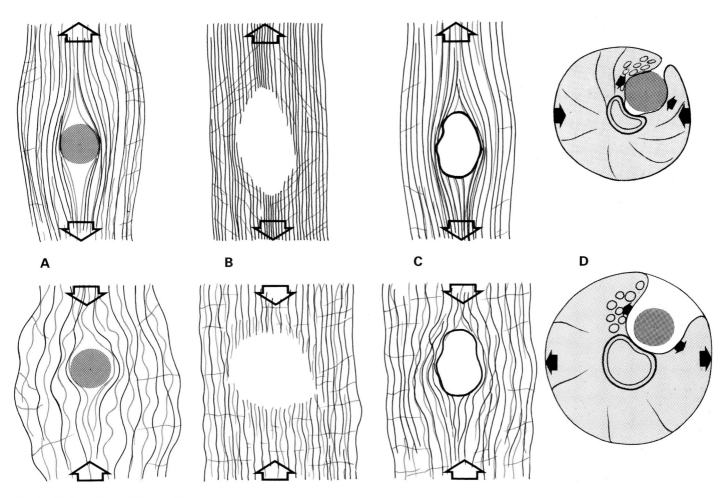

Fig. 78. Deformation of the cord tissue produced by various pathological changes and giving rise to tension on flexion of the spine; recovery on relaxation of the tissue obtained by extension. Analysis by photoelastic experiments.

A–C, coronal or sagittal section; D, cross-section.
Upper row. Stress fields set up on flexion.
Lower row. Resolution of the stress fields on extension.

A. Unyielding body exerting an outward thrust (tumour, scar, calcification, etc.).

B. Internal cavity without circumscribing membrane—for instance, malacic cyst (182).

C. Cavity lined with a membrane and filled with fluid (a walled cyst, organized haematoma, etc.).

D. Deformation of the tissue by a firm intramedullary body.

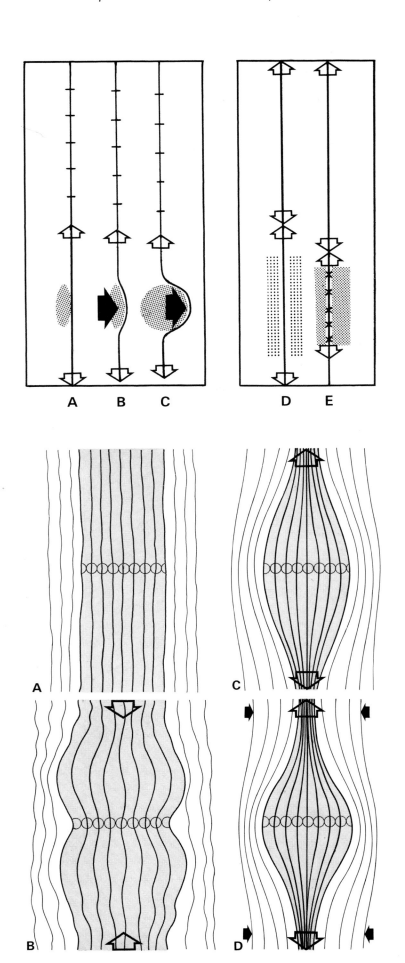

Fig. 79. Effect of the presence in the stretched cord of an unyielding structure: on a single nerve-fibre passing outside the structure (A–C) **and on one passing through it** (D, E).

A. Unaffected nerve-fibre outside the structure.

B, C. Various degrees of over-stretching depending on the size of the structure and the thrust exerted by it.

D. A nerve-fibre passing freely through the structure.

E. During flexion elongation of a nerve-fibre at the site where it is adherent to the structure is prevented, but there is over-stretching above and below this site.

To emphasize the effects of the tension in the nerve-fibres they are represented as following a straight course instead of a convergent one (Fig. 88).

Fig. 80. The effect of an inelastic scar, circumscribed oedema or the like, on axis-cylinders running axially in the white matter (*dark shading*), **and on cylinders outside the scar, oedema etc.** (*fine black lines*).

A. The rings denote the rigid scar. The axis-cylinders passing through the scar are shown as continuous lines to indicate their continuity (and any residual conductivity). In the *neutral posture* of the spine the parallel cylinders outside the scar are not under tension.

B. The undulating course of the cylinders in *extension*. As the scar remains undeformed one would expect them to show an hour-glass deformation at this level. This would result in some deflection of the cylinders along the periphery of the bulging areas (*fine black lines*). Since these cylinders are slack this phenomenon would probably not generate symptoms.

C, D. On stretching of the cord in moderate *flexion* the elastic axis-cylinders involved in the scar form a gradually narrowing spindle (C), which becomes accentuated in full flexion (D). It is conceivable that artificial synapses (15, 116, 163) may arise in situations analogous to (D) at the point of greatest tension.

When the cross-section of the stretched cord narrows (*black arrows*) in full *flexion* the intact axis-cylinders surrounding the spindle will be subjected to increased tensile bending, which will probably impair their conductivity. Experience has shown that when the axis-cylinders are relaxed in extension the neurological symptoms decrease.

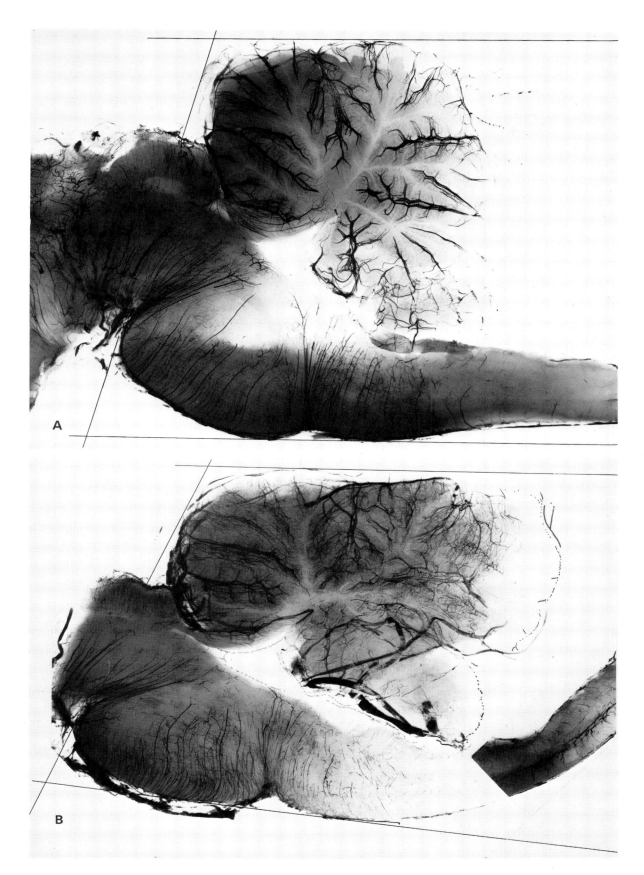

Fig. 81. Deformation of hind-brain and fourth ventricle induced by artificial increase in supratentorial pressure (112, 133).

Microangiograms of 5 mm midsagittal sections through the mid- and hind-brain.

A. After a small increase in supratentorial pressure with the head and neck *flexed*. Note shape of fourth ventricle.

B. After a greater increase in pressure with the head and neck *extended*.

Stippled lines show the boundaries of the deformed fourth ventricle and the moderate cerebellar pressure cone. Photomontage of the upper part of the cervical cord.

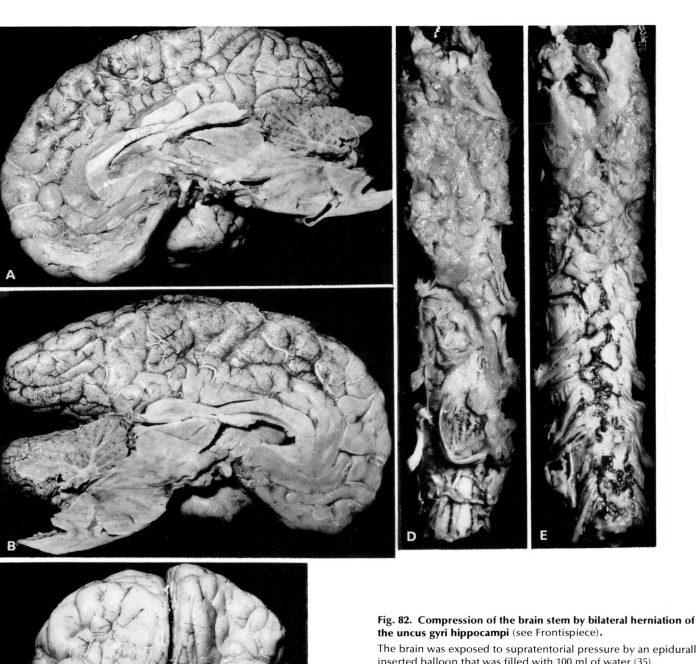

Fig. 82. Compression of the brain stem by bilateral herniation of the uncus gyri hippocampi (see Frontispiece).

The brain was exposed to supratentorial pressure by an epidurally inserted balloon that was filled with 100 ml of water (35).

A. Right half. B. Left half. C. From below.

The high pressure produced extreme deformation due to mass displacement; besides the formation of a tentorial pressure cone and uncal herniation, the tissue of the decussatio brachii conjunctivi has been forced forwards and upwards so that it bears against the corpus callosum; the great masses of bilateral herniated uncal tissue have compressed the mid-brain and pons, thereby squeezing and displacing them in the vertical direction. This is also evident from the microangiogram in Fig. 83.

Another striking effect of this pressure is the extrusion of all the caudal part of the cerebellum, part of it down and around the upper cervical cord: D, anterior view; E, posterior view. The caudalward shearing force has denuded the basal aspect of the pons of its pia mater, and the basal artery has been torn away.[1]

[1] In the case of a high pathological pressure in the posterior cranial fossa the pons and oblongata may be pressed against the clivus and thus squeezed (flattened) so that a pathological axial tension is set up in them. On flexion of the spine this tension is augmented by the physiological tension in the pons–cord tract; if the total tension is then transmitted to the mid-brain mesencephalic neurological manifestations will probably result (p. 188).

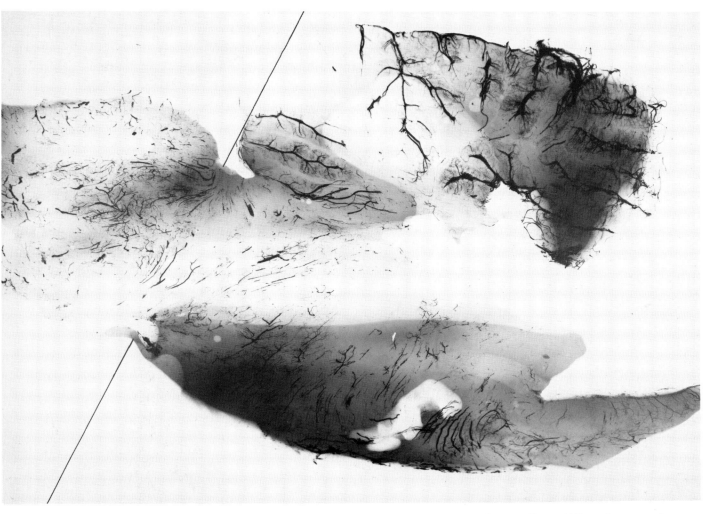

Fig. 83. Effects of bilateral compression on the microvasculature of the brain stem.

The axial distension of brain tissue between the clivus and calvaria has resulted in extensive rupture of vessels. Microangiogram of a 5 mm mid-sagittal section through mid- and hind-brain shown in Fig. 82.

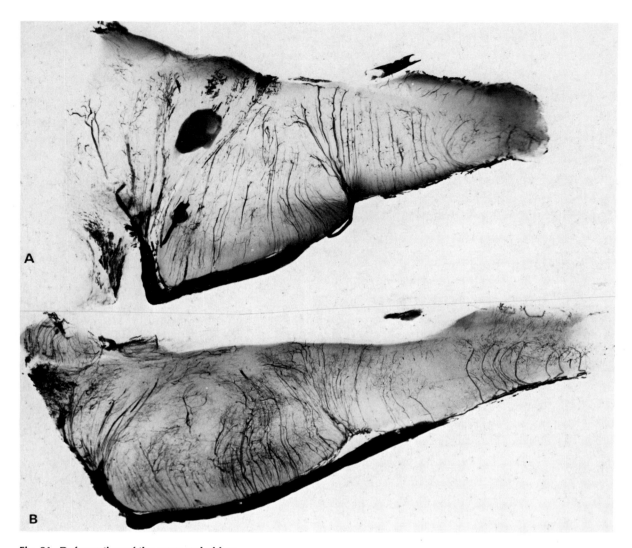

Fig. 84. Deformation of the pons and oblongata resulting from increase in supratentorial pressure.

Microangiograms of 4 mm sections through the mid-brain, pons and medulla oblongata. ×2.0.

A. A supratentorial expanding lesion has led to a haematoma in the pons, the cavity of which has been filled with contrast medium (see *Frontispiece*).

B. Another specimen with a supratentorial space-occupying lesion where obviously no uncal herniation developed: the resulting bilateral compression would otherwise have produced vertical distension of the pons and over-stretching and rupture of the vessels, as in A.

Courtesy of Ove Hassler, M.D., University of Umeå, Sweden (133). With kind permission of the Editor of Neurology.

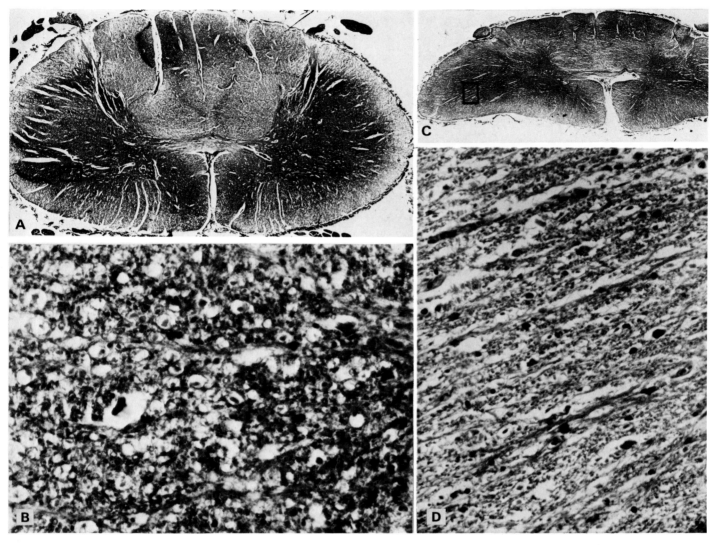

Fig. 85. Histodynamic effect on the cervical cord tissue of anteriorly located osteophytes.

A. The cervical cord, formaldehyde-fixed *in situ*, with the spine in the *neutral* posture (transverse section at the C_5/C_6 level. ×6.0).

Along the anterior aspect of the cord the fibres are oriented in a palisade formation in the anteroposterior direction.

B (*framed area in A*). The tissue has an amorphous reticular or honeycombed appearance.

C. In full *flexion* the cervical cord was exposed to pressure on the anterior aspect of the cord, stretching of the cord over the osteophytes and oblique anterior traction on the attachments of the dentate ligaments. Consequently a transverse tensile field is set up. *In situ* formaldehyde fixation. Transverse section at the same level as the specimen in A. (×4.2).

D (*framed area shown in C, corresponding to the framed area in A*). Because of the transverse tensile field, discrete transverse strata are seen. In spite of the marked antero-posterior constriction of the cord there is ample interstitial space between these elements; they are closest together parallel to the axis of stress, which is directed towards the attachment of the dentate ligament.

As a result of the increase in width of the cord the ganglion cells and the transversely sectioned axis-cylinders have separated (*cf.* B).

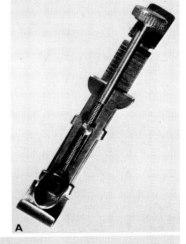

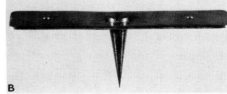

Fig. 86. Mechanical aids used for producing artificial deformation of the tissue.

A. An instrument for graded compression of, for instance, peripheral nerves. By means of a screw action a curved metal surface compresses the nerve, which is held in a curved metal cradle.

B. A metal cone which is inserted in the cord so as to distend the tissue (Figs. 88 and 89).

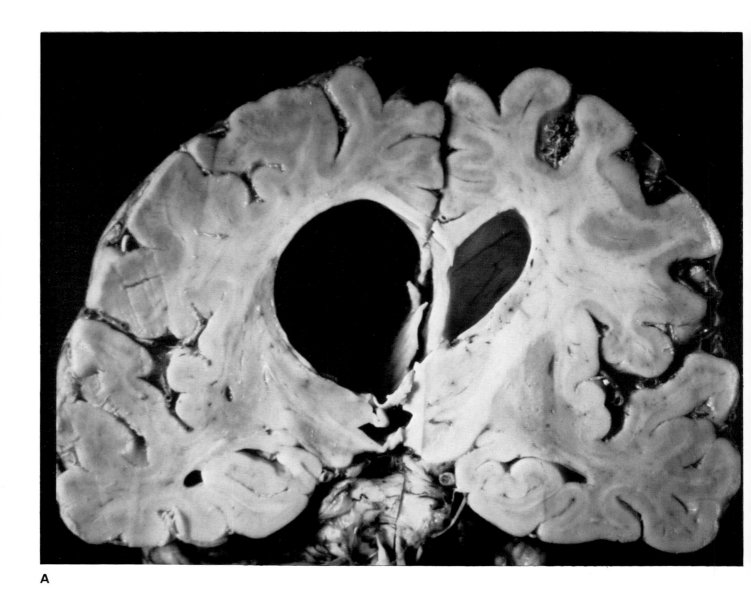

A

Fig. 87. Histodynamic stress in the brain tissue due to hydrocephalus.

A. Unilateral hydrocephalus produced in the cadaver *in situ* by inflating a thin rubber membrane placed in the left lateral ventricle through the posterior horn.

The pressure on the ventricle wall is transmitted to the contiguous structures, including the left internal capsule. The nerve-fibres and blood-vessels are subjected to compressive stress (specimen B) and are thus lengthened. Tension set up in this way may well account for impairment of conductivity of the nerve-fibres in a patient with internal hydrocephalus where a similar deformation exists.

B. Peroxidase stained section through human brain with severe hydrocephalus (Brodmann's area 39) (×28).[1, 2]

C. Peroxidase-stained section through human brain with no hydrocephalus (Brodmann's area 39) ×28.[1]

[1] Courtesy of O. Hassler, M.D., Department of Pathology, University of Umeå, Sweden (131). With kind permission of the Editor of Acta Neuropathologica.
[2] When the amount of fluid in the ventricles increases and their walls thus expand, the brain substance is clamped between the rigid skull and the fluid encapsulated in the ventricular system. As a result a stress field is set up in the brain tissue. Because of the curved shape of the clamping surfaces and the softer consistency of the white than of the grey matter, the distribution and magnitude of the resulting tensile stresses are difficult to determine. The stress pattern in the tissue, however, can be analysed in the microangiogram from the deformation of the blood-vessels: the direction in which the pressure acts is the prevailing direction

of the telescoped vessels; the direction of the tensile stresses that in which the vessels deviate. *Pressure:* In coronal and sagittal sections through the brain the capillary network in the grey matter tends to be displaced towards the skull and the arteries passing eccentrically through the cortex are telescoped. *Tension:* The tension in the brain substance is zero at the rigid surface of the skull and increases steeply in the direction of the expanding ventricular wall. The effect of this reactive tension is evident in the deep grey matter, where the compressed meshes of the capillary network are drawn taut, producing a denser texture. The severe stretching continues throughout the white matter. The arterioles leading from the large arteries at the base of the skull (which normally radiate into the white matter perpendicularly) are pulled taut along the outer margins of the ventricles (119); there is also evidence of fragmentation and extravasation. The resulting narrowing of the lumina of these arterioles reduces the oxygen supply to the over-

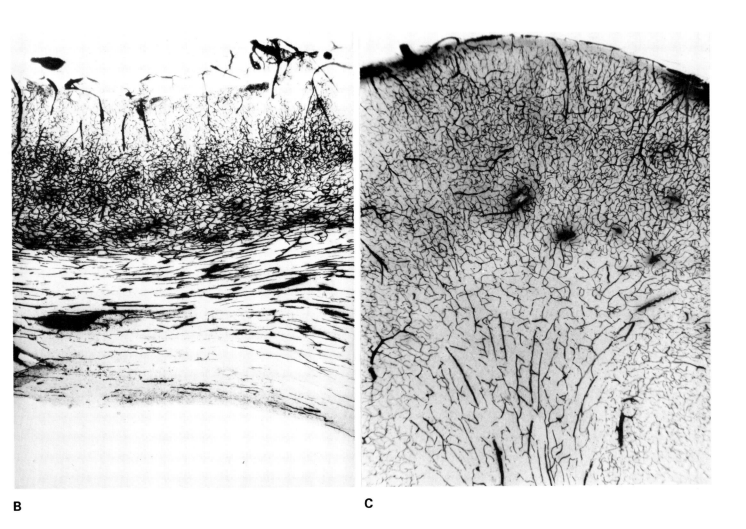

B

C

stretched nerve-fibres in the grey matter and further impairs their conductivity.

Relaxation of nerve-fibres and blood-vessels in the internal capsule—a beneficial bio-mechanical effect of procedures for shunting of cerebrospinal fluid from the cerebral ventricles (see *Frontispiece*).

Cerebral neurological manifestations are often evoked by distention of the cerebral ventricles, and morphological analyses have shown that the nerve-fibres and blood-vessels in the internal capsule are then over-stretched (Fig. 87 A). Moreover, other paraventricular fibre systems might also be affected by such intracerebral tension.

   That neurological effects also occur in low-pressure hydrocephalus is probably due to an alteration of the visco-elastic properties of the paraventricular tissues. When, for example, in the ageing brain the elasticity of cerebral nerve-fibres and blood-vessels is reduced by processes leading to *softening* of the brain substance in circumscribed areas within, or close to, the ventricular walls, even a small increase in the intraventricular pressure would probably result in over-stretching of these cerebral structures and thus in impairment of their conductivity. This may well explain in some measure the beneficial effect of shunting procedures even in low-pressure hydrocephalus. If, on the other hand, the normal resilience of the nerve-fibres and blood-vessels in these areas is reduced through the *hardening* processes of oedema or gliosis,[3] there would again be an increase in the intraventricular pressure, which might well lead to compensatory over-stretching of neighbouring nerve-fibres and blood-vessels. By lowering the intraventricular pressure by means of a shunt operation the freshly inflamed or chronically over-stretched nerve-fibres and blood-vessels would be relaxed and the neurological manifestations in some measure alleviated.

[3] At autopsy of a multiple sclerosis patient suffering from left-sided symptomatic trigeminal neuralgia (the tic douloureux attacks of which could be precipitated also by bending the neck forwards) the cerebral foci of demyelinization were found to be localized predominantly around the most laterally projecting recesses of the anterior, posterior and inferior horns of the lateral ventricles.

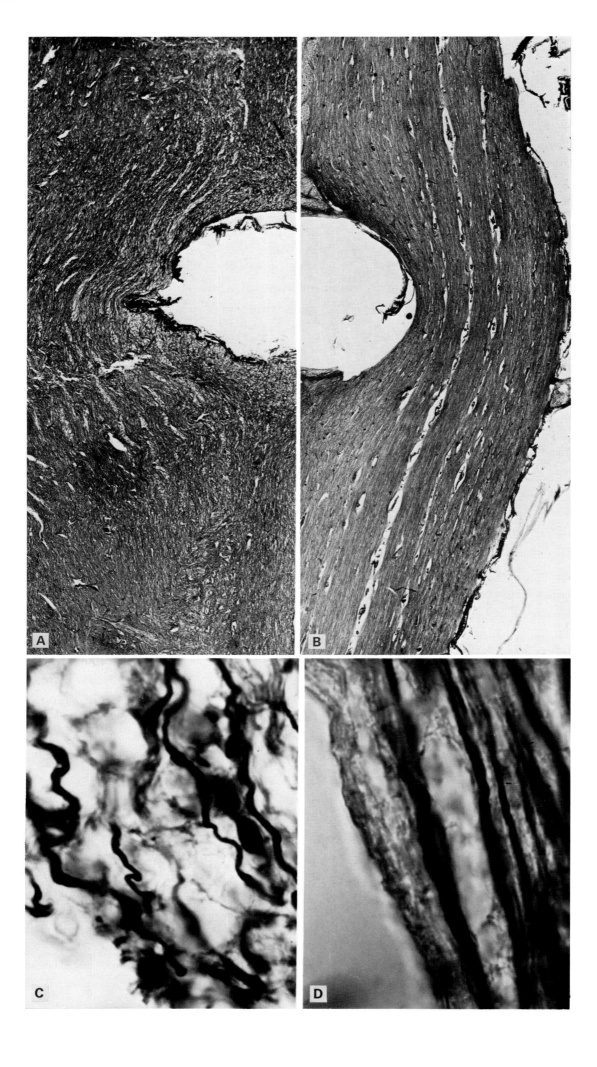

Fig. 88. Histodynamic effect of a rigid cone inserted in the cervical spinal cord tissue.

A metal cone 3 mm in diameter was inserted in the transverse plane from the anterior aspect *in situ* with the cord in the relaxed state, after which the spine was *flexed*. The cord was then fixed in formaldehyde for 24 hours *in situ* and, after dissection, fixed again for a fortnight. Coronal section in front of the anterior commissure, ×13.8.

B. The stress field around the cone of the stretched cervical cord tissue. The direction of this field is reflected in a spindle-shaped deformation of the fibres of the tissue network around the cone. The fibres nearest the cone have been pressed together to form a pseudo-membrane, which has been torn from the surrounding tissue.

A. Resolution of the stress field (in another subject) on relaxation of the tissue by *extending* the spine with the metal cone still in place. The relaxed fibres have moved away from the obstruction and assumed an undulating course. Preservation procedure as above.

High magnification (×1900) of the pseudo-membrane (in B and A).

D. The stretched and tightly packed fibres of the pseudomembrane. Though subjected to pressure, the axons do not actually come into contact, probably because of the intercellular fluid and the intervening glia.

C. Relaxed fibres bounding the cavity (*left*) after extension.

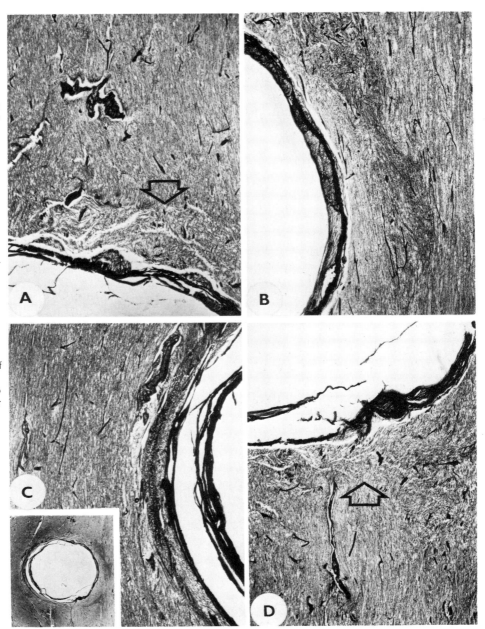

Fig. 89. Histodynamic effect of a rigid cone inserted in the cervical spinal tissue.

Preparation of specimen (Specimen no. 7, Table 2).

B, C. Visible stratification in the tissue produced by deflection and stretching of the fibres by the cone.

Inset.—The defect in the cord due to the cone (×3.4).

A, D. All fibres running axially are telescoped and fissures (*arrows*) are produced (×3.8).

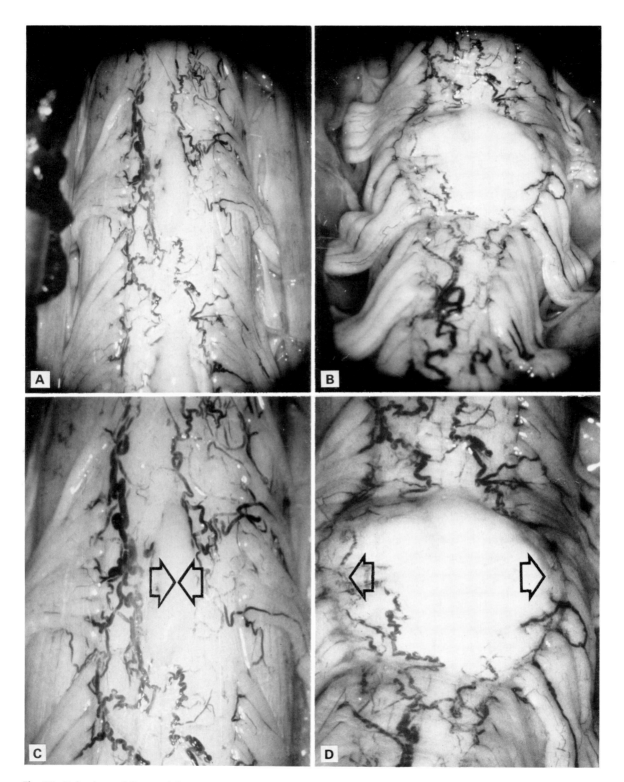

Fig. 90. Behaviour of the cord tissue on stretching and relaxation, shown by means of a posterior sagittal incision in the cervical cord (*in situ*).

A. General view—the incision, about 1 cm long, is visible in the upper two-thirds of the picture (operating microscope).

B. Owing to the telescoping of the cord when the cervical spine is extended, the borders of the incision separate to form a deep groove.

C. Higher magnification of A. When the spine is flexed an axial tension is set up in the cord, and the cut surfaces are pressed together. (The forces acting toward the cord axis are manifested in the bulging of a small central strip of tissue.)

D. Higher magnification of B.

Photo: Stellan Linzander, M.D., Stockholm.

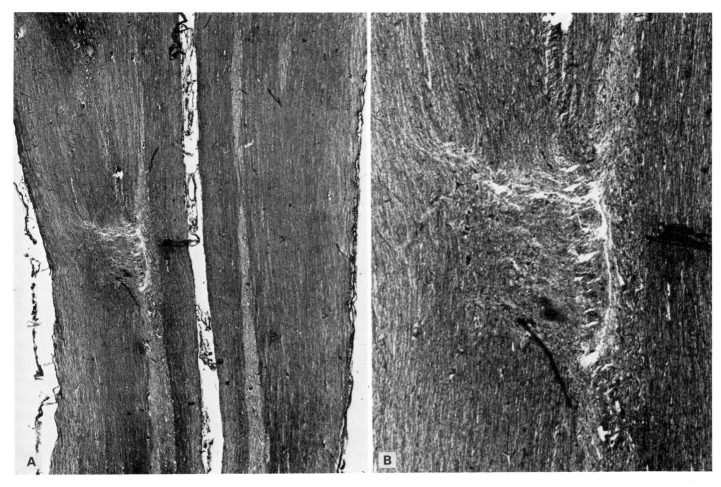

Fig. 91. Evidence of the stress in the stretched spinal cord tissue surrounding an artificial cavity.

Longitudinal sections of the cord in which a cavity was produced *in situ* by punching out a cylindrical piece of tissue from one-half of the relaxed cord with the cervical spine in *extension*.

A. The coronal section obtained after fixing the stretched specimen *in situ* lies in front of the anterior grey commissure, and thus shows two halves of the spinal cord. (×8.5).

B. Enlargement of A. According to the photo-elastic model, A in Fig. 76 and its graphical interpretation in Fig. 76', when the fibres are stretched on flexion, a large increase in tension in those running tangentially to the cavity would be expected (Fig. 78, B in upper row); this is confirmed in this experiment where the tissue was displaced into the cavity; the requisite force can have originated only from a greatly increased axial tension in the fibres surrounding the cavity (×25.6).

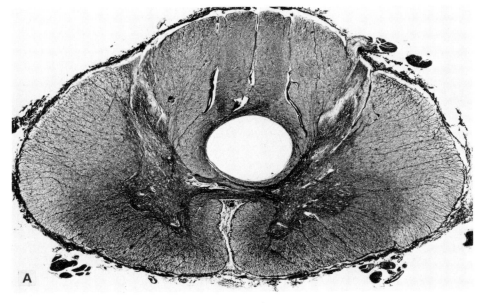

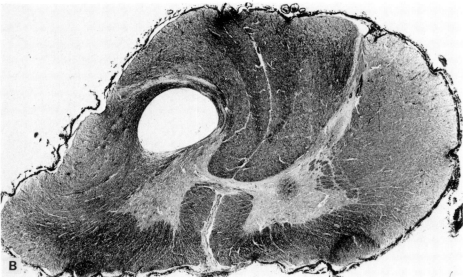

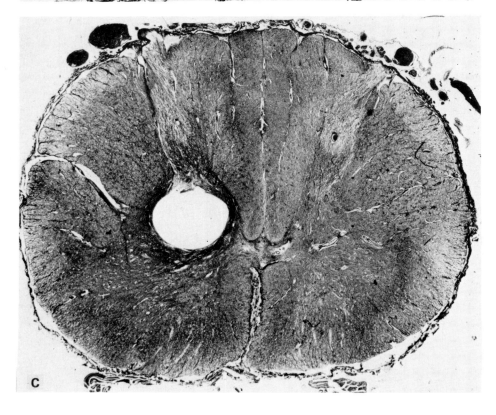

Fig. 92. Stress set up by a cylindrical body in the cord in the stretched, neutral and relaxed states (transverse sections; ×11.5).

A. *Neutral.* Histodynamic effect on an isolated cervical spinal cord specimen that has been formaldehyde-fixed when unstressed in the neutral posture of the spine. The cylindrical body, inserted in the sagittal direction, was located between the posterior horns, just behind the posterior grey commissure.

The compression of the tissue is greatest in the immediate vicinity of the cylinder, where there is evidence of a pseudomembrane. The tissue of the posterior columns has been subjected to slight anteroposterior pressure, which is reflected in the somewhat tortuous course of the vessels and the slightly increased cross-sectional area of the perivascular spaces. At the same time the posterior contour of the posterior columns has been pressed posteriorly (Table 2, no. 4).

B. *Stretched.* Cord fixed under tension corresponding to full flexion of the spinal column. The cylindrical body, which was inserted lateral to the right posterior horn, has produced marked compression of the tissue, which is evident over practically the whole cross-section. The bending tensile stress in the transverse plane due to the thrust of the cylinder is most pronounced in the fibres (glial and commissural elements and blood-vessels) belonging to the pathways located adjacent to the cylindrical body (Table 2, no. 5).

C. *Relaxed.* Cord fixed in total relaxation corresponding to extension. The cylindrical body has been placed slightly anterior to its position in B.

The compression of the tissue is restricted to the immediate vicinity of the cylinder, but the half of the cord containing it is slightly wider than the other half (Table 2, no. 6).

PART TWO

Clinical implications of adverse tension

Neurological symptoms generated by flexion of the spine

That neurological symptoms may be evoked by movements of the spinal column is well established and many are the studies concerned with the nature of the mechanical forces generated by these movements in the presence of pathological structures and lesions. These may consist of osseous, cartilaginous and ligamentous alterations in the spine or extra-, peri- and intra-medullary indurative, hyperplastic or neoplastic processes. That intramedullary lesions may also give rise to neurological symptoms is evidenced by Lhermitte's sign in multiple sclerosis. Lhermitte and others have proposed that the electrical sensations are due to 'lashing' of demyelinized lengths of the cord against the inside of the canal as the cervical spine is flexed (177). This commotional theory and many other unconfirmed hypotheses illustrate the reliance on baseless suppositions to account for the mechanical forces. So far as multiple sclerosis is concerned the nature of these forces has commanded little more than casual interest, and the possibility of diminishing, to say nothing of eliminating, them appears never to have been considered.

With advances in the technique for extirpation of herniated lumbar discs (258) that brought the cervical spine within the scope of this area of surgery came recognition of the practical value of a better insight into the mechanical background of the neurological symptoms produced by movements of the spinal column. While this knowledge had been lacking reliance had to be placed on local surgical methods. A change in this situation has come about with the discovery that the elongation of the spinal canal accompanying flexion gives rise to forces which are transmitted throughout the dural theca and the pons–cord tract (35). We are, however, still at the beginning of this new approach to functional neuroanatomy (55) and neuropathology and many mechanical and histodynamic factors in the precipitation of symptoms require careful investigation. Two paths have been available, one of them *via* detailed clinical observations, and the other *via* exact experimental biomechanical analyses. To the latter belong observations conducted on postmortem specimens and on patients during operations. In clinical observations or the interpretation of anamnestic data it is necessary to rely on indirect inference. Direct information is obtained from the examination of tension and relaxation phenomena in the soft tissues of the spinal canal during surgery—for example, by using an adjustable head-rest that enables the curvature of the spine to be varied and hence also the tension set up in the tissues (Fig. 141).

The history as a guide to the cause of signs and symptoms

It is obvious that so long as we have to rely on a purely clinical analysis, the search for the possible mechanical causes of the neurological symptoms can be little more than guesswork. However, from the nature of the symptoms one may at least infer the site of action of the generating histodynamic forces.

The following clinical observations are intended as a point of departure. Attention will be restricted to flexion of the cervical column; this movement may be regarded as a rough triggering mechanism.

Long-standing spasticity in both the upper and lower extremities—for instance, in patients with cervical myelopathy, caused by protrusions into the spinal canal—may sometimes be sharply aggravated by flexion of the cervical column. If during flexion the patient immediately experiences pain, paraesthesia or stiffness of the neck, shoulder girdle or arms, and if at the same time fibrillary twitching of the muscles is observed, the mechanical source of excitation will most probably be located in the vicinity of the cervical cord, or more accurately, in the nerve-roots. If at the same time the patient is conscious of an uncomfortable sensation in the lower back (Hyndman's sign) or a radiating sciatic pain in one or both legs, the triggering tension will most certainly have been transmitted to the lumbosacral nerve-roots.

Sensory root symptoms

Neurological symptoms evoked simultaneously in a local and in a more remote region of the body by flexion of the head probably have a common pathological origin. Studying Frykholm's series of patients with cervical root-sleeve fibrosis (104) Torkildsen observed that on flexion of the cervical column some of these patients experienced not only uncomfortable sensations radiating to the head and arms but also sciatic pains (250). The association between the production of symptoms in the cervical and lumbar regions was so patent to him that he called this phenomenon 'brachialgic sciatica' (although he does not give an entirely adequate mechanical explanation). A similar but opposite phenomenon may be observed in patients with chronic cervical rhizopathy. If the test for Lasègue's sign is performed on the side where the brachialgia was previously manifest, pains similar to those experienced during the acute rhizopathy period will possibly be felt in the arm. One such patient that the author has observed had recently had a lumbar disc herniation on the same side as the earlier brachialgia. In Lasègue's test the patient experienced pains in both the leg and the arm—a phenomenon that might be referred to as 'sciatic brachialgia'.

Sensory and motor funicular symptoms

In certain cord lesions it is fairly common for motor funicular symptoms (possibly accompanied by radicular symptoms) to be evoked suddenly on flexing the cervical spine. In the patient with multiple sclerosis (Case 1, p. 228) transient motor funicular symptoms were evoked and also Lhermitte's sign. He found that he could provoke or increase spasticity in both legs by placing both hands behind the neck and bending it forwards as far as possible; the spastic rigidity in both legs increased immediately: mistaking it as an improvement that enabled him to stand on his weak legs, the patient frequently exploited this traumatizing stimulus.

In at least three patients with cervical myelopathy the author has also observed an increase in spasticity on flexion and a reduction on extension of the cervical spine. Patients with rapidly progressing spasticity who could not be operated on immediately were supplied with a supporting collar for the neck.

Maxwell & Kahn report a case of a young girl with severe kyphosis at the T_5 level for which laminectomy had been performed (at another hospital than the authors') for slightly increasing paresis in one leg (187). After the laminectomy there was not only a neurological deterioration caudal to the level of the operation but also a deficit at higher levels. At operation a marked increase in tension in the spinal cord had been confirmed. The following details show the complexity of the pathodynamic situation in this case: "Severe kyphosis at the T_5 level. After laminectomy complete spastic paraplegia with increasing atrophy of the legs, incomplete sensory loss below the T_9 level. After a second operation 3 months later there was weakness of both arms, increasing to spastic paraplegia, and a decrease in sensibility below C_5. Symmetric diaphragmatic paralysis necessitated respiratory treatment. Surgical exploration disclosed an atrophied spinal cord, stretched tightly round the apex of the kyphosis. When the cord was transected at the level of the protrusion of the kyphosis the intact part retracted craniad and there was spontaneous re-

covery of breathing." Evidently, the neurological deficits must be ascribed to traction on the cord due to its elevation by the kyphosis at the T_5 level, and to transmission of the pathological tension to the respiratory centres of the medulla oblongata (p. 180). The girl's paraplegia, which arose after the first laminectomy, was obviously produced by a pincer action on the cord.

Facial neuralgia (migraine cervicale)

Flexion of the head and cervical spine for shorter or longer periods has proved to be the cause of headache and possibly accompanying symptoms in about two-thirds of all attacks,[1] especially in cases of patent atypical facial neuralgia or migraine cervicale (12), manifested as radiating pains from the neck to different parts of the face. However, in only a small number of these patients have the pains appeared more or less immediately on bending the head forwards.

Idiopathic trigeminal neuralgia (tic douloureux)

In at least 75 per cent of a group of 24 patients with trigeminal neuralgia tic douloureux could be elicited by bending the head and cervical spine forwards (35, 42).[2] In a later series (Table 3) tic douloureux was evoked in 10 out of 40 patients on flexion of the cervical column, and in 27 by flexing the whole column from the neutral posture; the attacks could be consistently precipitated also by stimulating trigger zones in the face (Table 3). Just as it was not always possible to produce an attack by touching a trigger zone, so flexion of the column did not always provoke pain (no study of the refractory period for flexion has been carried out).[3]

In 5 other patients (not included in Table 3) with symptomatic trigeminal neuralgia due to various primary diseases, attacks of pain were consistently evoked by flexion; in 4 of them the attack could be precipitated also by touching a trigger zone. Two of these 5 patients had multiple sclerosis (man, 58: avoids flexion which almost invariably evokes pain; man, 49: for three years has had pains evoked by flexion; one year before the operation the pain could be banished by marked flexion of the neck). Another of these patients had atypical glossopharyngeal neuralgia (woman, 65:

[1] Frykholm, R.: Personal communication, 1969.
[2] Having confirmed that elderly ladies not infrequently experience trigeminal neuralgia (*tic douloureux*) when bending over their embroidery, a Stockholm neurologist suggested to them they would be better advised to turn to ornithology.
[3] When asked by another investigator what happened when they tried to tie a shoelace, some of the patients that had said that they had had no attack on flexion readily admitted that then there was, of course, pain. A patient with fresh tic douloureux who had flatly denied having an attack on bending forwards immediately had an extremely severe one on being asked to bend his head forwards.

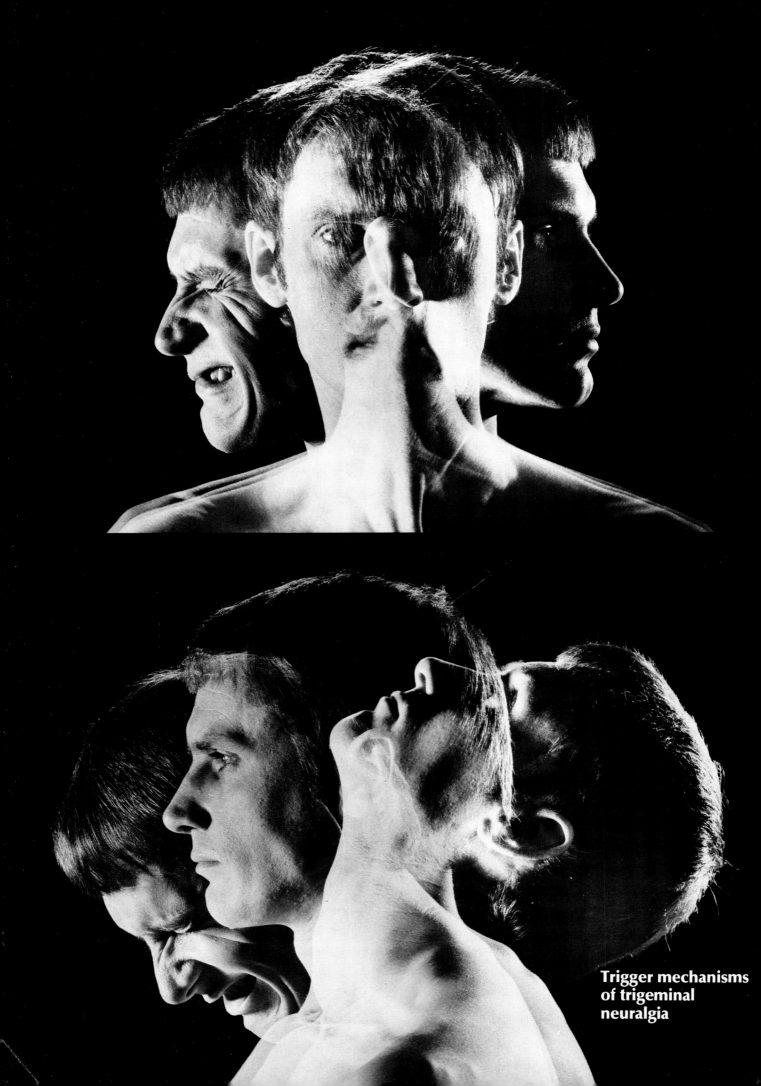

Trigger mechanisms
of trigeminal
neuralgia

TABLE 3. Precipitating stimuli in 53 unselected cases of idiopathic trigeminal neuralgia.

No. of patients	Sex	Mean age	Facial trigger points[a]	Cause of stretching of hind-brain and trigeminal nerve-root				Surgical findings	
				Bending of neck	Stoop-ing	Turning the head	Walking on uneven ground, etc.	Thickened fibrotic nerve-fibres adherent to trigeminal root-sheath	Condition of root not noted
Tic douloureux initiated by stimulation of trigger points and histodynamic irritation[b] of trigeminal nerve-root; 40 patients									
17	♂	68	17	3[c]	14	2	3	5	8
23	♀	62	23	7	13	1[d]	2	7	7
Tic possibly initiated by histodynamic irritation of the trigeminal root; 7 patients									
1	♂	71	1						
6	♀	63	6						
Tic not initiated by physiological stretching of the trigeminal root; 6 patients									
3	♂	69	3						
3	♀	67	3						

[a] In all these patients the second branch is involved.
[b] Bending tensile stress and notch stress acting within the Gasserian ganglion and the trigeminal nerve-root set up by postural changes.
[c] Pains also in neck and arms.
[d] Head turned away from the side of the neuralgia.

Intraradicular histodynamic trigger mechanisms of trigeminal neuralgia

Apart from the general phenomenon in which trigeminal neuralgia can be evoked by touching the skin of the face or the mucous membranes of the mouth, an attack of tic douloureux can often be triggered by the following movements of the spine and head:

1. By flexing the head and (cervical) spine when the trigeminal nerve-root is bent and stretched over a firm structure located beneath the root (31–5,206).

2. By rotating the head and cervical spine, when there is a firm structure located medial to the root on the side towards which neck and head are rotated (Fig. 96).

3. By involuntary vertical shaking of the head. The trigeminal nerve-root then probably rotates about an axis in the horizontal (coronal) plane and will be bent and stretched round any firm structure located either basal or cranial to the nerve-root; tension is thus set up in its tissue (*Frontispiece*).

In all three movements tic douloureux may alternatively be evoked by the tension set up within the nervous tissue around a fissure produced by fragmentation (15, 74, 107, 163, 229).

In a consecutive series of 324 patients collected over a period of 21 years Arthur Ecker, New York, has performed selective alcoholic Gasserian injection for tic douloureux. He says (personal communication, 1976): "Many of my patients with trigeminal neuralgia have symptoms produced by bending the head forward but a single exceptional case had neuralgia precipitated by bending the head backward."

pain triggered by pressure on leukoplakia in the fauces on the left side and by marked flexion of the cervical column). In one of the remaining 2 patients a tumour had been found in the middle fossa at the operation, and in the other there was an atypical arterial loop just below the trigeminal root; this has been reported by other workers (73, 74, 210).

From these observations it is evident that besides the stimulation of facial trigger zones there are other, hitherto overlooked, mechanisms for the precipitation of trigeminal neuralgia, amongst them the elongation of the spinal canal and stretching of the pons–cord tract accompanying flexion of the cervical spine or the whole column (Fig. 94), and rotation of the head with consequent stretching of the trigeminal nerve-root owing to displacement of the pons towards the side to which the head is turned (Fig. 96).

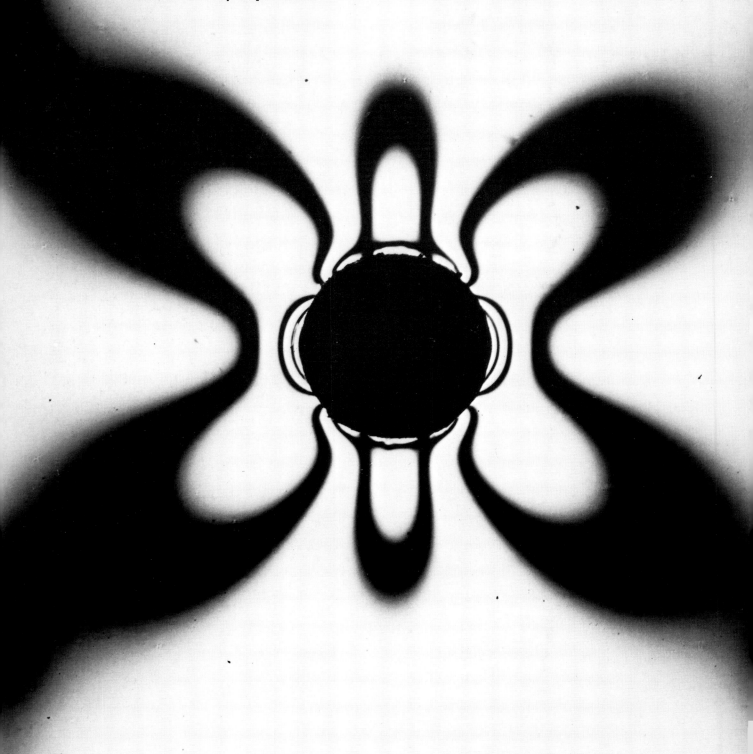

The histodynamic background to symptoms evoked by spinal flexion

Multilateral thrust

The histodynamic background to symptoms evoked by spinal flexion

The elongation of the spinal canal that occurs during flexion subjects the nervous tissue to physiological tension throughout the length of the pons–cord tract. Any pathological structures outside or within the tract that exert a thrust on the tissue might then over-stretch it and set up local *pathological* tension (Figs. 98–100), the magnitude of which will depend on the total axial tension acting in the tract and the size of the depression (Fig. 93). This local deformation is the fundamental cause of neurological symptoms (45, 237).

Pressure exerted by intramedullary lesions

Among the intramedullary lesions and structures that evoke neurological symptoms by exerting local pressure and setting up tension in nearby nerve-fibres and blood-vessels are the various space-occupying alterations; they include inflammatory, haemorrhagic, indurative, neoplastic and hyperplastic lesions and cysts. To elucidate their mechanical effect on the surrounding tissues a spherical mass may be taken as the simplest model. Provided that it is compact and hard enough to resist the reactive pressure of the investing tissue, the mass would presumably exert a pressure as soon as its diameter exceeds the distance between two adjacent nerve-fibres (Fig. 79). The effect of pathological structures larger than this on the medullary tissue should be examined in both the transverse and sagittal planes, since these are the predominant directions of the strata in the spinal cord, with the majority of the fibres oriented in the former plane in the grey substance and in the latter plane in the white. So long as the spinal cord is relaxed and the slack fibres can fold within the pia and the cord septa, the lesion may be relatively large before appreciable tension is set up in the transversely and sagittally disposed tissue elements.

The amount of tissue that can be displaced in the neighbourhood of an unyielding lesion is determined in some measure by the structure of the myelin sheaths and the neuroglial fibres, and especially their function as a supporting substance between the nerve-fibres. These fibres appear to follow a helical path between the sagittally and transversely oriented nerve-fibres (Fig. 85). There is thus a 'glia reserve', so that when the cord is elongated the respective nerve-fibres can extend freely. There is, moreover, reason to believe that at maximum elongation of the spinal cord the glia spirals, just as the pia, lose their resilience. When the spirals are folded, with consequent separation of the nerve-fibres, they will probably be unable to yield further on maximum shortening of the spinal cord, and if the axial compression is increased kinking will result.

As is evident from Fig. 17, the neuroglial fibres running transversely are also folded. The stiff fibres that emerge from the pia and surround the funnels of the transversely coursing blood-vessels are a direct continuation of the rhomboid network of inelastic fibres in the pia. When the funnels shorten due to stretching of the cord the stiff fibres impinge on the surrounding tissue (Fig. 25); this may be of significance in the presence of an expanding lesion. In the relaxed state of the pons–cord tract, a firm intramedullary lesion thus interferes less with both the nerve-fibres and the blood-vessels (Figs. 78, 92 C, 99). As soon as the tension in the pons–cord tract is augmented, however, the picture changes. Elongation of the spinal canal results in an increase in the magnitude and range of the axial tension, and hence in the pressure exerted by the unyielding lesion on the investing tissues (Figs. 88, 93). The tension in the nerve-fibres of the white substance around the lesion also increases, as does the pressure on the transverse nerve-fibres in the grey substance, so that these, too, are possibly subjected to tension.

Whatever the nature of the intramedullary lesion (182) it will always give rise to adverse pressure on and tension within the surrounding nerve-fibres and blood-vessels. However, the distribution and magnitude of the tensile forces vary with the location and configuration of the lesions.

When the canal is elongated an intramedullary firm lesion not only gives rise to a local bending tensile stress but it also increases the axial tension in the pons–cord tract (Figs. 93, 99). As these components of tension are additive there is an increase in the local axial and transverse tension, with a consequent intensification of the symptoms from the lesions; the increase in the axial tension may in its turn evoke neurological symptoms from other sections of the pons–cord tract.

The occurrence of neurological symptoms at the moment when the column is flexed is a clear indication that they are produced by elongation of the spinal canal and pons–cord tract and the resulting increase in tension in the pia and the nervous tissue. Scarring both superficially and within this tissue interferes with the normal elastic elongation and is likely to lead to compensatory intramedullary over-stretching and bending tensile stress. Symptoms elicited on flexing the cervical canal may well be due to stretching of the axis-cylinders over superficial or intramedullary scars.

Tension triggering tic douloureux

In many cases of trigeminal neuralgia, *tic douloureux* can be triggered by stretching and bending of the trigeminal nerve-root over a firm pathological structure (132,

206, 210), and possibly also by notch stress and bending tensile stress *within* the tissue of the trigeminal nerve-root (15, 163, 229) or in the pons. Among his multiple sclerosis patients with trigeminal neuralgia, the cause of which was unknown during their lifetime, the author recalls one in which autopsy disclosed a glial scar at the point where the trigeminal root entered the pons. While it is true that the descending tract of the fifth nerve communicates with the substantia gelatinosa Rolandi in the cornu posterius at the level of the second cervical sensory nerve-root (217), it is improbable that intrapontine tension in these pathways can account for symptoms of trigeminal neuralgia; the pons is fairly thick, its normal elongation is comparatively small and the intramedullary changes probably greatly restrict further local stretching. Any unyielding structure or lesion will therefore be unlikely to exert appreciable intrapontine tension. Instead, the normal or pathologically increased axial tension will be transmitted *via* the oblongata and pons to the trigeminal nerve-roots. Accordingly, it would seem that its over-stretching is due to pathological changes within the actual trigeminal nerve-root or the surrounding structures; its nerve-fibres may then be either pressed against, for instance, the ridge of the petrous bone (134, 206), the loop of an artery (15, 74) or calcifications in the surrounding tissues (132), with consequent exposure of the root-fibres to both pressure and tension, or they may be subjected to bending tensile and notch stress, the former produced by vacuolizations and scars and the latter around fissures in the ganglionic and nerve-root tissue (15, 163).

Tension evoking pyramidal and sensory funicular symptoms

Spasticity and impaired sensibility, the latter if it involves the whole lower half of the body, are often indicative of intramedullary tension. Clinical experience shows that so long as the elasticity of the relevant pathways is not exceeded and the blood supply is not compromised, relief of the tension can result in abolition of the neurological symptoms and signs (226) and fairly complete recovery of their conductivity (Case Reports, pp. 207–31).

Possible sites of tension responsible for bladder symptoms

It is sometimes difficult to decide whether neurological symptoms have been evoked by tension in intramedullary pathways in the vicinity of the basic lesion or whether they derive from remote nerve-roots. Bladder symptoms provide a good example, for the pathways responsible for micturition run the length of the cord in the reticulospinal tracts of the lateral columns (199, 200).

Are the bladder symptoms that occur in cases of foramen magnum tumours, cervical and thoracic myelopathy, multiple sclerosis and other intramedullary lesions produced by tension in the section of the spinal cord tract adjacent to the basic lesion, or are they produced by over-stretching of the sacral nerve-roots the effect of which is transmitted through the length of the spinal cord? In either case the nerve-roots are pulled strongly against the pedicles, and are thus subjected to adverse pressure and tension. Even quite small deviations from the normal arched form of the pedicles, especially those due to osteophytes, can obviously give rise to symptoms (187). It has been observed that they do in fact originate in both these ways. From experience of patients with herniated lumbar disc it would seem likely that pressure on the sacral nerve-roots and an increase in the tension in them may elicit some form of bladder symptoms. Moreover, in patients with tumours of the foramen magnum region and in the case of osteophytes at the anterior wall of the cervical canal in patients with cervical and thoracic myelopathy, both sciatica and bladder symptoms not infrequently disappear quite soon after removal of the tumour and extirpation or neutralization of the protrusion (p. 207). Being a specific root symptom from the fifth lumbar or the first sacral nerve-root, sciatica cannot have an intramedullary origin. If the symptoms from the lumbar and sacral nerve-roots are eliminated by extirpation of a tumour in the upper cervical region that is exerting a local pressure on the cervical cord and thus over-stretching it, then the tension responsible for these remote symptoms will also have been relieved. If bladder symptoms disappear at the same time as the sciatica, they, too, will most probably have originated in the sacral nerve-roots. That the reduction of the tension in the sacral nerve-roots can be responsible for this beneficial effect is also evident from the radiographic examinations in extreme functional positions of the spinal column, which show that slackening of these nerve-roots accompanies the relaxation of the cervical dura, dentate ligaments and cervical spinal cord (49, 53).

In spinal cord injuries and multiple sclerosis, too, clinical observations suggest that bladder symptoms may be evoked both as a direct mechanical effect of scars or other lesions on the intramedullary pathways, and by over-stretching of the sacral nerve-roots. In both spinal cord injury and multiple sclerosis the possibility of such tension in the sacral nerve-roots being part of the pathological picture and of it being responsible for the symptoms will evidently depend on the extent of the intramedullary damage and glial scarring, and the consequent reduction in elasticity. If there is total interruption of the conductivity within the cord any over-stretching of the sacral nerve-roots will, of course, be of no practical significance; but otherwise cord tension transmitted to the sacral nerve-roots may be at least partly responsible for the bladder symptoms. This must be borne in mind when contemplating surgical measures for relief.

Tension evoking symptoms from the autonomic nervous system

Excitation and deficit symptoms from the autonomic nervous system may presumably also be evoked by tension set up either intramedullarily in the pathways of the lateral columns or in the nerve-fibres of the sympathetic trunk (263). Because flexion of the extended leg at the hip-joint results in stretching of the intrapelvic lumbar sympathetic trunk (Figs. 131, 132), osteophytic spurs on the anterolateral aspect of the vertebral bodies might exert pressure on it and set up tension. Relief of sympathetic symptoms due to removal of a herniated disc may sometimes be attributed to relaxation of the trunk.

Flexion of the cervical spine might likewise generate tension in the sympathetic plexus around the carotid and vertebral arteries, on which spondylarthritic spurs protruding from the uncovertebral joints are impinging (234). Flexion also stretches the nerve-roots in the upper cervical section of the tract and in the posterior fossa; quite small pathological structures—such as arachnitic adhesions resulting from haemorrhage and inflammation—can then produce tension in these nerve-roots. In this way the symptoms typical of upper cervical syndrome (43) or migraine cervicale (12) may be produced. In these syndromes the action potentials would appear to be transmitted along the pathways between the posterior cervical roots and the trigeminal nucleus (217), since sensations within the area innervated by the trigeminal nerve are typical of these syndromes, especially migraine cervicale. In the production and transmission of the objectively recordable phenomena in migraine cervicale (12) other pathways than these two may conceivably be involved.

Rehabilitatory athletics and physiotherapy

Limitations and contraindications

The rapid spread of interest in athletics for the handicapped in recent years stems largely from Ludwig Guttmann's idea of linking competitive athletics for certain groups of such persons with the Olympic Games. Not only do the efforts that the participants make in these activities satisfy their urge to improve their performance, thereby increasing their self-respect; their progress and example can also serve as encouragement to their less fortunate companions, and constitute for them a much-needed stimulus.

The generally beneficial and well-documented value of athletics for the physiological condition of the handicapped is not in dispute. The question that we are concerned with here is whether the athletic events include certain movements that might be potentially harmful. The answer to this question has important implications in view of the evidence that specific movements, such as flexion of the spine, can jeopardize residual neurological functions in the case of certain injuries to the central nervous system.

When a handicapped person who is suffering from sequelae, not of damage to the central nervous system, but instead of muscular, skeletal or organic disorders, performs a movement or a sequence of movements that is harmful to the affected part of the body, there is usually pain or some other manifestation either immediately or a little later. In the case of certain lesions of the central nervous system, however, no such warning signals are emitted if the handicapped should perform adverse movements such as flexion of the spinal column (p. 110). Where the person notices, say, loss of power or precision in certain actions he may mistakenly ascribe them to fatigue or some other transient phenomenon, and he may then try to compensate for this deficiency by making more strenuous efforts. There is ample evidence that when a person with a pons or cord injury persists with actions that involve flexion movements of the spine he may further impair the functional capacity of the nervous system—possibly to the point of causing irreversible damage.

Such a deterioration was observed in practically all those patients whose histories have been presented in various sections of this book and who are known to have performed flexion movements of the spine. These patients, it will be recalled, were suffering from cervical, thoracic and post-traumatic myelopathies, multiple sclerosis, para-pontine and para-medullary tumours, certain kinds of disc herniation and various diseases of the nervous system. In every case the reason for their deterioration could be traced to a single factor, namely, the presence of firm structures of different kinds that impinged on the pons–cord tract, the cranial nerves or the nerve-roots (p. 231). When the tract is stretched on flexion of the spine all these structures, which are less yielding than the surrounding nervous tissue, exert a thrust on the tract; this sets up tension in the nervous tissue. The resulting pathological stress is capable of producing symptoms of neurological deficit or excitation and hyper- or hypofunction of various organs (pp. 207–31).

Another purpose of athletics for the handicapped, and perhaps the most important one of all, is the rehabilitation of persons suffering from the sequelae of a compressive spinal cord injury. After such injuries, too, there is intramedullary scar formation (p. 88). Any forward or lateral flexion of the column may then cause the scar to exert an outward thrust on adjacent nerve-fibres that may have remained unaffected or suffered only minor damage. In patients with relatively large cross-sectional lesions who are confined to a wheel-chair the possibility of insidious impairment of the conductivity of such nerve-fibres that have been over-stretched or even torn through flexion of the spine is unlikely to be detected if the perhaps subtle neurological manifestations are masked by more prominent symptoms of deficit or excitation. Of the types of progressive impairment that may occur, a change in sensibility is probably the easiest to detect. In the patients mentioned above a positive Lhermitte's sign, for example, invariably indicates the presence of a thrust on the cord tissue.

The observations made so far in this new field of neurology do not constitute a firm enough basis for judging which adverse concrete effects are likely to result from the thrust exerted on the nervous tissue by flexion movements over a period of time in the individual patient. We do know, however, that symptoms from a localized lesion may be relieved to a greater or lesser extent when the pons–cord tract is rendered slack. In the light of our new insight into the obviously adverse effect on some of the neurological functions of spinal flexion and bending of the head, it must be regarded as an urgent task to re-examine the general programmes of rehabilitation exercises for the handicapped. This applies to flexion movements involved in actions performed by the handicapped himself and to passive such movements effected by the physiotherapist. For effective rehabilitation these undesirable and possibly traumatizing movements and postures must be avoided. It would then obviously be an advantage if the physiotherapist is acquainted with the normal and pathological biomechanics of the pons–cord tract.

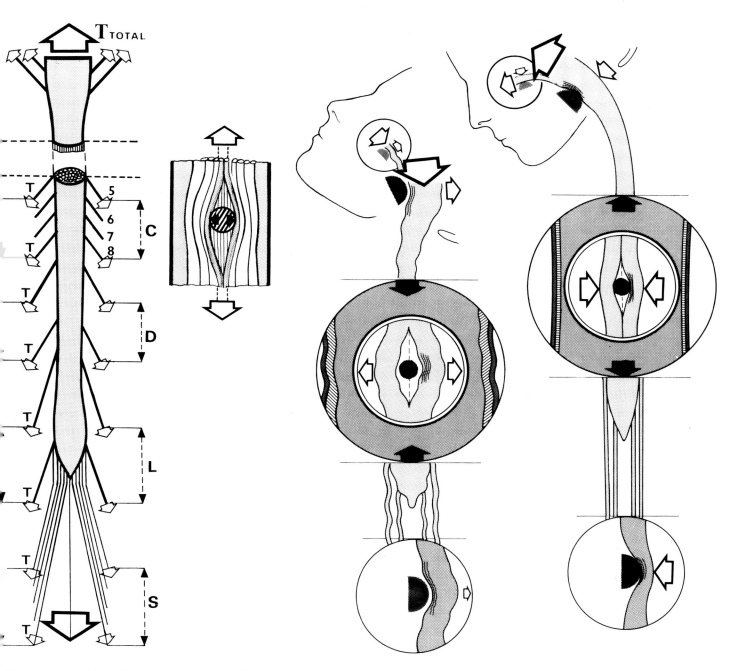

Fig. 93. The cranialward increase in tension set up in the spinal cord on flexion.

The total force (T_{total}) focused in the upper part of the pons–cord tract is the resultant of the component forces acting in the individual nerve-roots (T).

Inset. The higher the level of a pathological structure in or beneath the cord the greater is the tension it produces. The resulting increase in the total force will be transmitted practically undiminished to the lumbosacral nerve-roots (53, 250). The cranialward tension produced by a herniated lumbar disc, on the other hand, cannot exceed about one-thirtieth to one-twentieth of the tension produced in the lumbosacral nerve-roots by a similar protrusion located at the cervical level.

Fig. 94. The origin and elimination of stress produced by impinging bodies *(hatched shading)* **at various levels of the pons–cord tract.**

Right. Bending tensile stress set up in the nervous tissue in the vicinity of impinging bodies on elongation of the spinal canal accompanying *flexion*.

Left. The stress is eliminated throughout the tract by relaxation of the cord produced on *extension*.

Top, in the circles. Impingement may arise from the margin of the petrous bone (206), calcified tissue (132), a tumour or the like (15, 74, 163, 210), all located near the trigeminal nerve-root.

Below the circles. Clivus tumour or anteriorly located foramen magnum tumour, or the like.

Centre right (magnified). An intramedullary firm body (Figs. 88, 99) setting up a bending tensile stress in adjacent nerve-fibres.

Centre left (magnified). The relief of this tension by relaxation of the cord.

Bottom right (magnified). Stress set up in a nerve-root by a herniated lumbar disc.

Bottom left (magnified). Relief of this tension by relaxation of the nerve-root.

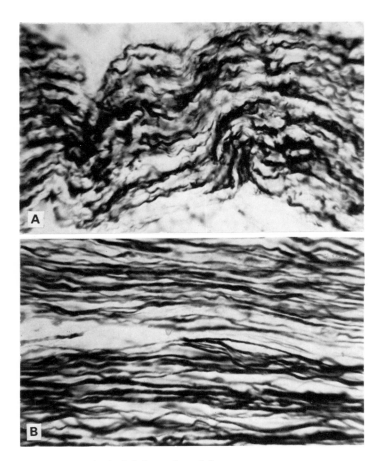

Fig. 95. Physiological deformation of the fibres in the trigeminal nerve-root.

A. With the head and cervical spine of the cadaver *extended*, the pons–cord tract was fixed for 24 hours by subarachnoid injection of formaldehyde *in situ*. The nerve-fibres are obviously slack in this position.

B. Similar procedure with the head and cervical spine *flexed*. Nerve-fibres under normal tension.

The trigeminal nerve-roots apparently behave just as the other roots of the pons–cord tract. The thrust of a body impinging on them may therefore be compared to that of a herniated disc; the neurological symptoms evoked by pathological tension in the trigeminal nerve-root—that is to say, tic douloureux evoked by irritation of the C-fibres—may likewise be ascribed to bending tensile stress in its nerve-fibres.

For 'Deformation of the trigeminal nerve-root between its attachement to the pons and its ostium at the entry into the central fossa, due to flexion and extension movements of head and spine' *see* Fig. 105 in (35): Biomechanics of the Central Nervous System. Almqvist & Wiksell, Stockholm, 1960.

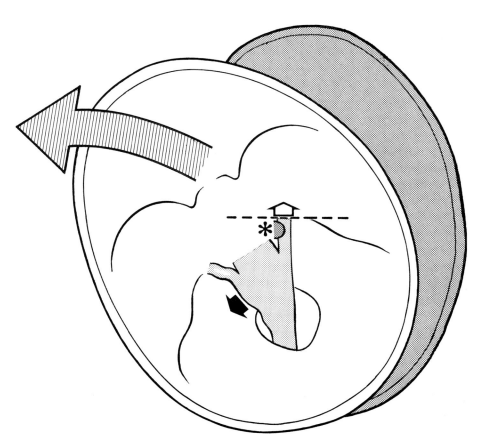

Fig. 96. The internal trigger mechanism of tic douloureux on rotation of the head.

For internal trigger mechanism on flexion of the head and spine, see Fig. 94, *right (top in the circle)*.

For survey of the internal trigger mechanisms known to date, see Table 3 (p. 113).

Shaded. Head facing front.

Light. View into the base of the skull when the head was turned to the left (*large hatched arrow*). Only the oblongata and pons with the trigeminal nerve-roots have been drawn in.

Black arrow. Leftward deviation of the pons and oblongata. *Small white arrow.* The attachment of the right trigeminal root and the force stretching it, produced by the leftward displacement of the pons. Of the resulting deformations only the normal stretching of the right trigeminal root and the relaxation of the left root are indicated.

Asterisk. Structure impinging on the medial side of the right trigeminal root.

When the head is turned the trigeminal nerve-root located on the side to which the head is turned is relaxed, while that on the opposite side is stretched.

Histodynamic features

Clinical observations suggest that the thrust on the trigeminal nerve-root can be produced by an unyielding structure located either outside the nerve-root (elevated margin of the petrous bone (35, 206), a tumour, arachnoidal calcification (132), etc. The myelin fragmentation in pathological Gasserian ganglia and trigeminal nerve-roots—as seen in electron microscopical pictures (15, 163)—includes fissures, as in Figs. 68, 69. Notch stresses will arise around these fissures and contribute to the neurological symptoms.

In the presence of a structure impinging on the medial side of the stretched nerve-root a bending tensile stress is set up in its

nerve-fibres which can evoke tic douloureux attacks. If the head is turned in the opposite direction, however, the relaxation of the trigeminal nerve-root can itself abolish the triggering potential of the impinging structure (or the fissure). When an attack of pain has once been elicited by this internal trigger mechanism, it can be most reliably alleviated by extension of the cervical spine, which produces the greatest, and therefore most effective, relaxation of the nerve-root at the same time as of the whole pons–cord tract.

In the case of an applied force of fairly large magnitude and short duration no evidence of an artificial synapse was found, there nowhere being a critical approximation of the non-demyelinated axis-cylinders (Fig. 88, C, D). In view of the symptom-producing effect that is characteristic of histodynamic lesions it is hardly necessary to look for a critical interaxonal distance, a repelling surface charge, etc. (107).

Causes of adverse tension; its effect on neurological function

Survey of the pathological situations responsible for histodynamic tension

Tension set up in the brain, spinal cord and nerve-roots through the presence of a pathological structure or lesion located within or outside the tissue is a prominent cause of neurological signs and symptoms. This is evident from analyses of the histological and micro-angiographical deformation of such tissue that has been fixed *in situ* while being subjected to the action of forces exerted by such structures (Fig. 97).

Three common pathological situations responsible for symptom-producing tension are the following.

1. *Scarring lesions*

When the pons–cord tissue tract is stretched scars and other sclerotic lesions, such as in multiple sclerosis, exert a thrust and produce tension in the surrounding normal tissue. These structures, moreover, give rise to potentially harmful tension both in the relatively immobile supratentorial brain tissue and, to a more marked degree, in the mobile tissues of the hind-brain and spinal cord. In electron microscopical studies of Gasserian ganglia and trigeminal nerve-roots, tissue rupture has been found together with demyelinization and induration (15, 163). Physiological stretching of the trigeminal roots as well as pathological over-stretching can then set up a secondary tensile stress—a 'notch stress' —concentrated around the ends of the fissures.

2. *Increased interstitial fluid pressure*

Accumulated fluid—in, for instance, haemorrhage and hygroma—that has penetrated the tissue along more or less bizarre routes can exert pressure and set up tension which may lead to diverse neurological pictures, depending on the resulting deformation and the function of the affected tissue. (For potentially adverse effects of circumscribed oedema on neural conductivity see Fig. 100.)

If anatomical cavities, such as the lateral ventricles, are expanded through excessive production of fluid the nerve-fibres and blood-vessels in the surrounding internal capsule will be stretched (119, 275); this typical deformation (low-pressure hydrocephalus in the adult) produces fairly constant symptoms, namely, dementia, spasticity of the legs, ataxia and urinary incontinence.

A reduction of the pressure obtained by shunting the fluid will relax the nerve-fibres and restore their conductivity (51, 120).

3. *Space-occupying lesions*

Neoplasms.—The operating microscope often discloses evidence of superficial deformation of the brain and spinal cord by tension exerted by a tumour. On making an incision in the region of the deformation a gap opens up, thus confirming forces acting in the tissue, including the nerve-fibres and blood-vessels. By conducting morphological examination this tension can be traced to the cell membranes and the cytoplasm, and its deleterious effects analysed. Such an examination has been made of the rupture of the microvasculature produced on experimental compression of the spinal cord in the monkey (82).

From a study of the histological and microangiographical pictures in different planes it is evident that also in biological material any type of force produces its own characteristic stress field, whose configuration and range depend on the magnitude, direction and other properties of the responsible force. So far it has been possible to identify the following kinds of stress in the brain, cord and nerve-root tissue:

1. Bending tensile stress—when the tissue is stretched and bent round a firm protruding structure.

2. Short-range axial tensile stress in the tissue, acting perpendicular to the plane of a pincer mechanism.

3. Notch stress—set up by tensile forces acting on intact fibres in the vicinity of ruptured tissue around the end(s) of a fissure. (The sites where these types of stress may arise are shown in the *Frontispiece*.)

From the microscopical picture presented by the tissue and the membranes of the nerve-fibres subjected to tension it would seem possible to analyse the biomechanical conditions and effects also at the ultrastructural level (97, 128).[1]

---

[1] On basic mechanical grounds it is logical to suppose that when a nerve-fibre is bent and stretched round a firm structure the molecules of its membrane are drawn further apart on its convex than on its concave aspect. This unequal separation will result in a difference in osmotic permeability and hence in the resistance of the membrane to ionic migration; this in turn will probably result in alterations of the axon potentials.

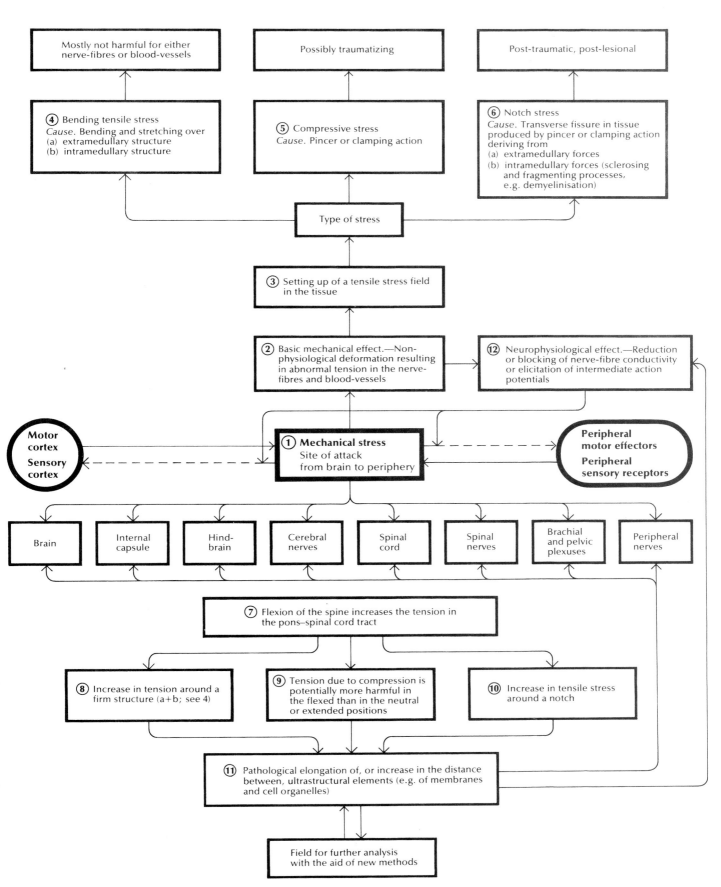

Fig. 97. Histodynamic stress in the nervous tissues, the essential cause of symptoms in all deforming lesions.

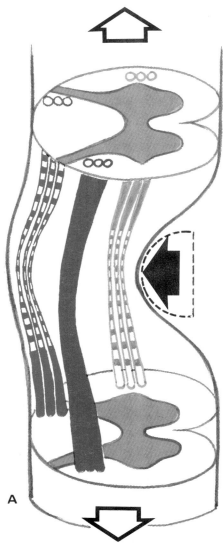

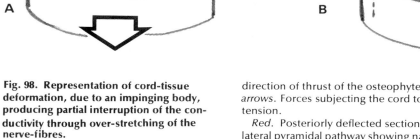

Fig. 98. Representation of cord-tissue deformation, due to an impinging body, producing partial interruption of the conductivity through over-stretching of the nerve-fibres.

The diagram has been drawn from histological sections through various levels of the fully flexed cervical cord, subjected to the thrust exerted by an osteophyte located on the anterior wall of the canal.

A. The anterior surface of the cord is impressed, with resulting deflection of the axially coursing fibres. *Black arrow.* Main direction of thrust of the osteophyte. *White arrows.* Forces subjecting the cord to axial tension.

Red. Posteriorly deflected section of the lateral pyramidal pathway showing narrowing at the level of maximum stress, coinciding with the level of the centre of the impinging body.

Green. Spinothalamic pathway. Three deflected fibres narrowed most at the level of maximum deflection. The impaired (possibly abolished) conductivity of the fibres is indicated by the broken lines.

Yellow. The effect of the deflection of the centrifugal pathways for micturition (200) is similarly indicated.

B. *Small black arrows.* Forces set up by the impinging body (applied perpendicular to the plane of the diagram). *Large white arrows.* As in A.

Small white arrows. Transverse, deforming, forces acting within the tissue, and producing an increase in width. The deformation due to the thrust is countered by inelastic glial fibres (271), as indicated by the grey transverse lines between the yellow fibres, and between these and the pia mater.

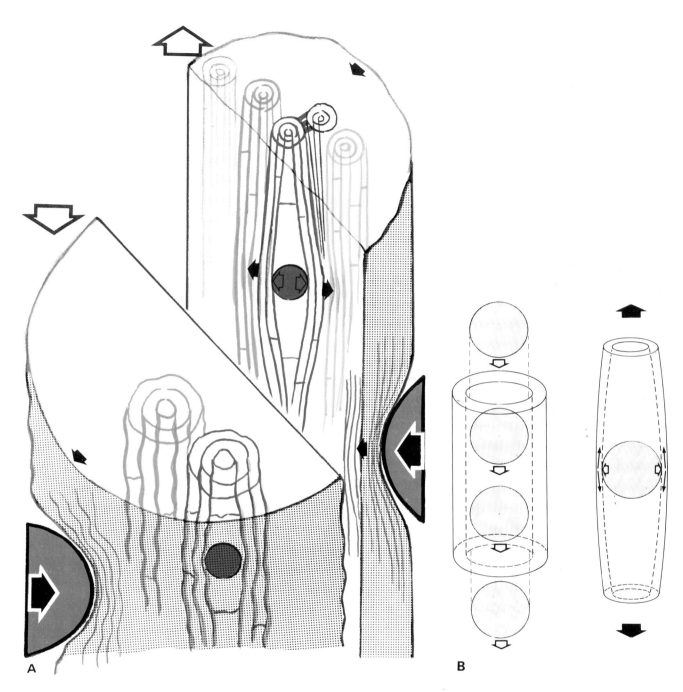

Fig. 99.

A. Representation of the thrust exerted on nearby pathways and axially oriented blood-vessels, etc., by:

Red discs. An intramedullary unyielding structure (glial scar, cyst, haematoma, incompressible circumscribed oedema, etc.).

Blue areas. An extramedullary protrusion (osteophyte, tumour, etc.).

Right. External and internal thrust to which the cord tissue is exposed on physiological stretching (35).

Left. Elimination of the outward and inward thrust obtained on relaxing the cord.

B. Diagrammatic representation of the effect on the walls of an elastic tube exerted by a ball within the tube when this is stretched.

The mechanical effect of a rigid intramedullary structure on the surrounding normal tissue may be illustrated by means of a simple model: a ball that is slightly smaller in diameter than the lumen of a rubber tube and that is just passing through the tube (*left*) is arrested when the tube is stretched (*right*). The ball then exerts a pressure from within, and deflects the tube wall. When the spinal canal is elongated on flexion of the spine the cord tissue is likewise stretched around any firm structure within the tissue (Figs. 88 and 90).

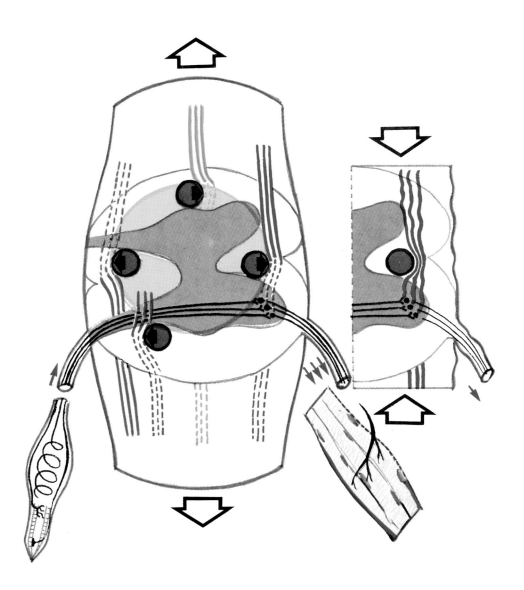

Fig. 100. Partial interruption (or blocking) of spinal cord conductivity due to distension of the nerve-fibres by internal gliotic and oedematous lesions (foci).

Left. During stretching of the pons–cord tract on spinal flexion in the acute and sub-chronic stage of disseminated sclerosis, the scars exert a thrust on the nerve-fibres in neighbouring pathways, thus setting up a bending tensile stress in them and impairing their conductivity (*broken lines*). In the chronic stage atrophy of the cord, too, contributes to the distension of the fibres. The outward thrust exerted on the cord tissue by either a single large unyielding lesion (*yellow*) or a number of such lesions (foci) (*grey circles*) is represented by the bulging of the cord. The latter foci are located near the following pathways:

Pathways conducting inhibitory impulses to the anterior horn (*red*), and the reflex arc (*black*) with the afferent fibres from the muscle spindles—γ-fibres, flower-spray ending, annulospiral fibres—to muscles. The pathological tension in the nerve-fibres set up by the impinging body prevents inhibitory impulses from reaching the anterior horn, with resulting spasticity in the legs (Case 1, p. 228).

Nathan and Smith's centrifugal pathways for micturition (*orange*).

Funiculus cuneatus (*green*).

Lateral and anterior pyramidal pathways (*red*).

Right. Background to the reduction in symptoms obtained through relaxation of the spinal cord. When the cord is slackened the thrust of all the impinging lesions (foci) on the involved intact or only slightly damaged pathways will be relieved, with resulting gradual recovery of their conductivity and hence partial or total regression of the neurological signs and symptoms.[1]

---

[1] On spinal flexion a conducting fibre is constricted only in the vicinity of tissue whose stretching is prevented. Among the most common lesions that reduce the capacity for elongation of the affected nerve-cells and -fibres is evidently local oedema. Dispersal of intramedullary oedema can often lead to restoration of the normal histomechanical properties of the affected cells and fibres. The local oedema around a relatively small intramedullary focus of myelitis (demyelinization) may indicate an extensive transverse lesion of the cord; however, after dispersal of the oedema the focus decreases in size and the conductivity of any remaining intact fibres may well recover.

Radiological diagnosis of tension in the pons–cord tract[1]

Under normal anatomical conditions the optimal lengths of the spinal canal, dura and pons–cord tract are exactly matched; during maximum elongation of the canal the dura, dentate ligaments and tract are accordingly stretched (Fig. 3). In the case of kyphotic angulation or osteophytic protrusions that produce pathological elongation of the canal and hence over-stretching of the dura and tract, changes in spinal posture, especially full flexion, give rise to contact pressure between any pathological curvature or protrusion along the anterior wall of the canal and the dura and spinal cord (45). The resulting pathodynamic conditions thus involve the whole pons–cord tract; for all these anatomical components are interdependant, and all segments of the spine comprise a functional unit.

A complete analysis of the individual case should therefore include a radiological examination of the whole spine in the neutral position, in full flexion and extension. If this is impracticable, radiographs should be taken at least with the spine in the extreme positions, in which the tract would presumably be exposed to detrimental forces. If it is impossible to take a single radiograph of the whole spinal column that visualizes the stress-generating situation it should be ensured that the posture does not change until all the exposures have been made. This applies especially to gas myelograms and tomograms.

Today, radiography is the only reliable basic diagnostic method for establishing whether pathological changes of the spine are liable to prove detrimental for any part of the dural theca and the tract. Experience has shown the need to check the mechanical effects of lesions on the spine itself, the dura and the cord in extreme functional positions. To view the pathodynamic situation in its entirety, radiological examinations of the whole pons–cord tract in extreme positions must be made, using plane films and preferably also gas myelograms; otherwise there is a risk of overlooking the full implications of pathological tension, whether due to some kind of protrusion into the canal, pathological curvature of the spine (39, 149), scarring and stretching of various sections of the dura, or pathological alterations in the dentate ligaments and the tract itself.

The object of the following survey is to point out some of the possibilities offered by special radiological techniques for recognizing and visualizing the mechanical conditions under which spinal lesions are likely to produce potentially harmful tension in the pons–cord tract. No claim for completeness is made, attention being confined to the more important mechanical features.

In recent years high kilovoltage and gas myelography have enabled clear and highly detailed pictures of the tract to be obtained. If enough air, oxygen or other gas has been insufflated into the subarachnoid space there is no difficulty in outlining the pons and medulla oblongata as well as the spinal cord. Films depicting changes in shape and position of the dura and tract provide a sound basis for an analysis of the responsible forces; there are, however, limits to the possibilities of reliable interpretation.

Radiological signs indicative of tension

Spinal flexion in the supine position

Observations of pathological changes in the shape of the subarachnoid space made under static conditions, without checks in optimal functional positions of the whole column, may easily lead to an incorrect assessment of their pathogenetic significance (150, 151, 155, 156, 158). Full flexion of the spine is the method most likely to reveal whether a particular protrusion is pressing on, and over-stretching, the tract. An X-ray examination that does not take advantage of this procedure, but merely shows that a clearly visualized anterior or anterolateral protrusion does not reach the surface of the tract, provides no basis for a diagnosis of the

[1] In this section only chronic lesions of the spinal cord and its encasing structures are considered; the author has not examined the effect of the fresh spinal cord injury on the biomechanical behaviour of the cord. In a recent myelographic study of patients that had sustained such an injury a frequently encountered feature was swelling of the cord, which persisted up to 6 days (228); however, no specific biomechanical or therapeutic inferences have been drawn.

dynamic conditions. The only examination of practical value is one that affords the possibility of ascertaining whether or not the suspected protrusion actually produces an increase in tension in the dura, tract and nerve-roots.

It is true that a fairly accurate impression of the mechanical effect of the protrusion can be obtained by having the patient adopt maximum flexion of the spine while in the lateral posture; but only in the *supine position*—when the stretched tract is raised against gravity to press on the protrusion from below—can it be established whether it is indisputably this protrusion that is exerting a force on the tract. With a biomechanically sound and objective radiographic technique at our disposal we are now in a position to perform a diagnostic assessment of the pathogenetic significance of a certain degree of spondylosis or kyphosis of the flexed cervical spine.

In gas myelography all fluid in the spinal subarachnoid spaces is replaced with gas, so that the contours of the canal and the stretched tract can be visualized; by cautious tilting of the body, gas may be retained in the spinal canal during flexion, so that it does not enter the cerebral subarachnoid space.

If, instead of using an objective method such as the proposed one for analysing the pathogenic effect of a protrusion, reliance is placed on suppositions, errors in diagnosis will be inevitable. For instance, with the column in the neutral posture one may suspect a protrusion that is seen nearly to make contact with the cord; but on full flexion of the whole spine it may be found that the cord is forced towards, and stretched over, two neighbouring protrusions one of them perhaps located cranial and the other caudal to the suspected one (Fig. 101). These two protrusions, which on static evidence appeared to be entirely innocuous, might actually prevent the suspected protrusion from making any contact with the cord, and themselves turn out to be the potentially harmful ones. Although flexion of the cervical spine will often stretch the tract enough to force it against the anterior aspect of the canal, in some patients with many degenerated discs and hence a shortened canal, axial stretching of the whole tract can be obtained only when the whole spine is fully flexed and the canal thus maximally elongated. Occasionally, it may even be necessary to flex both legs up to the trunk (as in the Lasègue's test), a measure that prevents retraction of nerve-roots from the pelvis into the spinal canal (Fig. 133) and thus holds the lower part of the spinal cord so that it cannot be drawn upwards.

The stretching due to each of several protrusions is, of course, additive. Evidence of tension produced by an impinging structure may sometimes be visualized radiographically as a depression in the spinal cord caused by the protrusion(s). Unlike any compression, this depression can be observed directly at surgery.

Where there are apparently no protrusions large enough to be potentially pathogenic, the presence of neurological symptoms should prompt a radiological search for other possible causes of stress. X-ray analysis in cases of, for instance, spasticity in the upper extremities, where the most striking feature is protrusion of the C_6/C_7 disc or a thoracic kyphosis, on closer inspection will probably reveal one or more firm structures at higher levels on the anterior aspect of the cervical canal, possibly strongly curved normal structures that exert contact pressure on the over-stretched pons–cord tract and produce a local axial and transverse bending tensile stress in this section of it.

If, with the body in the supine position, the head and neck are gradually extended, the cord will sag on to the posterior aspect of the cervical canal (153) (Fig. 102). On the television monitor a continuous and usually persistent gas layer will be seen in the subarachnoid space anterior to the cord. But if, even only on full extension, this gas stratum is no longer visible, and if the cord is found to contain a depression caused by a protrusion of any kind, a pincer or clamping action may be suspected (29, 216). The actual compression of the nervous tissue will be due to pinching between the pathological structure protruding from the anterior side into the canal, and the firm surface of the dura, supported by the ligamenta flava and the cristae arcorum (Fig. 45). If the radiological examination is not conclusive a measurement of the cerebrospinal fluid pressure in the extended position may provide an important clue by showing whether extension interferes with the transmission of CSF pressure generated proximally.

To establish the occurrence of detrimental forces in the thoracic and lumbosacral region the same methods and criteria are essential (154, 158), except for the measurement of CSF pressure. When a patient suffering from a spinal disorder of the thoracic region is examined in the supine position and the canal is lengthened by flexion of the whole spine, the cord is raised against any protrusions, kyphosis, angulations, spondylolisthesis, etc., and pressure (unilateral thrust) on the cord can result, giving rise to bending tensile stress in the tissue. The same applies if a patient suffering from neurological symptoms due to kypho*scoliosis* is examined in the lateral position; on lateral flexion of the spine produced by raising the shoulders and pelvis with pads, the cord is often forced upwards so that it bears on the lateral convexity protruding into the canal. The contact pressure thus produced can extend over a relatively long section of the pons–cord tract.

In pure scoliosis harmless contact with the cord not infrequently occurs at the levels of two consecutive convexities.

It is self-evident that in the thoracic region, too, actual compression can exist only when there is total displacement of the contrast medium on both sides of the cord. For technical reasons (a viscous opacifying fluid can be arrested where gas can still pass) only gas myelography can yield an unambiguous result.

While this is the method that gives the best results

in the upper sections of the spinal canal a water-soluble medium must be used in the lumbosacral region.

A continuous layer of this medium along the lateral contour of the lumbar or sacral nerve-roots rules out the possibility of compression by, for instance, a herniated disc (53). In this case the nerve-roots are usually stretched and pushed into the canal, though not so far as to make contact with the opposite wall. As they pass over the offending disc these roots describe a definite curve (Fig. 137). If they are further stretched on flexing the vertebral column the curvature will be shallower, and the pressure on the roots, and thus the bending tensile stress in them, will be increased (for use of Metrizamide as diagnostic aid *see* Fig. 119 and pp. 143, 227).

Spinal flexion in the visualization of tension

In patients with incapacitating neurological symptoms due to kyphosis or kyphoscoliosis where surgical measures must be considered, it may be desirable, if not essential, to ascertain whether the whole tract is over-stretched and sections of it are therefore being subjected to unilateral thrust and bending tensile stress.

It is impossible to judge the tension in a straight section of the cord. A reliable impression of the state of tension in any section of the tract can be obtained only from the degree of bending and elongation of the spinal canal and the consequent tension in the whole of the tract, the examination being performed without changing the spinal posture.

Over-stretching of the tract will immediately be suspected if the examination discloses a large firm structure, such as a herniated thoracic disc, which deflects the tract towards the opposite wall of the canal so that the cord is angulated over the protrusion. The deformation of the contour of the tract must be followed throughout the length of the canal in order to obtain a realistic overall picture of the pressure and the resulting tension and bending tensile stress.

When there are no firm structures and no deflection of the tract towards the centre of the curvature or movement of the posterior contour of the dura towards the centre of the canal—signs of stretching or, possibly, over-stretching—it may be difficult to decide whether or not a section of the tract is in fact under tension.

If, because of pathological alterations, a section of the spine or canal that would normally have assumed a curved shape remains straight, or becomes so, during flexion, while sections cranial and/or caudal to it bend in the normal fashion, the cord within the straight section of the dura and canal will follow a straight course. It may then be inferred from the elongation of the neighbouring cranial and/or caudal sections of the canal and dura that the straight section must also be under tension.

If it is necessary to avoid strenuous examination of the injured cord by gas myelography in extreme positions of the spine and different body postures, no picture of the state of tension in the pons—cord tract can be obtained, and one must rely on one's experience of the biomechanical behaviour of the tract in different positions of the spine.

Behaviour of dura and cord during spinal flexion

Full flexion of the whole spine produces tension throughout the dura and tract. In this position the curvature is most pronounced in the cervical section, and the cervical cord assumes the same strongly curved form (35). In the absence of suspensory apparatus (dentate ligaments and arachnoid septa) the cord that is under tension would tend to follow the shortest course through curved parts of the canal and thus invariably make contact with its convex sections; however, this tendency is counteracted by the dentate ligaments, which keep the cord near the middle of the canal and the dural theca.

Gas myelography during flexion of the cervical canal with the patient in the supine position visualizes the subarachnoid space on the anterior and posterior aspects of the *curved* cord. Under normal conditions the slight deflection of the stretched dura towards the

centre of the canal that may then sometimes be seen (157) does not appreciably affect the configuration of the cord. If, in full flexion of the spine and hence maximum elongation of the canal, a particular section of the stretched cord is seen to follow the curvature of the canal, the presence of gas in the surrounding subarachnoid space does not rule out the possibility that the pons—cord tract is under tension; in fact, these findings constitute evidence of normal elastic tension. This interpretation of the readily verifiable observations is inconsistent with the view that in flexion of the spine the cord always appears to be stretched, and that it follows the shortest route through the spinal canal (216). This will, however, be the case as soon there is pathological over-stretching of the dura and cord and yielding of the fibres in the epidural displacement layer (169) and the attachments of the dentate ligaments.

Pathogenetic significance of tension in the dura and cord

As a rule a forward displacement of the *cord* is found only at the level of a pathologically increased curvature of the spine—that is to say, in kyphosis or kyphoscoliosis—where the lengthening of the canal raises the tension in the cord.[2]

From the site of displacement of the *dura* through its over-stretching it may be possible to locate any mechanical injury to the cord due to pressure of the dura and perhaps compression. This displacement of a section of the dura toward the centre of the canal in severe kyphosis (Case 1, p. 227) is obviously indicative of a clamping action on a relatively long section of the cord (144, 274).

Avoidance of spinal flexion in spinal cord injury

Immediately after the trauma flexion must be avoided so as to prevent intramedullary tension and thus aggravating the damage to the cord.

In the vent of adhesions between the cord and the dura flexion would set up tension in the nerve-fibres immediately above and below the lesion and stretching of the nerve-fibres around the scar would impair their conductivity.

Behaviour of dura and cord during spinal extension

In extension of the spinal column, where the pons–cord tract is slack, the extent of its contact with the canal wall depends on the body posture. Contrary to what has been supposed, this contact has no pathogenetic significance. Acquaintance with this phenomenon is therefore necessary if misinterpretations are to be avoided.

In full extension of the whole spine, with the body in the *prone* position, the slackened cord sags on to the anterior surface of the canal under gravity. The cord tissue will be moulded around any protrusions and will also come into contact with any intervening plane surface of the dura (Figs. 32 B, 33 C, D).

As can be seen in the cadaver, in full extension of the whole spine or just the cervical part, with the body in the *lateral* position the slackened cord sags on to the lateral contour of the canal under gravity (Fig. 5). The lateral suspensory attachments of the dentate ligaments then yield under the weight of the cord. The area of contact between the cord and the dura varies considerably, depending on the widths of the cord and the canal; when the area is small, contact is visualized as a faint line; when it is large, a broad zone of contact is seen. On flexion of the cervical spine the cord is pulled towards the centre of the canal by the dura and the attachments of the dentate ligaments; this displacement, which occurs quite rapidly, is strikingly large and can amount to as much as 8–10 millimetres.

In the *supine* posture extension of the cervical spine results in sagging of the slackened cord on to the posterior surface of the dura and canal. The nerve-roots with their root-sheaths, which are not visualized by gas myelography in this position, are then drawn out. The attachments of the dentate ligaments must then have yielded, together with the gossamer fibres that bridge

the subarachnoid space from the pia mater to the arachnoid (Figs. 10, 102).

Relaxation of the pons–cord tract can also be induced by lateral flexion of the cervical spine, the lumbar spine or the whole column. If it is difficult to obtain functional gas myelograms in the prone and supine positions an attempt should be made in the lateral position of the spine, with especially the cervical section flexed away from the table. The resulting considerable shortening of the upper concave wall of the canal slackens the dura and dentate ligaments on the upper side so that the relevant section of the cord falls under gravity on to the lower wall (Figs. 5, 6).

Assessment of degree of therapeutic cord relaxation

The effect on the injured tissues that can be obtained by slackening the pons–cord tract is best examined by extending the cervical spine; this check is indispensable, firstly, for ascertaining the type and severity of the traumatic damage to the tract—such as adhesions and stiffening—and secondly for finding the potential slack that may be exploited in the treatment. Extension of just the cervical spine will usually suffice provided that it is unaffected by disease and its mobility is normal.

[2] Unlike the pathological curvature of the canal, deviation of the dura from its normal path as a possible cause of neurological symptoms has received relatively little attention from radiologists. Relatively recently, however, displacement of the dura through stretching has been demonstrated in the cervical canal (157).

With full extension or lateral flexion of the cervical spine the site, extent and, possibly, the state of the injured part of the cord[3] may be visualized under favourable conditions.

If the damaged cord is slack it will then be possible, by rotating the examination table (99), to follow its deformation under gravity in the subarachnoid space, now empty of fluid. The displacement of the relaxed cord and the nerve-roots accompanying postural changes can indicate to what extent slackening also of the injured part of the cord can be induced.

At the site of a lesion there is often adhesion of the medullary tissue to the dura or bone, and the slackening of the cord obtained by extension or lateral flexion of the cervical spine may not be visualized. However, an impression of the biomechanical state of the damaged tissue may be obtained by observing whether, and to what extent, the slackened tract just caudal and cranially of the affected part sags under gravity in the supine, prone and the two lateral positions.

In view of the established benefits derived from slackening the dura and the pons–cord tract in the treatment for several kinds of chronic myelopathy and spinal cord injury, it is reasonable to suppose that this technique will be used to a greater extent in the near future; it will then be increasingly important to be able to detect tension in the cord and—despite prophylactic immobilization of the cervical spine in slight extension—to assess the degree of any persistent stretching or over-stretching by radiography prior to surgery. It will also be necessary to ascertain the extent of the slackening that can be obtained in different sections of the tract. The examinations required for this purpose must be performed under well defined, standardized and stable mechanical conditions, since the phenomena to be observed, whether normal or pathological, occur most distinctly in maximum functional positions of the spine and the body posture.

During surgery, X-ray television monitoring can be used to check whether the intended extension of the cervical spine will suffice to ensure the necessary slackening of the pons–cord tract. Gas myelography may also be advisable during the operation so as to ensure that the slackening extends to injured parts of the tract inaccessible to direct observation. After the operation a radiographic examination is required to check that cervicolordodesis or other surgical measures have not produced undesirable mechanical changes of the spine.

[3] This does refer to other pathological changes in shape than the above-mentioned state of oedema.

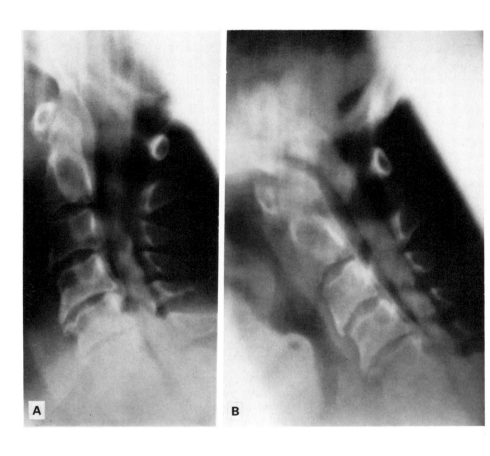

Fig. 101. Midsagittal tomographic gas myelograms in extreme postures of the cervical spine with the patient in lateral position.

A. *Extension.* Though deflected by the protrusion at the C_4/C_5 level, the cord is not under tension.

B. *Flexion.* In its stretched state the cord almost loses contact with the protrusion, and is instead pressed against, and stretched over, another at the C_5/C_6 level; it is here that the tension in the tissue responsible for the neurological symptoms is set up (bending tensile stress).

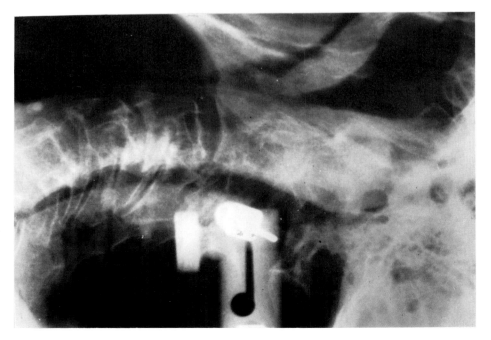

Fig. 102. Effect of gravity on the cord in extension of the cervical spine (gas myelogram).

Under gravity the slackened cervical spinal cord of a patient in the supine position with the neck extended has sagged on to the posterior aspect of the canal.

Courtesy of The Good Samaritan Hospital, Los Angeles.

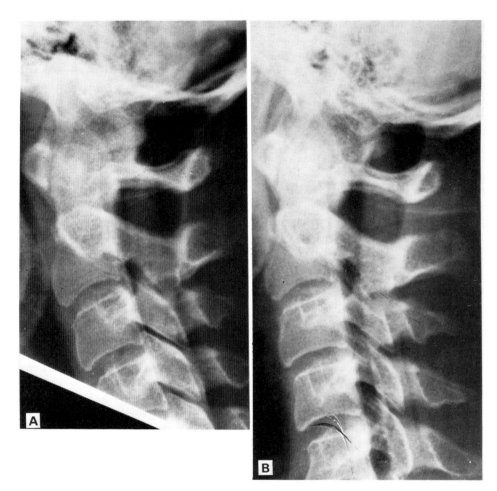

Fig. 103. Effect of gravity on the cord with the cervical spine in neutral position (gas myelogram).

A. With the patient *prone* the cord and the medulla oblongata are in contact with the soft tissues along the upper, posterior border of the odontoid process and the posterior border of the third vertebra.

B. In the *supine* position the cord sags on to the wedge-shaped posterior border of the C_2 and C_3 arches. Remote from the point where it was in contact with the tip of the odontoid process the cord now curves rostrally.

Postural reduction of fractures of the cervical spine

Fractures and dislocations of the vertebrae can often be reduced by applying traction to the spinal column. In the case of a fracture comparison of successive radiographs during traction therapy may show the progress towards partial or complete approximation of bone fragments. This is due to the generation of tension in the anterior and posterior longitudinal ligaments (so long as they are intact) and the pressure that they then exert from the anterior and posterior direction on loose or mobile bone fragments. A similar mechanism accounts for the correction of a dislocation.

Besides the intended reduction of the fracture, traction on the vertebral column can, however, lead to additional trauma to, and tensile ischaemia in, the damaged spinal cord or brain stem, especially during the first weeks after the trauma. Traction must then be avoided at all costs. A technique that has been found to be effective in reducing vertebral fractures at any levels, and that avoids the risk of damage to the cord, is to place the patient on a support that extends the section of the column containing the damaged vertebra or vertebrae and holds it stable.

It would seem that in the lordosed posture of the spine there are two main interacting mechanisms that tend to reduce a fracture. One of them is the stretching of the uninjured anterior longitudinal ligament—though less so in the posterior ligament—when the spine is extended, and the other is the pressure from behind exerted by the support on the vertebral arches and, *via* them, on the vertebral bodies (so long as the arches are intact). The forces tending to reduce a vertebral fracture are thus similar to those acting during therapeutic traction.

Using this method of postural reduction of vertebral fractures the author has obtained good reduction and consolidation of such spinal fractures in a score of patients where, to judge from the moderate displacement of the fragments, there was probably no gross damage to the ligaments. Postural reduction of fractures of vertebral bodies, pedicles or arches (of the latter at their junction with the vertebral body) were effected in the lumbar and thoracic regions, and in the cervical region even in the case of fracture of the axis and atlas vertebrae (see Figs. 106–8).

The advocated induction of lordosis also results in therapeutic relaxation of the pons–cord tract; this is especially indicated where the spinal cord has suffered damage.

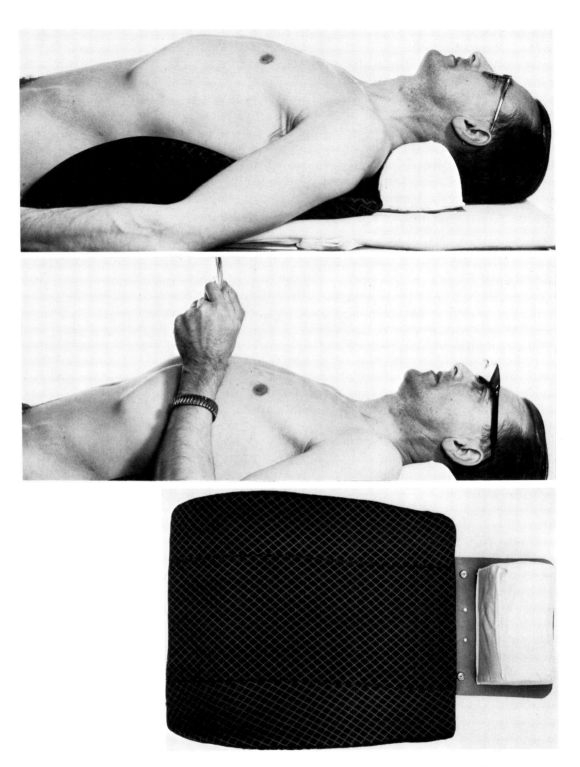

Fig. 104. Spinal supports for maintaining extension in the supine patient.

The supports consist of a neck bolster to accommodate the slightly extended cervical spine, and a back rest[1] for producing lordosis of the lumbar spine. They ensure that the spine is extended in all regions. But to achieve maximum relaxation in the spinal canal, the hips and knees should be kept flexed and the feet plantarflexed. The patient is wearing prismatic spectacles to allow reading without cervical flexion.

The same relaxed posture can be obtained with a variety of aids (53, 190). In practice it has often proved effective in the short or long-term treatment of patients with (*i*) dislocation and fracture (Figs. 106–108); (*ii*) neurological symptoms from the spinal cord and nerve-roots due to various extra- and intramedullary pathological lesions (from the posterior cranial fossa to the sacral canal (Fig. 94); and (*iii*) disc herniation. (For anatomical reasons, however, (Fig. 32 H) the relaxation method is more or less ineffective in lesions located at the entrance to, or within, the intervertebral canal.)

In the case of a pathologically narrow canal the physiological bulging of soft tissues occurring on extension of the vertebral column and the consequent reduction of the lumen of the canal can aggravate neurological symptoms.

[1] "Sana" model, Kifa Co., Stockholm.

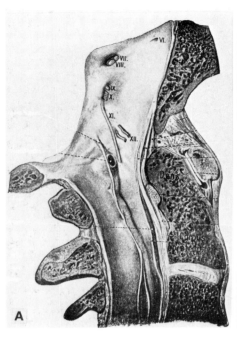
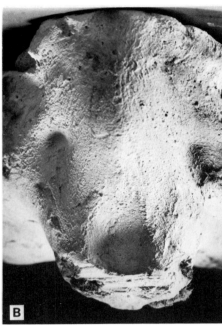

Fig. 105. The part of the posterior fossa on which the pons and oblongata bear.

A. Mid-sagittal section through the atlanto-occipital junction.

B. Plaster cast of the floor of the posterior fossa, including the upper cervical canal at the level of the odontoid process. Corresponding to the keel-shaped form of the clivus there is a broad medial elevation, and corresponding to the prominence of the odontoid process, a marked impression in the cast.

  The pons and oblongata fit exactly into this impression of the clivus.

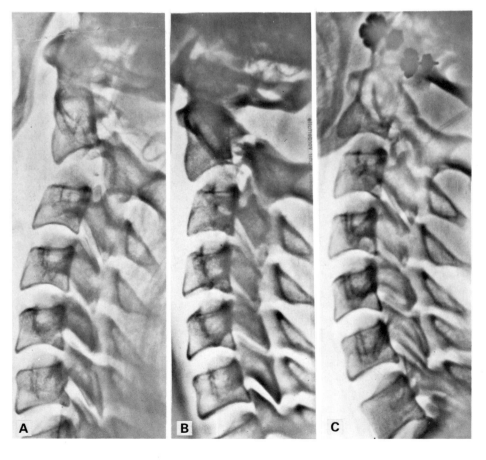

Fig. 106. Reduction of fractures of various parts of the cervical spine by extension of the head and cervical spine.

A. Bilateral fracture of the arches of the axis just anterior to the articular facets, with displacement of its body, carrying with it the atlas and the head. Apart from neck pain, the young female patient suffered from only minor neurological symptoms.

B. Twenty-four hours after supporting the neck on a round bolster with the head slightly extended (Fig. 104), the fracture gap was clearly reduced.

C. Reduction was practically complete within 3 days (X-ray not available). It was maintained by keeping the patient on this support for the next month. This X-ray was taken 30 days after the accident. The patient was then allowed up wearing a collar (Fig. 107 B) for 3 weeks to maintain the slight extension of the neck. Thereafter full mobility of the neck was recovered and all symptoms vanished.

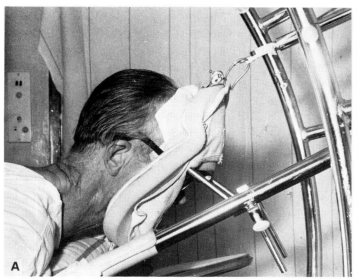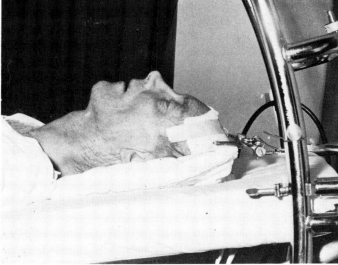

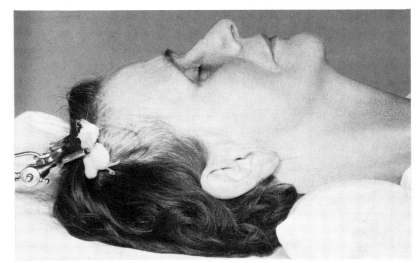

Fig. 107. The reduction of fracture of the odontoid process by extending the head and cervical spine.

A. The treatment for the fracture consists simply in placing the neck on a round bolster. The sole purpose of the Crutchfield's forceps, anchored in the *frontal* bone and loaded with a weight of about 0.5 kg, is to keep the head and neck slightly extended.

Left. Prone position.

Right. Supine position. (The patient is nursed in a Circ-O-Lectric bed.)

B. *Upper.* Patient with fracture of the odontoid process treated as in A.

Lower. For long-term immobilization of the cervical spine in the slightly extended position a supporting collar is used. The collar is made of a light plastic material and consists of an anterior and posterior part, which are strapped together (and also around the chest); it is thus readily adjustable. A cotton pad under the chin prevents abrasion.

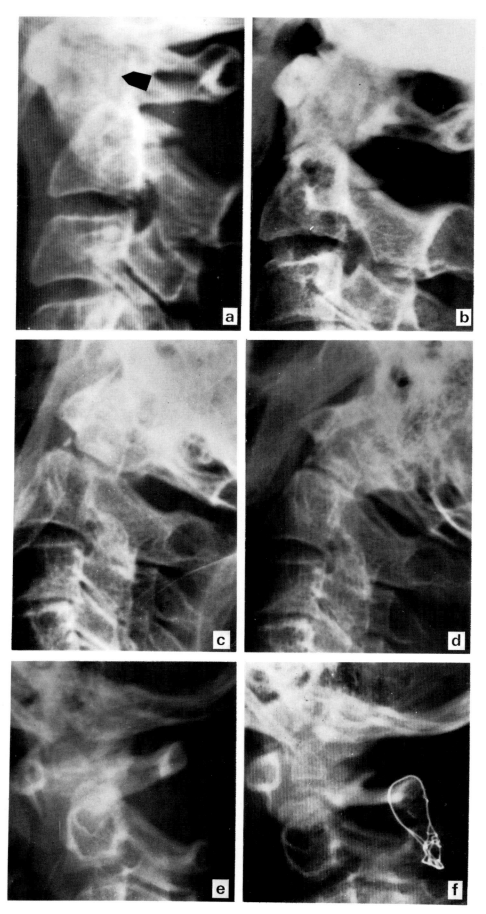

Fig. 108.

A. Fractures of the odontoid process before and after reduction by the postural method, in which the head and cervical spine are kept extended by the support.

Upper.
a. Anterolisthesis. The atlas arch together with the fractured odontoid process is displaced forward (*arrow*).
b. Spontaneous reduction of the fracture secured by extension on the support.

Middle.
c. Retrolisthesis. The arch of the atlas together with the fractured odontoid process is displaced posteriorly.
d. Spontaneous reduction of the fracture secured by extension on the support.

Lower.
e. Anterolisthesis. Before reduction of the fractured odontoid process.
f. After reduction retained by cerclage, osteosynthesis and extension on the support. (The periosteum of the arches of the atlas and axis was removed and their surfaces roughened; a bone graft was then held in contact with them by means of the wire. The patient was a 10-year-old Egyptian girl treated by the author, 1962, in Cairo.)

B. Fracture of the odontoid process treated by skull traction.

Fracture of the tip of the odontoid process in a middle-aged woman. Skull traction immediately after the injury (Crutchfield's forceps loaded with a weight of 3.5 kg) resulted in a pseudarthrosis. An X-ray check at 10 year follow-up disclosed no consolidation.

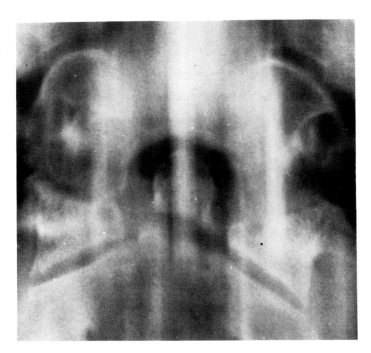

Cervical myelopathy

Histodynamic background

Cervical myelopathies stand out as a typical example of neurological disorders having their origin in tension in the spinal cord tissue, and the resulting distortion of both nerve-fibres (59, 60) and blood-vessels (246). The investigation reported above throws some light on the forces acting on the tissues of the cervical spinal cord during flexion of the cervical spine in the presence of osteophytes along the anterior aspect of the canal. These structures exert a unilateral thrust on the cervical cord and thus increase the axial tension throughout the pons—cord tract, the extent depending on how far they protrude into the canal, and on the degree to which the spine is flexed. Further, the thrust of an osteophyte sets up a local bending tensile stress field in the cord tissue, the transverse component of which is increased by virtue of the fact that the cord is anchored by the attachments of the dentate ligaments (Figs. 32, 34); severing contralateral ligaments reduces this component of the stress (160). The axial and the transverse components are both responsible for the neurological symptoms and signs. The forces producing the transverse component of the tension in the cervical cord also result in stretching of the lateral branches of the central arteries (54); these vessels follow a transverse course and supply the lateral pyramidal tracts (255, 256), and it is thus evident that their stretching can account for the spasticity typical of myelopathies (142).

Besides the local bending tension and long-range axial tension in the pons—cord tract due to *flexion* of the cervical spine, short-range axial tension can be set up in the cervical cord tissue by a pincer or clamping action on the cord during *extension* of the cervical spine (28, 29, 91). Manifestations of this tension are the familiar persistent neurological symptoms experienced after 'hyperextension' injury (245). The pincer action is produced by osteophytes approaching the canal's posterior wall, consisting of the dura, the ligamenta flava and the vertebral arches, and it occurs either when a large osteophyte projects into a cervical canal of normal width or also when a relatively small osteophyte projects into a shallow canal. The magnitude and direc-

tion of the forces involved in a pincer (or clamping) action differ from those in a unilateral thrust; moreover, the axial tension set up by the pincer action is *not* transmitted throughout the tissue tract. However, unlike the relatively moderate tensile forces generated by the unilateral thrust, this localized axial tension can be so great as to cause tearing of nerve-fibres and even blood-vessels (56).

The fact that the neurological symptoms can usually be relieved simply by slackening the cord suggests that protruding osteophytes seldom cause lasting damage. It would thus seem that the symptoms associated with osteophytes in a spacious cervical canal are due to the unilateral thrust of these structures rather than to a pincer action.

The degree of extension at which the pincer action starts and neurological symptoms are evoked will depend on the distance that the osteophytes protrude into the canal. In the case of a *spacious* canal a pincer action may not occur at all; on the other hand, where the canal is *narrow* or otherwise abnormal in shape, a pincer action may start quite early on in the extension movement.

In a paper read at *Journée Internationale sur les Myélopathies Cervicales* in Paris in November, 1974, the author summarized this view on cervical myelopathy as follows: An indispensable condition for the development of chronic symptoms from the cervical myelon is disturbance of the normal biomechanical function of the spinal cord by pathological alterations in the canal. Today, it is established beyond reasonable doubt that the neurological symptoms are generated chiefly by forces of external origin (abnormal loading of the nervous tissue). Cervical myelopathy is characterized by a constantly changing pathological state of tension in the tissues of the cervical spinal cord. This intramedullary tension has been identified as the basic cause of the neurological signs and symptoms.

For *surgical treatment* of cervical myelopathy, see p. 250.

Thoracic myelopathy

Surgical problems involving the thoracic section of the pons–cord tract and nerve-roots are relatively uncommon; they are nonetheless clinically significant. For not only is the thoracic cord at risk from any lesion encroaching upon the spinal canal, but the thoracic region of the spine is frequently the site of deformities that are a major cause of pathological tension in the soft tissues of the canal.

Over-stretching of the pons–cord tract and local bending tensile stress in its tissue assume special significance in thoracic kyphosis resulting from trauma, or in vertebral collapse due to tumours, infections or osteoporosis.

Thoracic spinal deformities of less acute onset—whether idiopathic, osteogenic or congenital—fall in a different category, if only because of the more generous time factor. The slow development of deformities allows time for adaptation, through growth, of nerve-fibres, blood-vessels, supporting tissues and dentate ligaments. Only when nerve-fibres are constricted by compression is the effect of adaptation inhibited.

Whatever the type of lesion responsible for the over-stretching of the thoracic cord, the neuropathological effects are governed chiefly by *cervical* posture and movement. Before dealing with some of the clinical syndromes, their histodynamic analysis and surgical treatment, the biomechanical behaviour of the thoracic spinal canal and its soft tissues under normal conditions will be outlined.

Normal biomechanics of the thoracic spine

The position of the spinal cord and dura mater in the thoracic spinal canal in the normal range of movement of the thoracic spine is greatly dependent on the posture and movements of the cervical and lumbar regions (35, 154). Because of its small sagittal mobility there is comparatively little change in length of the thoracic canal from extension to flexion. In lateral flexion the elongation on the convex side and the shortening on the concave become somewhat greater as the intersegmental mobility of the thoracic vertebrae approaches that of the lumbar vertebrae. The thoracic mobility is absolutely greatest on axial rotation, when no lengthening of the canal itself takes place.

When the canal is lengthened on forward or lateral flexion of the whole spine, the dura mater and pons–cord tract shift a few millimetres cranially in the toracic canal in relation to the vertebrae (Fig. 28). Moreover, they take a slightly shortened route—not the shortest route, however, for both epidural and subarachnoid spaces remain patent on the concave side, while the epidural space is maximally widened on the convex (157, 158). The epidural space is not occluded on the

concave side because of fatty tissue, which, unlike the venous plexus, is incompressible. The subarachnoid space remains patent on either side of the cord because tension in the dentate ligaments constrains lateral shift, and their posterior direction prevents anterior displacement of the cord towards the dura mater (35, 169) On axial rotation of the thoracic spine, the dentate ligaments become taut and there is some deformation and decrease in circumference of the cord (35).

Kyphosis

In thoracic kyphosis the length of the spinal canal is greater than normal, and during cervical and lumbar flexion there is a tendency for over-stretching of both dura and cord. This may, however, be offset to some extent by a progressive reduction in cervical and lumbar flexibility as the kyphosis increases with age. The thoracic dura mater and cord take a straighter and relatively shorter route (28, 155) and the epidural space becomes wider posteriorly (155, 158). Because of the pathological increase in tension in the dura and pons–cord tract caused by the kyphosis, the cervical spinal cord shifts posteriorly, so that the anterior subarachnoid space is widened in the neck (Fig. 117 C).

In every case of kyphotic myelopathy the gas myelogram shows that the cord is pressed against the anterior wall of the canal, with the anterior subarachnoid space obliterated at the apex. This is usually caused by pathological tension in the pons–cord tract; in patients with far advanced kyphotic deformity a pressure may be exerted on the posterior surface of the cord by the stretched and anteriorly displaced dura (135, 185, 231, 274). When, in such a case, the posterior dura is split sagittally at operation, the two portions separate and slip in the anterior direction on either side of the cord (185, 231, 274). It is notable that in those cases of kyphosis without signs or symptoms of myelopathy the anterior epidural and subarachnoid spaces are still visible.

The appearance of the epidural space on the myelogram depends very much on the applied technique. During drainage of cerebrospinal fluid and insufflation of gas the space diminishes noticeably in the lumbar region (126), and the contour of the dura is generally smooth. This contrasts with the defects visible when barium myelography is performed experimentally in the cadaver (39). It is essential to be able to determine from the myelogram the area of contact between the cord and the anterior surface of the spinal canal. For a given degree of kyphosis the pressure between cord and canal resulting from the tension varies inversely with the area of contact. Thus, with a small such area the pathological tension would set up local intramedullary bending tensile stress, whereas, with a sufficiently large, smooth area, no such histodynamic stress would be generated. In general, the greater the curvature the greater the likelihood of neurological signs and symptoms of myelopathy.

The presence of epidural fibrosis and underlying ligamentous bulging, or the occurrence of arachnoidal proliferation, is likely to modify the myelographic picture. It is obviously of great value to perform the myelography dynamically, so as to observe the effects of movements of the thoracic spine and neck; it is just as important to have functional radiographs taken at the extremes of sagittal mobility (28, 158). The mere visualization of a straightened cord is not necessarily evidence of tension.

Scoliosis

Scoliosis alone rarely generates neurological manifestations. As seen from anteroposterior and lateral projections, scoliosis is a simple deformity of the spine in the frontal plane (93, 231) with no elongation of the canal. Thus, the gas myelogram of a scoliotic patient contains no evidence of tension in the pons–cord tract unless there is also kyphoscoliosis (Figs. 114, 117). In a large series of cases of pure scoliotic deformity neurological involvement was recorded in only 0.35 per cent (231).

In one severely affected patient there was reportedly myelographic block at the apex of the curve (231), probably with cord compression. In such cases the dura mater may be deflected away from the convex side, to press the cord against the pedicles, which, like the neural arches on the concave side, are hypertrophied. In most cases of *true* scoliosis the reversal of the curve above and below the main deformity prevents pathological tension developing in the pons–cord tract, as there is no increase in the total length of the canal. However, on applying therapeutic traction to the spine in order to straighten the scoliotic curvatures pathological tension may be set up in the soft tissues in the spinal canal that can lead to neurological deficit (see below).

Kyphoscoliosis

For a given magnitude of pathological tension in the pons–cord tract thoracic myelopathies are more likely to occur in kyphoscoliosis than in scoliosis because of the complexity of the curve and the greater number of points at which the spinal canal wall may impinge on the cord, and hence over-stretch it. It is difficult, however, to draw a general pathodynamic picture because of the variety of individual curves, and the variability in the size of hypertrophied spondylotic spurs and in the sites of epidural fibrosis or adhesive arachnoiditis.

The route taken by the spinal cord is rarely the shortest one, and careful scrutiny of lateral and anteroposterior radiographs is needed to determine it. In patients with diastematomyelia the complexity may be increased

by the presence of a protruding bony ridge, which divides the cord (Figs. 109, 110). On flexing the spine the two cord halves are stretched and bent over this ridge and intramedullary bending tensile stress is set up in both halves of the cord. The actual site of contact between cord and bony ridge would then determine which pathways are affected and hence the nature of the symptoms and signs of neural deficit so evoked. As can be seen from the deformed cross-section of the cord at the level of the scoliotic curvature in a patient with kyphoscoliosis and diastematomyelia (Fig. 113), the tension in the dentate ligament and the site of thrust on the cord may combine to determine the nature of the deformation; the effect in this case is to over-stretch the lateral pathways and the lateral branches of the central arteries.

Treatment

The aim of any form of treatment for thoracic myelopathy is to relieve pathological tension in the pons–cord tract and remove any pinching or clamping structure causing local over-stretching of the cord. Discriminating appraisal of the myelographic appearances is essential. For instance, obliteration of the anterior subarachnoid space in kyphosis is not in itself a sign that an operation is necessary, but when the posterior space, too, is not visualized, surgical intervention is more likely to be justified. The most compelling indication is the deterioration from spasticity to flaccidity of the legs. Otherwise, the indications for surgery are the familiar signs and symptoms and the constraints that the condition imposes on the patient's routine activities.

Local space-occupying lesions, such as tumours or prolapsed thoracic discs, also present intrinsic histodynamic problems. For successful relief of the local pathological tension set up in the medullary tissue, and to avoid a momentary and potentially harmful increase during extirpation of such lesions, there are two vital requirements of the surgical technique. First, when laminectomy is chosen as the measure for relieving compression of the cord at the level of the lesion a protective method should be used, so as to avoid any instrumental intrusion into the canal. Second, in surgical measures on an extra- or intramedullary lesion the relaxation technique should be used; when exploring an extradural lesion on the anterior wall of the canal this technique enables both dura and cord to be drawn aside. If this is impracticable a lateral approach should be considered (261).

The presence of pathological tension in the pons–cord tract can create major difficulties during an operation. The posture of the patient is important: in order to reduce tension at the site of operation it is essential to obtain maximum relaxation of the tract; this may be accomplished by extending the neck and the lumbar spine and flexing the hip- and knee-joints. However, in many cases where permanent slackening is required this can be achieved by creating a shorter route for the over-stretched tissues (144).

Satisfactory treatment of kyphotic myelopathy by laminectomy has been reported (185, 274), but many patients are not helped. It is conceivable that in the successful cases the thoracic spine has been unwittingly extended through the removal of the neural arches from a spacious canal so that the intact arches are brought closer together and the degree of the kyphosis is reduced. In many cases the kyphosis itself cannot be modified, and then sagittal incision of the dura is an alternative measure (231, 274). This procedure may be the logical one—certainly it is when the kyphosis has set up excessive tension in the cervical dura and the neck is already compensatorily extended, so that nothing is to be gained from cervicolordodesis. Another tentative approach, with the object of obtaining maximum slackening of the dura and cord, is 'laminectomy à distance' (2), performed in the cervical spine with removal of many neural arches.[1] The benefits offered by this technique are limited, although it can be of value when cervical spondylotic protrusions are exerting a pincer or clamping action at many levels. Nerve-roots are tethered in the intervertebral foramina by epidural root-sleeve attachments, and it has been shown that on full extension the distances between dural attachments of the dentate ligaments are unchanged by cervical laminectomy, however extensive it may be (35). There is thus little to be gained by *laminectomy à distance* that cannot be achieved by the relatively minor surgical procedure of cervicolordodesis. The successful outcome of this operation in a man with kyphotic myelopathy is fully described in a Case Report (p. 227).

When more radical surgery is called for in order to create a shorter route for the cord (144) the posterior part of the vertebral bodies must be resected. The author has attempted this only in cases of trauma, when comminuted fragments of a vertebral body had been displaced posteriorly in the epidural space. A technical problem in such operations is to achieve adequate relaxation of the dura and pons–cord tract; this can be accomplished by careful positioning of the body with the spine extended, in particular through cervical extension using a self-adjusting head-rest (Fig. 141). Another means of obtaining full extension of the spine in cases of ankylosing spondylitis—where the flexion deformity rather than a myelopathy is the disability—is to perform a laminectomy and a spinal osteotomy with interbody fusion (172); but this is still only a theoretical solution.

Finally, a word about the dangers of applying tractive forces to the spine. Crutchfield's forceps, haloes or calipers are of value in stabilizing the posture of the neck (181), but their use in traction may increase tension in the dura and pons–cord tract to the point of overstretching. Irreparable damage to the brain stem is known to have resulted from applying halo-pelvic traction in kyphoscoliosis;[2] and paresis has been reported in a patient with scoliosis (231).

---

[1] Unless a protective method is used also this extensive type of conventional laminectomy incurs a risk of immediate damage to the cord (194); moreover, it incurs a long-term risk of uncontrollable kyphosis and scoliosis with potential damage to the cervical cord and nerve-roots.

[2] Winter, R. B., Haven, J. J., Moe, J. H., Lagaard, S. M.: Diastematomyelia and congenital spine deformities. J Bone Jt Surg 56A: 27–39, 1974.

From Discussion: . . . distinct association between diastematomyelia and congenital deformities of the spine . . . an incidence of 4.9 per cent; . . . correction of a scoliosis . . . involves stretching . . . perhaps the cord as well . . . cord injury is a realistic possibility . . . recommend that Harrington instrumentation be avoided in congenital scoliosis unless diastematomyelia has been proved to be absent . . . one patient with congenital scoliosis and a hair patch [additional sign for midline bone spur] . . . became paraplegic with . . . instrumentation.

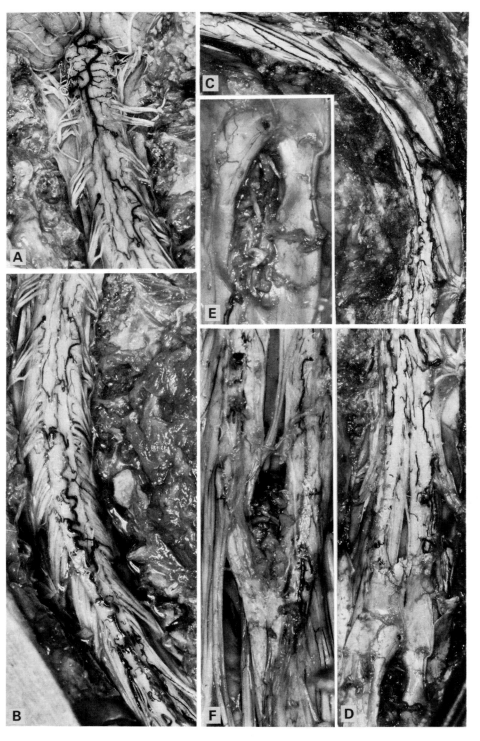

Fig. 109. Deformation of spinal cord and nerve-roots in kyphoscoliosis.

Severe kyphoscoliosis, diastematomyelia and hydromyelia. Before exposure the spinal cord was injected with contrast medium *via* a vertebral and the great anterior medullary artery and fixed *in situ* with the body in the neutral position by subarachnoidal injection of formaldehyde.

A. Lower part of the hemispheres of the cerebellum with the posterior inferior cerebellar arteries, medulla oblongata and upper cervical cord.

B. Cervical and upper thoracic cord displaced towards the right, shortened, wall of the canal. The nerve-roots and dentate ligaments along the left, elongated, wall are under tension, while those along the right wall against which the cord bears are slack.

C. Thoracic cord stretched over the left, shortened, wall of the canal. The nerve-roots and dentate ligaments are now stretched on the right, elongated, wall.

D. The region of diastematomyelia at lower thoracic levels with an initially common dural theca for the two separated halves of the cord. Lowermost in the figure, not far from the medullary cone, the dura is also divided.

E. Bony spur surrounded by blood-vessels and connective tissue, projecting between the two halves of the dura.

F. Dura removed. The nerve-roots leaving the cauda equina are exceptionally thick.

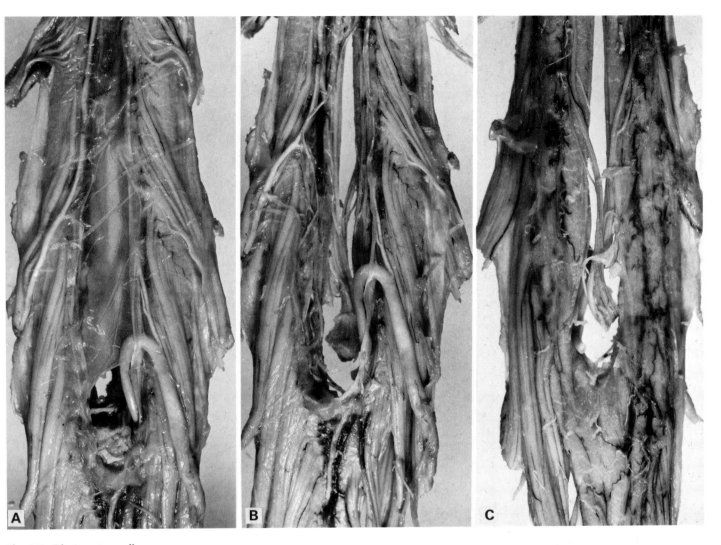

Fig. 110. Diastematomyelia.
(Specimen removed from cord in Fig. 109)

A, B. Anterior view of the diastematomyelia with the great anterior medullary artery on the right. In A the greater part of the arachnoid membrane remains and is particularly well developed between the two halves of the cord. In B the membrane has been removed. The great anterior medullary artery gives off only one, relatively fine, branch in the cranial direction. The main trunk of the artery turns back caudalward, and apparently supplies the cauda equina.

C. Posterior view of specimen. The great anterior medullary artery is torn away.

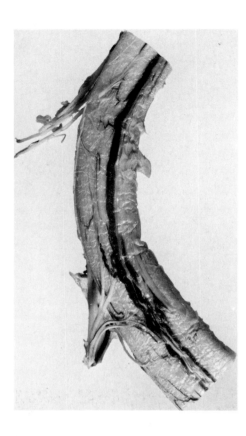

Fig. 111. Part of the thoracic cord (in Fig. 109), anterior view, showing the effect of unilateral thrust exerted in scoliosis by the stretching of the cord over the kyphosis.

The left half of the cord (on the right in the figure) is telescoped and appreciably narrower than the right half; the extensive folding is a result of axial shortening.

The other side of the cord is stretched, the nerve-roots thus leaving at a greater angle than normal. The angle of the roots varies round the curve at the apex.

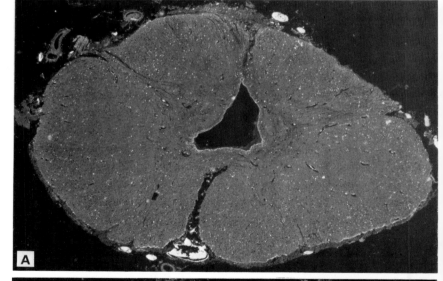

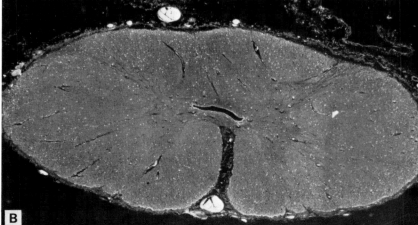

Fig. 112. Histodynamic effect of kyphoscoliosis on the thoracic cord which results in increased axial tension.

A. Transverse histological section through the cord (same specimen as in Fig. 109), seen from below, in the region of its maximum leftward curvature. There is simultaneous transverse stretching of its right half and of the nerve-roots and dentate ligaments. The central canal shows cystic widening (hydromyelia). The left half of the cord, which had been pressed against the canal wall, is appreciably narrower than the right half, the anteroposterior diameter thus being greater than on the right.

B. A tranverse section taken at a slightly lower level, just above the bifurcation of the cord.

Fig. 113. Histodynamic stress in the tissue of the thoracic cord in kyphoscoliosis.

Deformation of the cord tissue at the level of the scoliotic curvature, protruding into the thoracic canal from the right. Because of the pathologically increased axial tension in the pons–cord tract the curvature exerts pressure on the right half of the cord (*left black arrow*). This sets up anteroposterior tension (*upper and lower open arrows*). The lumina of affected blood-vessels (of both the external and internal circulations) will thus be reduced (*pair of straight lines, bottom left*), while the vessels running in the transverse direction are folded, and their lumina are possibly widened (*pair of wavy lines on left*). Because of the displacement of the right half of the cord towards the scoliotic curvature, the nerve-roots and the dentate ligament on this side are slack.

The left half of the cord, on the other hand, is kept in transverse tension by the stretched nerve-roots and the attachment of the dentate ligament (*right black arrow*). This tension results in transverse stretching of the tissue of the left half of the cord (*left and right open arrows*). The deformation of the blood-vessels is then the opposite of that in the right half (*pairs of straight and wavy lines*). The axially directed nerve-fibres and the blood-vessels of this half of the cord are therefore subjected to marked, and those in the right half to moderate, bending tensile stress.

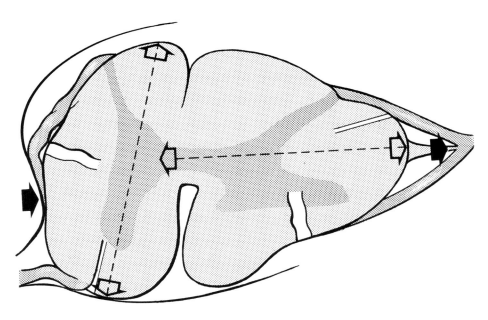

Fig. 114. Radiograph in a woman, aged 49, with severe kyphoscoliotic deformity. Gas myelograms.

A. Lateral view of the thoracic spine showing fairly marked kyphosis.

B. Anteroposterior view. At the T_6/T_7 level— that is, the level of the scoliosis with rightward convexity—there is contact between the cord and the left wall of the thoracic canal. Corresponding situation at the T_{12}/L_1 level with the compensatory leftward scoliotic convexity.

Histodynamic features. The contribution of kyphosis to the pathological lengthening of the canal is the reason for the pronounced tension in the cord that stretches it along the scoliotic curvatures.

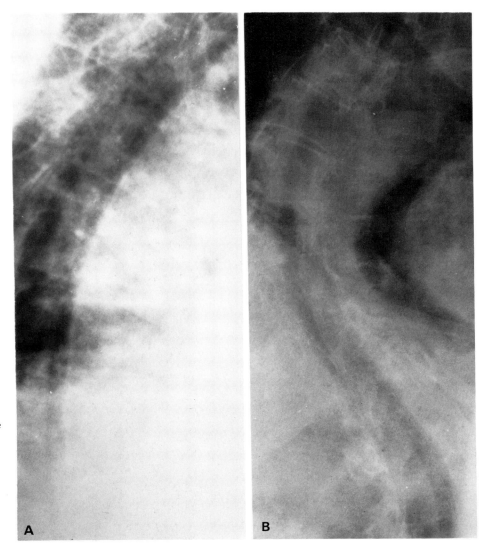

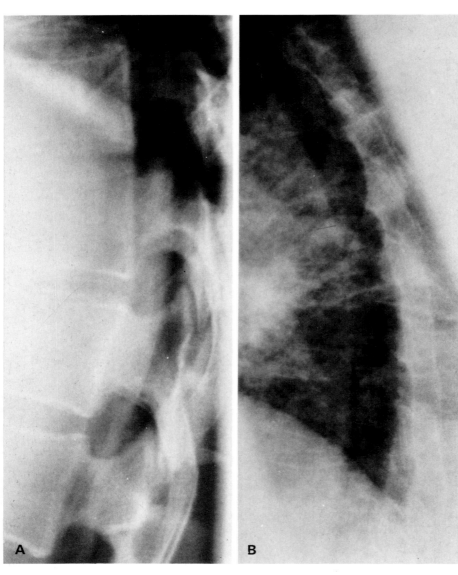

Fig. 115.

A. Radiograph in a woman, aged 55, with kyphosis giving rise to symptoms from the cervical nerve-roots and long pathways.[1]

Gas myelogram. At the level of the kyphosis of the spine, T_6–T_7, the cord is in contact with the posterior aspect of the vertebral bodies, and is narrower than elsewhere. It is, however, mobile, and in the supine position it does not make contact with the vertebral bodies.

B. Radiograph in a man, aged 65, with kyphosis of unknown origin.[2]

Gas myelogram. Fairly marked kyphosis at the level of the intervertebral discs T_9–T_{12}, which were reduced in height. Here the thoracic cord is in direct contact with the anterior wall of the canal and is narrower than elsewhere.

[1] *Neurological symptoms elicited histodynamically.* For 3 years the patient had been suffering from nuchal pain radiating to the arms; numbness in the middle fingers. Babinski's sign positive on the right.

It is not known whether any change in the diameter of the thoracic cord was observed during flexion of the spine, but this should in principle have been the case, since axial tension in the cord would produce a transverse tensile stress and hence a reduction in its anteroposterior diameter. The stress field thus set up in the cord tissue reduces the lumina of the branches of the central arteries supplying the lateral pyramidal pathways (Babinski's sign positive). It is likely that the cervical symptoms also may have been due to the axial tension.

[2] Admitted for suspected compression of the thoracic cord. No other neurological information. Histodynamic features probably similar to those in the patient under A.

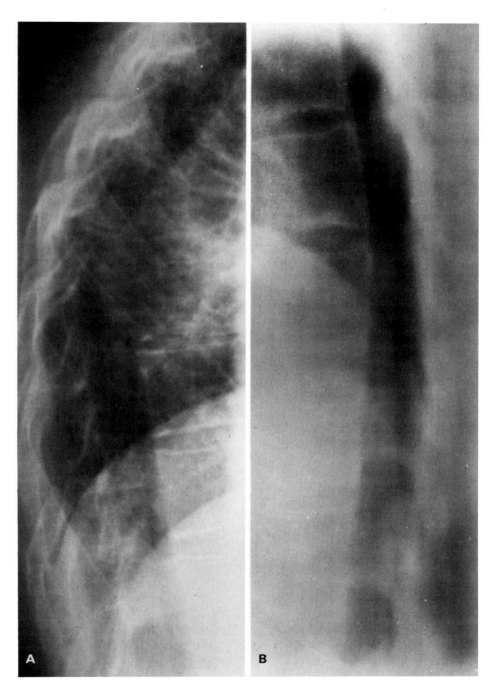

Fig. 116.

A. Radiograph in a woman, aged 27, with thoracic gibbus after traumatic compression of the vertebral body T₇.[1]

Gas myelogram. At the level of the compressed body T₇ the subarachnoid space is considerably narrowed by a soft-tissue shadow, protruding from its anterior aspect. There is no gas in front, or on the right, of the thoracic cord, which is greatly deflected at the level of the compressed vertebra.

B. Radiograph in a man, aged 65, with kyphosis after a road accident 2 years previously.[2]

Gas myelogram. At the level T₁₁–T₁₂ there is marked kyphosis and the cord makes close contact with the anterior wall of the subarachnoid space, indicated by absence of a radiolucent strip.

[1] *Neurological symptoms elicited histodynamically.* Four years earlier (cause not mentioned) there had been pain in a zone between the mammae and the umbilicus and this had increased in severity in the last 6 months. Pain on coughing and sneezing; numbness in the toes. No mention of other neurological features.

Histodynamic features. A local gibbus (in an otherwise normal spinal canal) exerts a thrust on the cord, producing a stress field within the tissue around the protrusion. This tension can be relieved either by surgical removal of the protrusion while the cord is relaxed or by cervicolordodesis. Since the relaxation also extends to the nerve-roots, though only to the region for the entry of the intervertebral canal (Fig. 138), it might possibly exert a beneficial effect also on the root symptoms.

[2] *Histodynamic features.* As in A.

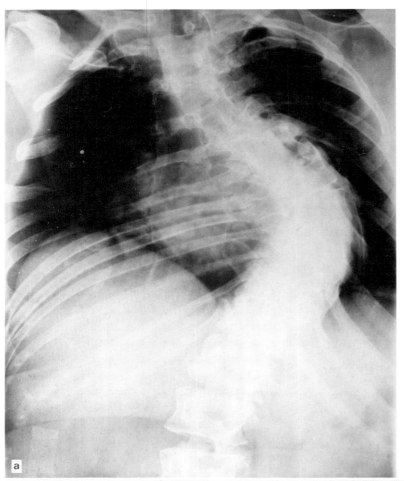

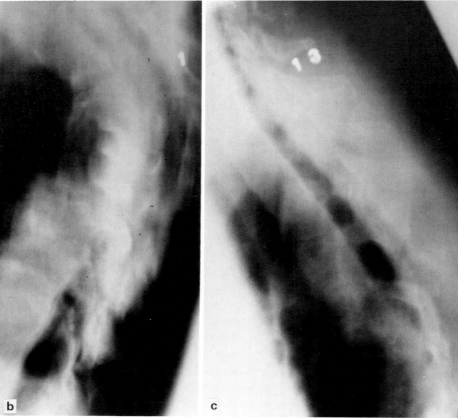

Fig. 117. Radiograph in a woman, aged 44, with severe kyphoscoliosis, developing after a birth injury.

a. Gas myelogram. *Anteroposterior* view.

b. Gas myelogram. Tomographic *lateral* view of the *thoracic* spine.[1]

At the level of the apex of the kyphosis, T_6–T_9, the spinal cord is in contact with the anterior wall of the spinal canal. Owing to marked stretching over the kyphosis the cord is flattened; the gas-filled subarachnoid space posterior to the cord is thus widened. (While screening and rotating the patient, the anterolateral subarachnoid space on the concave side was invisible for 7–8 cm.)

c. Gas myelogram. Tomographic *lateral* view of the *cervicothoracic* spine.[2]

Above the level of kyphosis the over-stretched cord is displaced toward the posterior aspect of the canal (and is possibly pressed against the C_2 and C_3 arches, thus widening the gas-filled anterior subarachnoid space.

[1] *Neurological symptoms elicited histodynamically* by the kyphoscoliosis in the *thoracic* region. Marked spasticity with cloni in both legs, positive Babinski's sign; atactic gait; left leg weaker than right—tension more marked in left pyramidal tract; superficial sensibility reduced below T_{12}; loss of deep sensibility in legs.
[2] *Neurological symptoms elicited histodynamically* in the *cervico-thoracic* region. Increased reflexes in arms, hands, finger-tips with increasing stiffness of hands (right more than left), due to increased tension in the cord and nerve-roots (more marked on right than left side).

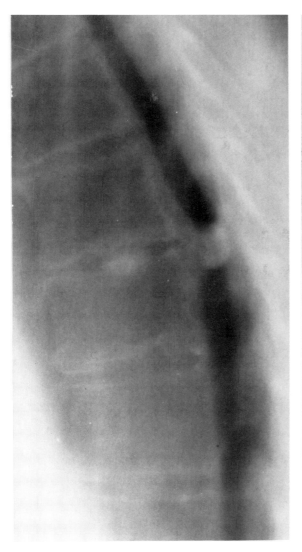
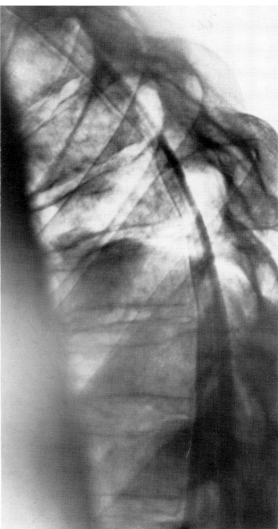

Fig. 118. Radiograph in a man, aged 66, with a calcified herniated thoracic disc.[1]

Gas myelogram. Corresponding to the T_7/T_8 intervertebral disc, which is lowered and displays a central calcification, is a pea-sized partly calcified discal hernia. The thoracic cord is clearly stretched over the protrusion, and hence presents a straight anterior contour above and below.

[1] *Neurological symptoms elicited histodynamically.* For the previous 18 months there had been increasing weakness and spastic paresis in the right leg, with positive Babinski's sign. Reduced sensibility on right side of the body below T_9. The neurological symptoms pointed to an impinging body on the right side of the spinal canal, producing a tensile stress field within the right half of the cord. The symptoms on this side resulted from the stretching of the nerve-fibres in the lateral pyramidal pathways, and the vessels supplying them and the posterior columns.

Fig. 119. Radiograph in man, aged 51, with angulation of the thoracic spine at 2 levels following 20 years' work demanding stooping posture with trunk flexed.

Myelogram with positive contrast medium (Metrizamide). Angulation of the spinal canal at T_7–T_9 with obliteration of the anterior subarachnoid space at the two intervertebral spaces. Cord appeared to be narrowed at both levels, to almost half its anteroposterior diameter at T_7/T_8. The whole dural theca is displaced in the anterior direction, though the posterior subarachnoid space remains well visualized.[1]

[1] *Neurological symptoms elicited histodynamically,* see Case Report, p. 227.

Pathodynamics of the lumbar spine

Normal biomechanics

In an analysis of the causes of pathologically elevated tension in the lumbar dura, cord and nerve-roots a number of factors pertaining to the normal mechanics of the system must be borne in mind. Unlike the thoracic spine but in common with the cervical portion, the lumbar spine is highly mobile in the healthy subject, and the soft tissues are therefore very adaptable. The lumbar subarachnoid space is occupied by a caudally decreasing number of nerve-roots, instead of, as the space in the cervical and thoracic regions, by the spinal cord. Moreover, to a much greater extent than the cervical and thoracic roots are affected by movements of the arms and trunk, the lumbar roots are influenced by the posture and movement of the legs, particularly at lower lumbar and sacral levels. Another difference of major pathological significance is that, whereas cervical movements affect the tension in both lumbar dura and nerve-roots, *via* the dura and cord, lumbar movements obviously only produce a reaction cranially, *via* the dura.

Variation in length of the lumbar spinal canal

On flexion, the lumbar *spinal canal* lengthens, particularly along its posterior wall; from full extension to full flexion the central axis can increase in length by as much as 20 per cent. Between the right–left extremes of lateral flexion the lateral wall of the canal changes in length by up to 15 per cent.

Because of this great variability the *dura* will be stretched during forward flexion of the lumbar spine; during lateral flexion the convex side is stretched, while the concave side is slackened. On the other hand, in extended postures the dura is relaxed and folded – more on the posterior than the anterior side. The dural root-sleeves make a larger obtuse angle with the axis of the extended spine than they do in the flexed posture, when they are taut; in lateral flexion they make a larger obtuse angle on the relaxed, concave, side of the curve. The lumen of the *subarachnoid space* is greater in flexed than in extended postures. On extension of the spine and on its concave side in lateral flexion, where the canal is shortened, the dura and ligamenta flava are folded and thus encroach on the space, while in flexion the lumen is widened because the dura is under tension both axially and transversely (35).

Effects of leg movements on the lumbar and sacral nerve-roots

Leg movements are able to affect the tension in the lumbar and sacral nerve-roots directly through stretching and slackening of the popliteal and sciatic nerves transmitted *via* the sacral plexus, but indirectly through the change in posture of the lumbar spine. Thus, when the knee is extended with the hip-joint flexed, the increase in hamstring tension leads to lumbar flexion and hence an increase in the length of the spinal canal. The spinal nerves and the sacral plexuses are under the greatest tension when the straight leg is raised as far as possible with the ankle dorsiflexed.[1] They are fully slackened when the ankle is plantarflexed, the knee is flexed and the hip-joint is flexed through an angle of 15–30° (Fig. 128).[2]

On raising the extended leg the roots are drawn distally into the intervertebral foramina (35, 53, 109). At the S_1 root, where the range of movement is greatest, it may approach 1 cm, decreasing cranially to zero at L_3. The movement begins within the first 15°, and as it nears completion the increasing tension is transmitted by the dura in the transverse plane to the contralateral root, which is drawn medially into the canal (Fig. 134).

Effects of movement of the cervical spine on the lumbar dura and nerve-roots

The characteristic stretching of the cord and the increase in tension in the spinal dura occurring in flexion of the cervical spine have already been described under the heading *Biomechanics of the pons–cord tissue tract*. When the cervical spine is extended from the neutral position and the canal is shortened there is progressive relaxation of the lumbar dura, the conus medullaris and the nerve-roots of the cauda

---

[1] An additional factor is the degree of rotation of the hip, for on medial rotation the sacral plexus is stretched as the distance between the lesser trochanter and the sciatic notch increases.
[2] It may be noted that in an acute attack of sciatic pain the patient tends to lie on his side with the affected limb uppermost and flexed, and with the lumbar spine flexed towards the side of the pain, thereby relaxing the spinal dura and nerve-roots.

equina (53); in flexion of the cervical spine the tension in these structures increases as the cervical canal is lengthened, and there is a small but definite reduction in the calibre of the dural theca and the conus medullaris. From full extension to full flexion the dura, root-sheaths and cord move cranially by about 3–4 mm in relation to a reference point on the caudal margin of a vertebral arch of the immobile thoracic spine, 6 cm cranial to the conus medullaris (53) (Figs. 27, 28, 94).

Variation of the lumbar canal lumen and the intervertebral foramina

When the lumbar spine is extended or when it is flexed laterally the annuli fibrosi bulge on the concave side of the spinal curve and encroach on the lumina of the canal and the intervertebral foramina. In extension the canal lumen is further decreased as a result of the slackening and folding of the dura and ligamenta flava.

Because of the relative movements of the adjacent vertebral arches the lumbar intervertebral foramen may undergo a marked variation in diameter. On extension the vertical height of the foramen may be reduced by one third (137, 176). The cross-sectional area of the foramen is also reduced by approximation of the superior articular facets of the subjacent vertebra to the inferior margin of the vertebral body and further reduced on ipsilateral flexion by posterolateral bulging of the annulus fibrosus. Thus, over the normal range of movement the space giving passage to the emergent lumbar root, with the dorsal root ganglion, the radicular artery and the grey ramus communicans, varies by a factor of at least two.

Pathodynamic effects of changes in lumbar posture

The pathological conditions that interfere with the normal mechanical behaviour of the spinal meninges and the nerve-roots during postural changes may be grouped according to whether they are caused by deforming lesions, compression, or tension due to adhesions.

Tension set up by deforming lesions

Any pathological structure encroaching on the lumbar canal or the intervertebral foramen will increase the tension in the tissues so deformed by an amount depending on the extent of their deformation. The first to be affected will be the vascular and fatty tissues in the epidural space, followed by the spinal dura. If the lumbar dura is slack the increase in tension will be purely local, but if it is already under tension because of a flexed spinal posture, the local increase in tension will be transmitted axially above and below the site of deformation and also in the transverse plane.

The spinal dura behaves as any other elastic tube under tension. It thus obeys Saint-Venant's law, according to which a tensile force applied in the longitudinal direction at a given point on the tube is distributed so that it becomes uniform around the circumference within an axial distance equal to three times the diameter (p. 43). The axial component of the tensile stress —that is, the tensile force per unit of area—thus diminishes with axial distance from the site of deformation. Accordingly, when the tension in the dura is ultimately transmitted around its whole circumference it is then uniform both cranially and caudally.

The axial tension in the lumbar dura is also transmitted to the nearby dural root-sheath, especially when the deforming force is lateral in direction. This is reflected in a cranialward retraction of the lumbar nerve-root into the spinal canal (the 'tissue-borrowing phenomenon' illustrated in Fig. 134). The transverse component of the increase in the tension in the lumbar dura is transmitted laterally on both sides and to both dural root-sheaths at the level of the affected segment. There is therefore a tendency for the two sheaths to be drawn medially. It should also be noted that when the axial tension is increased by flexing the spine the transverse component will also increase and its effects will be enhanced. Within the spinal canal and the root-pouch the deforming pathological process will probably deflect the nerve-root, with consequent angulation and increased stretching. This effect will be amplified if the root is pulled taut round the pedicle, and a bending tensile stress will be set up in it, the physical manifestations of which are illustrated in Figs. 135 and 136; these include a potential loss of conductivity in the nerve-fibres (184).

Compression

Because of the thrust it exerts on the tissue of a nerve-root, a deforming pathological structure initially produces a local increase in tension and more pronounced angulation. The interstitial pressure within the affected tissue is, however, not raised uniformly (Fig. 135). Only if the thrust is resisted by an unyielding structure, thus producing an equal and opposite force of reaction, can there be compression. The interstitial pressure is then uniform and it results in intense local axial tension, with consequent displacement of tissue elements. Compression of a lumbar or sacral nerve-root can be caused by, for example, a sequestred piece of disc lodging in the intervertebral foramen; it may also occur when the lumen is reduced by movements in the presence of arthritic spurs at of the apophyseal joints (92). Typically in the stenotic lumbar canal,[3] the cauda equina is compressed on extension (89, 159, 215, 258, 276).

Tension due to adhesions

One consequence of adhesions that has far-reaching clinical and biomechanical implications is the restriction of the normal range of movement of the lumbar dura and roots in relation to the vertebral column. A partic-

ular movement then produces a local increase in tension, the clinical manifestations of which are generally observed distal to the adhesion. The tethering effect may also restrict the mobility of the lumbar root within the subarachnoid space owing to arachnoidal proliferation—either within the space itself or in the dural root-sheath. Alternatively, the adhesions may be epidural, located within the spinal canal or the intervertebral foramen; they may then be due to disorders of the apophyseal joints, defects in the vertebral arches, or disc disease. They appear to form as a result of non-specific inflammatory reactions when nerve-roots and dural root-sheaths are subjected to pressure or excessive tension.

The prolapsed lumbar disc

An intervertebral disc herniated posteriorly or postero-laterally protrudes into the spinal canal and exerts local pressure on the anterior or anterolateral surface of the dura. The dura is then deformed and subjected to tension which has both axial and transverse components. Part of this tension is resisted by the fibres in the epidural space, which attach the dura to the periosteum on the anterior wall of the spinal canal, and to the posterior longitudinal ligament. The transverse component of tension stretches the dura at the site of the herniated disc and hence the dural root-sheath on each side. The fine fibres attaching the nerve-roots to the arachnoid membrane in the root pouch will also be stretched. The magnitude of this transverse tension in the root-sheaths and nerve-roots is dependent on the axial tension and the lengthening of the dura; the latter varies with posture. As soon as the cervical or lumbar spinal canal is lengthened, the axial component of the tension in the thoracic dura comes into play. Thus, the general increase in axial tension throughout the spinal dura resulting from flexion of the cervical spine is super-imposed on the local axial and transverse components of tension caused by the disc. Conversely, the tension in the dura set up on spinal flexion is itself increased by the herniated disc. The increase in tension in the dura augments the pressure exerted by the disc on the lumbar dura, and on any part of the individual dural root-sheath and nerve-root with which it is in contact. As it is stretched round the pedicle the deflected nerve-root is thus subjected to forces that result in a bending tensile stress, and in some cases to other forces. Some of the effects of the combined tensile forces acting in the nerve-root have been visualized radiographically (53) (Figs. 137–140).

It is commonly thought that the neurological symptoms produced by herniation and exacerbated by certain movements or postures are always due to com-

pression, but in fact this is seldom the case. Back pain elicited on bending the head forward (Hyndman's sign) is attributable simply to an increase in *tension* in the dura and root-sheaths and the resulting bending tensile stress in the root(s) at the site of the lesion(s). Similarly, the manoeuvre in the test for Lasègue's sign depends on the increase in tension in the dural root-sheath and nerve-root produced on stretching the sciatic nerve and sacral plexus. Again, the symptoms evoked on performing Fajerstajn's test (273), in which the sound leg is raised, are due to transmission of the tension generated by raising the extended leg, to the contralateral nerve-root at the site of the lesion.

For true compression to occur, the structure to which the deforming force is applied must be pressed against a firm surface. In the presence of a herniated disc the lengthening of the spinal canal on flexion results in a pathological increase in tension in the dura, widening of the subarachnoid space and a reduction in the calibre of the stretched nerve-root. Moreover, flexion tends to reduce the hernia, and this, together with the widening of the subarachnoid space, diminishes the likelihood of compression. When the spine is extended and the canal thus shortened the disc, the ligamenta flava and the dura tend to bulge into the canal, thus narrowing the epidural and subarachnoid spaces; the intervertebral foramina are also narrowed through the approximation of the articular processes (137, 176). True compression of the nerve-roots is therefore much more likely to occur in extension than in flexion. The risk of such compression from a disc is greatest within the intervertebral foramen on extension and flexion to the side of the endangered root. If a sequestrum of a pro-

[3] Jacobson, R. E., Gargano, F. P., Rosomoff, H. L.: Transverse axial tomography of the spine. Part 2: The stenotic spinal canal. J Neurosurg *42:* 412–419, 1975.

lapsed disc should be the firm surface against which the nerve-root is pressed on extension, the probability of compression increases with the distance caudally, it being greatest in the sacral canal. Compression by a disc in flexed postures is rare and is then usually due to other lesions (125).

Not infrequently a patient adopts a posture representing a compromise between the need to minimize tension in the dura and root, and the need to reduce the bulge of the prolapsed disc. There are some postures in which the nerve-roots would be relaxed but for the large hernia. It is not uncommon to see a patient with a flattened lumbar region flex the spine forwards to minimize the herniation and also ipsilaterally to relieve tension in the root. A typical instance is that in which a L$_5$ root is displaced laterally by a herniation medial to it (i.e. an 'axillary' herniation of the L$_4$/L$_5$ disc), which also tends to draw the root taut round the pedicle. In such cases, and any others in which the root is subjected to forces giving rise to bending tensile stress, the root is drawn upwards into the canal so that the tension distally in the spinal nerve is greatly elevated. The patient tends to adopt certain postures and to restrict leg movements so as to avoid further stretching of the nerve-root or sacral plexus. However, in some cases of central discal herniation, and also of lateral herniation when there is a spacious intervertebral foramen, the roots escape involvement and no bending tensile stress is set up. Sometimes the tension in the root produced by the hernia is balanced by the reduction in local tension in the dura due to advanced degeneration of the disc and a consequent decrease in the height of the intervertebral space.

The increase in tension in the dura due to the herniation of a lumbar disc might conceivably involve roots at the level of the suprajacent vertebra; but in any case this is not common, probably because of the operation of Saint-Venant's law (p. 43). The diminution of axial tension with distance from the point of traction on the dural tube where it is maximal, to the level at which it is distributed circumferentially is probably complete within the distance between intervertebral segments.

In contrast, a cranially produced increase in tension in the dura may exacerbate even a minor local pathological tension in a root located caudal to the source. For example, an extradural tumour situated at the anterior border of the foramen magnum will produce tension in the dura; if a herniated disc is already causing tension in a lumbar nerve-root, cervical flexion may then evoke symptoms that were not experienced before the tumour appeared (Case 1, p. 207). It is thus more likely that a tumour at a higher level or, for instance, a cervical spondylotic spur will trigger radicular symptoms from a prolapsed lumbar disc than that the lumbar disc will evoke symptoms at higher levels. In such cases the combined effect of tension in the dura and cord on the sacral roots may be indistinguishable from the effect of a large central discal herniation on the cauda equina (80).

A similar form of pathological tension can arise in cases of spondylolisthesis with advanced slip, when the sacral roots are sharply angulated as well as under tension. Common to all such conditions are paraesthesia and urinary dysfunction and leg pain and weakness brought on by walking and relieved by sitting down. The same tension in the nerve-roots is responsible for the more severe symptoms of pain (27), paresis, intermittent claudication (23, 276), incontinence (4, 90, 165, 227) and possibly impotence (27, 227). They may be relieved by neurosurgical relaxation.

Adhesions—a cause of tension in the lumbar dura and nerve-roots

Stretching of the soft tissues in the lumbar canal due to the thrust of a pathological structure is almost invariably reduced, if not eliminated, on shortening the canal by extending the spine or by flexing it towards the affected side. Acute discal herniation is, however, accompanied by non-specific inflammation and venous stasis; the pH is lowered (197) and there may be oedema of the dura and root-sheath. The epidural oedema, vasodilatation and consequent scarring may then anchor the dural root-sheath to the herniated disc (53). The sheath, which will already have been drawn up into the canal, is prevented from moving inferolaterally by the tension produced by the hernia; moreover, the transforaminal fascia (110) prevents any further cranial movement. The nerve-roots, too, are immobilized within the root pouches by the arachnoid fibres at the entry of the pouch. The conditions are now conducive to the deposition of fibrin in the affected tissues, and the development of a pathological state similar to cervical root-sleeve fibrosis (104). There are perineurial inflammation and degenerative changes of the nerve-roots, arachnoid proliferation and cyst formation (223, 224). The retraction of the nerve-root into the canal prior to the formation of adhesions increases the tension below the adhesion so that the root may become fixed and remain so even if the original cause of the tension has been eliminated. This leaves a permanent tension which cannot be relieved by any change of posture.

Root adhesions in the absence of manifest discal her-

niation are relatively common; they are a typical autopsy finding (224). Occasionally, the cause is apparent
from radiographs. The adhesions may have resulted
from a L$_4$ vertebral arch defect in a case of spondylo-
lysis or from hypertrophy of the apophyseal joints
in degenerative spondylolisthesis (203); but in many
cases the cause is suspected only after exploration of
the disc has proved negative (183). Adhesions are
frequently associated with stenosis of the spinal canal,
especially where there is narrowing of the lateral recess
(92), but in a proportion of cases they appear to have
their origin in comparatively minor changes in the
apophyseal joints.

Surgical relief

In the majority of cases of discal herniation which are
treated surgically, the removal of the herniated material
and the clearance of adhesions lead to relief of the
symptoms, and recovery. Evidence that all the adhesions have been broken and that tension has thus been
relieved is the return of pulsation and normal colour
of the dura, distention of the dural pouch by the CSF,
and mobility of the root in the foramen in response to
passive movements of the neck and legs. If removal
of disc prolapse and adhesions are not enough to
free the nerve-root it must be explored laterally, performing a partial facetectomy or foraminotomy to obtain
adequate exposure. This is more likely to be necessary

when disc degeneration has already narrowed the
foramina or if massive quantities of disc are removed.

The removal of the vertebral arch and the intervertebral joints may result in instability (252), and it may be
necessary to perform anterior interbody, lateral mass or
posterior fusion. To ensure a satisfactory result adequate time for osseous healing must be left before the
column is loaded. Weekly X-ray checks for the first
few weeks are essential to establish that osteosynthesis
has occurred in the correct extended posture.

In some techniques for lumbar interbody fusion the
vertebral bodies must be distracted so that substantial
bone grafts can be inserted (68). As with Cloward's
technique for cervical interbody fusion (66) there is a
risk that in maintaining disc hight, and thus the lumen of
the intervertebral foramina, the final position may be
overflexed and thus increasing lumbar dural tension
locally but in practice this seldom if ever occurs (100).

Nucleolysis by injection of chymopapain into degenerated discs has been tried with considerable success
in North America. Clinicians experienced in its use
found a marked loss in height of the disc space within
a few days of the injection. It is clear that, whatever the
fate of herniated disc material following nucleolysis,
this reduction must be accompanied by a corresponding relief of tension in the dura and roots. A major
relaxation of the lumbar and sacral roots has been
achieved by experimental resection of the whole L$_5$ vertebra (Fig. 38). This confirms that the greater the reduction in the intervertebral distance the greater is the
relaxation of the dura, root-sheaths and nerve-roots.

Closing remarks

Concerning the pathodynamics of the lumbar spine
there are two basic principles that have very wide implications. The first is that the tension produced by a
pathological process in the spinal dura is not only
local but is transmitted above and below the site of
origin. Any spinal movement that normally lengthens
the canal and stretches the soft tissues within it will
therefore exacerbate the manifestations of local tension. The second principle is that the effects of tension
in the lumbar region are not transmitted to higher
levels to the same extent as the effects of tension
in the cervical region are transmitted to lower
levels. Although tension originating in the lumbar
region may increase the stress throughout the dura, it
seldom produces a deleterious effect on the suprajacent
roots or on the cord. The pathological stress in the roots

and any consequent inflammatory reaction and loss of
conductivity are most likely to be manifested distally.

There is a wide variety of surgical techniques for
relieving tension in the dura and roots, all of which
depend on basic mechanical laws governing stress in
biological tissues. To this extent the surgical procedure
can be planned and the outcome predicted; however,
to relieve tension due to epidural and perineurial fibrosis is not so straightforward a matter, as a pre-operative
assessment of the local irritation or loss of function due
to adhesions and scarring may not be feasible. There is
therefore an obvious need for techniques to test the
mobility and extensibility of nervous and meningeal tissues by inducing movements of the spine and legs not
only at operation but at a neuroradiological examination.

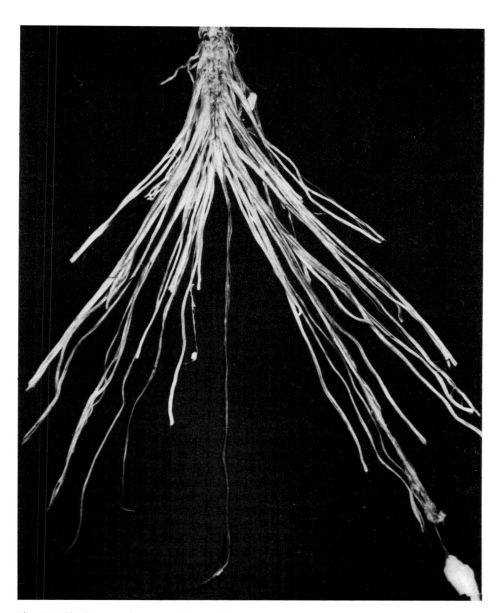

Fig. 120. The increase in amount of restraining tissue from the end of the sacral canal to the medullary cone.

The cauda equina and the filum terminale spread out to illustrate the cranial increase in the total amount of tissue available to transmit tension between the sacrum and the conus medullaris. Plaque-like calcification of the arachnoid membrane is seen at two sites—at bottom right and between the sensory and motor nerve-roots at the top of the figure.

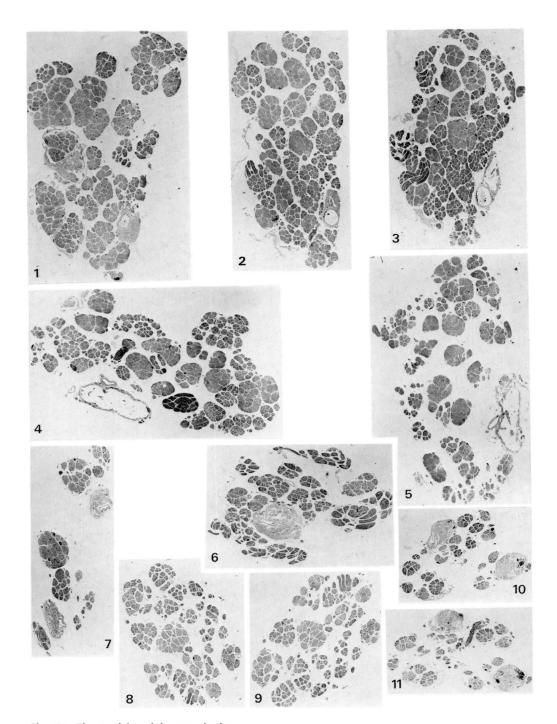

Fig. 121. The caudalward decrease in the number of nerve-roots composing the cauda equina, and the corresponding lowering of its resistance to stretching.

Serial transverse sections (nos. 1–11) through the nerve-roots of the cauda equina. Section no. 1 is located at the tip of the medullary cone, where the number of nerve-roots in the cauda equina is greatest.

Each successive section is taken at a level where the number of nerve-roots was diminished by one pair. (In theory, section no. 11 should therefore consist only of the filum terminale. However, the sections were not always precisely located at the required level.)

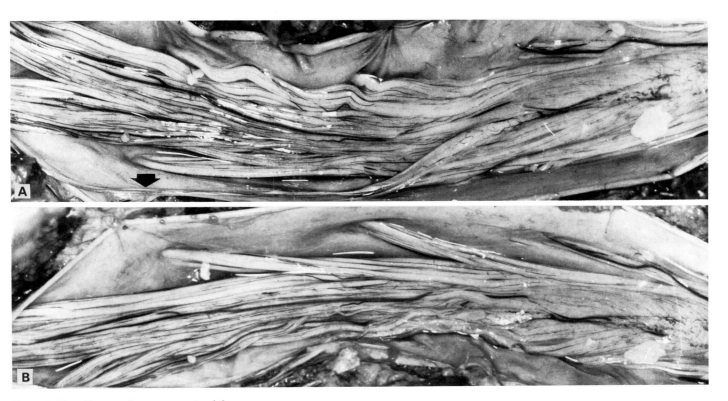

Fig. 122. The effect on the nerve-roots of the cauda equina of flexing the thoracolumbar spine to the left (A) and to the right (B).

(Cadaver in right lateral position.)

A. The medullary cone and the filum terminale have been drawn to the side in order to visualize them (*black arrow*).

B. The nerve-roots on the elongated side of the canal are stretched and those on the shortened side are slack.

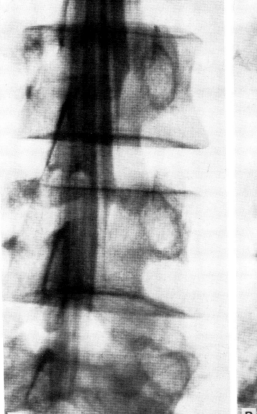
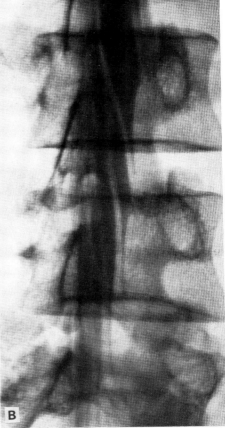

Fig. 123. Propagation of the tension (A) and slackening (B) of the pons–cord tract as far as the lumbosacral nerve-roots.

The nerve-roots form a smaller angle with the margins of the vertebral bodies in extension (B) of the cervical spine than in flexion (A), and are slackened and stretched, respectively. Water-soluble contrast medium injected into the lumbar subarachnoid space of a patient (53).

With kind permission of the Editor of Acta radiologica (Stockh.).

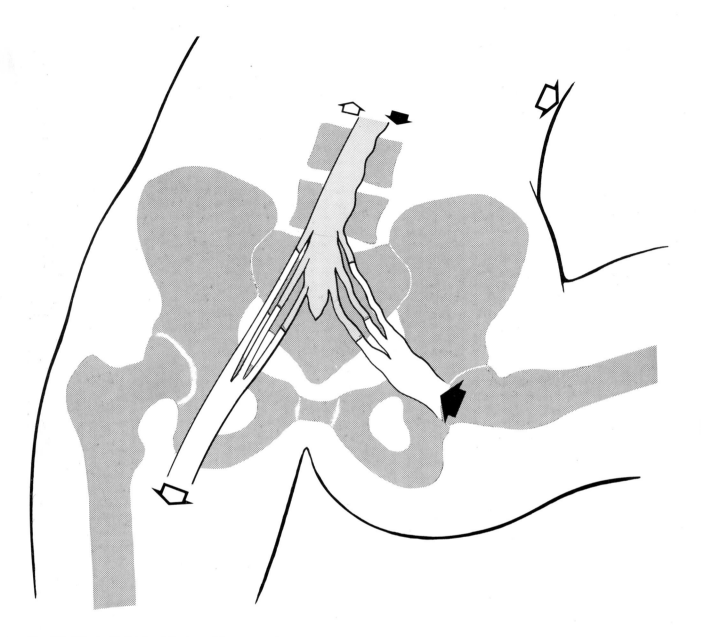

Fig. 124. Effect of left lateral flexion of the column on the sciatic nerve and the sacral plexus.

Shaded. The dura and root-sheaths.
Unshaded. The sacral plexus and the sciatic nerve.

Owing to the shortening of the lateral wall of the spinal canal on the side towards which the vertebral column is flexed, there is slackening of the lateral aspect of the dura together with the root-sheaths and the nerve-roots (not shown), and of the sciatic nerve together with the sacral plexus. The elongation of the opposite wall of the canal results in stretching of all the structures on this side (Figs. 122, 125).

Fig. 125. Effect of lateral flexion of the column on the spinal cord, nerve-roots, dentate ligaments, sacral plexus and sciatic nerve.

A. Sacral plexus and sciatic nerve in the pelvis with the body in the neutral position.

B. Effect of *flexion to the right* of the column on the sacral plexus and sciatic nerve.

C. Effect of *flexion to the left* of the column on the respective structures.

D. With the cadaver lying on its right side the middle of the column is flexed away from the table so that its left lateral aspect assumes an outward directed convexity; the resulting elongation of the left side of the spinal canal then stretches the dura along this surface, together with the nerve-roots and the dentate ligaments. The lumbar cord is thus raised to the middle of the canal and its left side is slightly convex.

So long as the thoracolumbar column is kept in this position the sacral plexus of the left side is stretched and resists attempts to

displace it with instruments inserted between the bone and the plexus (B), which has moved laterally towards the great sacrosciatic foramen (*white arrow* in B).

E, F. The trunk on its right side, the whole spine laterally flexed, to show the effects of stretch on the right side combined with the effects of gravity on the slackened structures on the left side of the canal. While the medullary cone (through the attachments of the lower dentate ligaments, the lower-most one of which follows an almost axial course—*black arrow* in F) is still held so close to the middle of the canal that it is out of contact with the right lateral aspect of the dura, the nerve-roots of the cauda equina sag so much that the ones situated farthest to the right rest on the dura.

The plexus tracts on the left side of the pelvis are now so slack that they can easily be displaced in any direction in the great sacro-sciatic foramen (C).

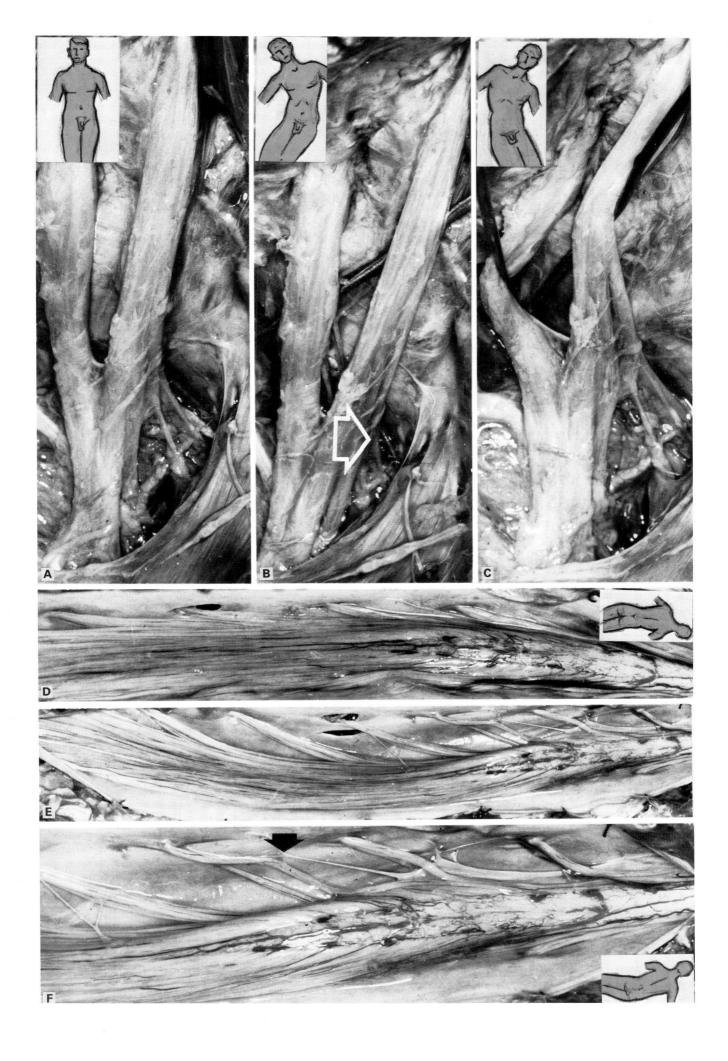

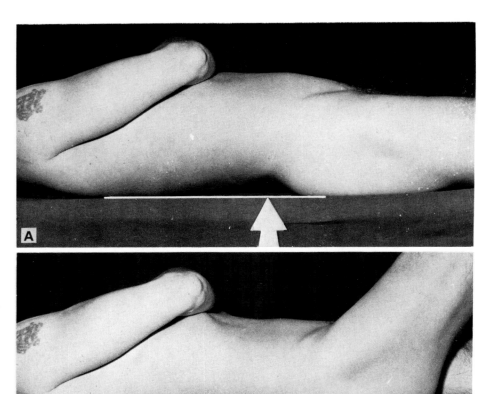

Fig. 126. Flattening of the lumbar spine produced by raising the extended leg.

A. With the patient placed on a firm table, the right leg is extended. The lumbar lordosis is clearly evident from the contour of the back.

B. When one extended leg is raised the lordosis of the lumbar spine is reduced, and flattening is visible.

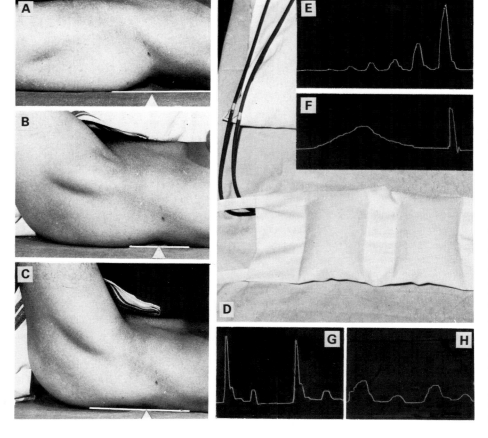

Fig. 127. Effect of change in leg position on the pressure between the lumbar spine and its supporting surface. Kymographic registration.

A. Subject supine.

B. Straight leg raising to 45°.

C. Straight leg raising to 80°, the lumbar spine now being flexed and flattened against the table.

D. Two rubber cuffs each connected by a tube to the recording unit of the kymograph. They are placed so that the cuffs are on either side of the spine, in contact with the erector spinae muscles.

E. Increase in pressure on the cuff with the extended leg raised 10, 20, 30, 70 and 90°

F. The shallow and steep curves (*left* and *right*) were obtained on raising the extended leg slowly and rapidly, respectively, through 90°. (Registration in another patient.)

G and H. Pressure tracings from the right and left sides, respectively, from a patient with unilateral sciatica due to discal herniation. The marked differences are due probably to increased muscle tension on the ipsilateral side.

From these observations it is evident that for clinical detection of an increased muscle tension it suffices to press lightly with one hand on the suspected side of the lumbar spine, while raising the extended leg carefully until pain is first elicited; the increased muscle tension will then be felt immediately.

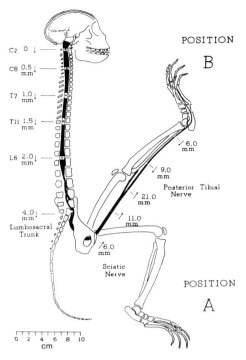

Fig. 128.

The displacement of reference points in the posterior tibial and sciatic nerves, lumbo-sacral trunk and spinal cord when the leg is extended and raised from position A to B. (The diagram was drawn from tracings of radiographs of *Macaca mulatta*.)

Courtesy of C. G. Smith, M.D., University of Toronto (238).

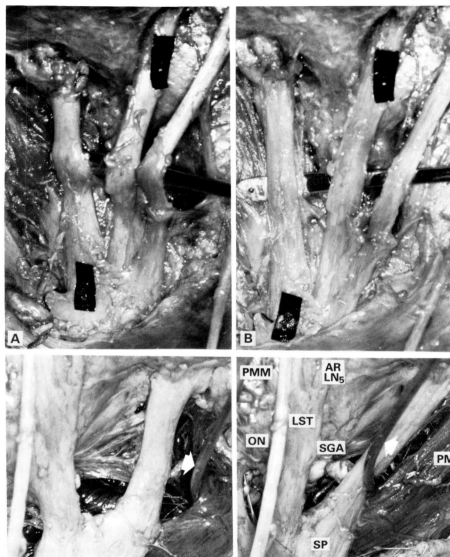

Fig. 129. Effects of extension and flexion of the column.

The stretching of the dura, the pons–cord tract, the nerve-roots (including the cauda equina) and the sacral plexus on flexion of the spinal column, and their slackening on extension, are transmitted on both right and left sides of these structures, whereas lateral flexion stretches them only on the convex and slackens them along the concave side (35).

A, B. Cadaveric specimens showing left sacral plexus.

A. When, with the whole vertebral column extended, both legs are flexed at the knee- and hip-joints, the sacral plexus is seen to be slackened so much that it can easily be raised with a dissector. The black paper marker then moves cranially from the left greater sciatic foramen.

B. On raising both extended legs, the tension in the sacral plexus becomes so great that the dissector is pulled back on to the bone; the black marker—stitched to the perineurium of the plexus—then moves toward the greater sciatic foramen.

C, D. Cadaveric specimen showing right sacral plexus and piriformis muscle.

Notation. PMM, psoas major muscle; *ARLN₅*; anterior ramus of the fifth lumbar nerve; *ON*, obturator nerve; *LST*, lumbosacral trunk; SGA, superior gluteal artery (76); *PM*, piri-formis muscle; *SP*, sacral plexus; *IGA*, inferior gluteal artery (76).

C. With the spine extended and hips and knees flexed (as in A), the pelvic muscles also slacken. The right piriformis muscle is easily displaced medially with a dissector (*white arrow*).

D. On raising the stretched leg the piriformis muscle—now under tension—moves laterally and resists displacement by the dissector (*white arrow*).

Biomechanics. As shown in Fig. 138, although neither stretching nor slackening of the dura has any *visible* active effect on the section of the root-sheath and the nerve-root located within the inter-vertebral canal, from the displacement of the sacral plexus at the exit of the intervertebral foramen it is evident that the stretching of the dura is in fact propagated to this point. Because of the firm attach-ments of the root-sheath to the periosteum within and at the exit of the intervertebral foramen, it can-not normally be displaced towards the pelvis. How-ever, so long as the sacral plexus is slack a dis-placement of the root-sheath into the spinal canal is possible (the 'tissue-borrowing phenomenon', Fig. 134). Owing to the propagation of the tension in the dura and the pons–cord tract to both sacral plexuses, on raising the extended legs, the fibres passing to the root-sheaths at the exit of the canals are stretched.

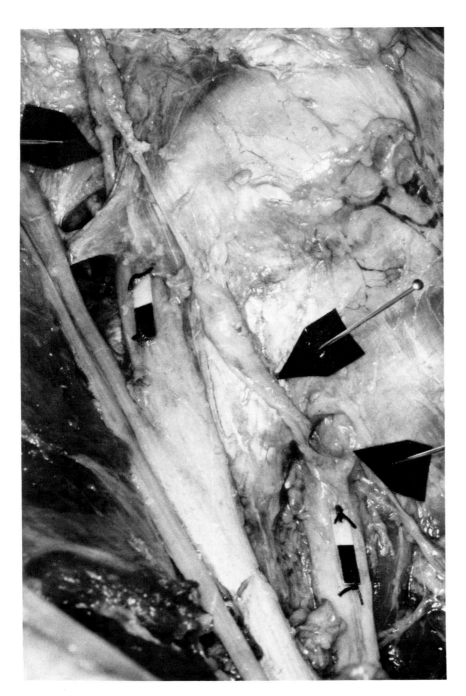

Fig. 130. Nerve-fibres and ganglia of the sympathetic plexus in relation to the uppermost nerves of the lumbosacral trunk.

Just below the uppermost black arrow, Golub and Silverman's ligament (110) is seen, dividing the outlet of the intervertebral foramen into two compartments; through the upper one a sympathetic nerve passes to the lumbosacral trunk (an artery that also ran through this compartment has been removed for clarity). Through the lower compartment passes a nerve belonging to the lumbosacral trunk.

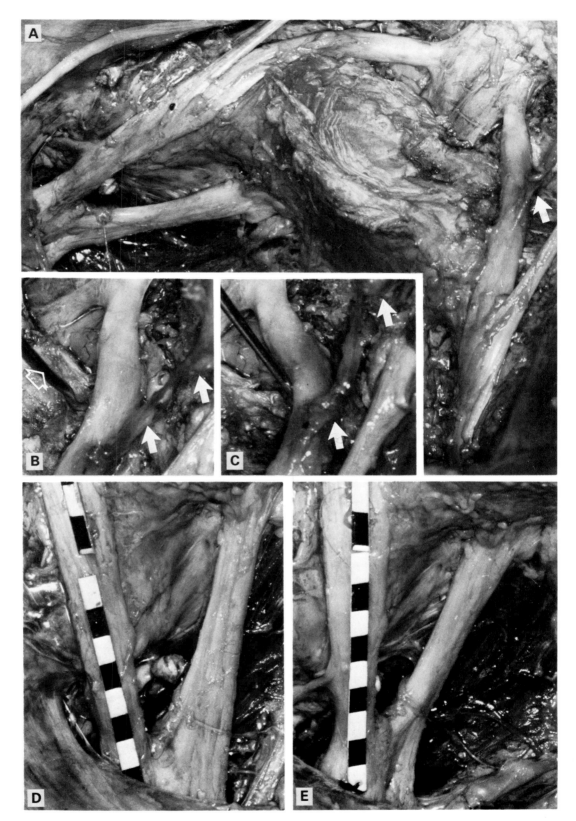

Fig. 131. The combined effect of flexion of the column and raising the extended legs, on the upper sacral portion of the sympathetic trunk and the L₄ and L₅ sympathetic ganglia, with other structures.

A. In front of the dura are the sacral surface of the cut L₅/S₁ disc and the backward sloping promontorium. (The L₅ vertebra has been removed.) The dura and the root-sheaths of the L₅ nerve-roots are under tension. *White arrow.* The stretched sympathetic nerve arising from the L₅ spinal nerve.

B. Position of legs and vertebral column as in A. On trying to displace the L₅ nerve-root laterally (*open arrow*) a definite resistance is encountered, and the sympathetic ganglionic chain is tautened. *White arrows.* L₄ and L₅ sympathetic ganglia.

C. Flexion of the legs at the knee- and hip-joints and extension of the spinal column result in slackening of the lumbosacral plexus, L₅ root-sheath and nerve-root, together with the sympathetic chain. All these structures can now be displaced laterally at will. *White arrows.* As in B.

D. On raising the stretched leg, the two paper markers (whose cranial and caudal ends have been sutured to the perineurium) move apart, indicating stretching of the plexus.

E. On flexion of the legs at the knee- and hip-joints the markers move together, indicating relaxation of the plexus.

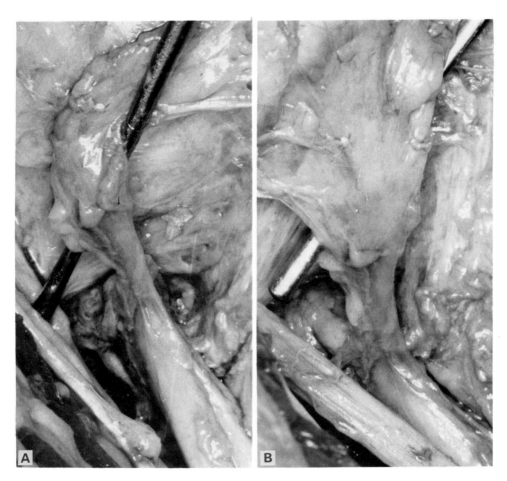

Fig. 132. Straightening and slackening of the ganglionic chain together with the L$_5$ sympathetic nerve in Lasègue's test.

A. When the legs are flexed at the knees and hip-joints, the ganglionic chain, together with the surrounding tissue, slackens and presents practically no resistance to displacement.

B. When the hip-joint is flexed with the legs straight, as on performing Lasègue's test, the sympathetic chain is stretched.

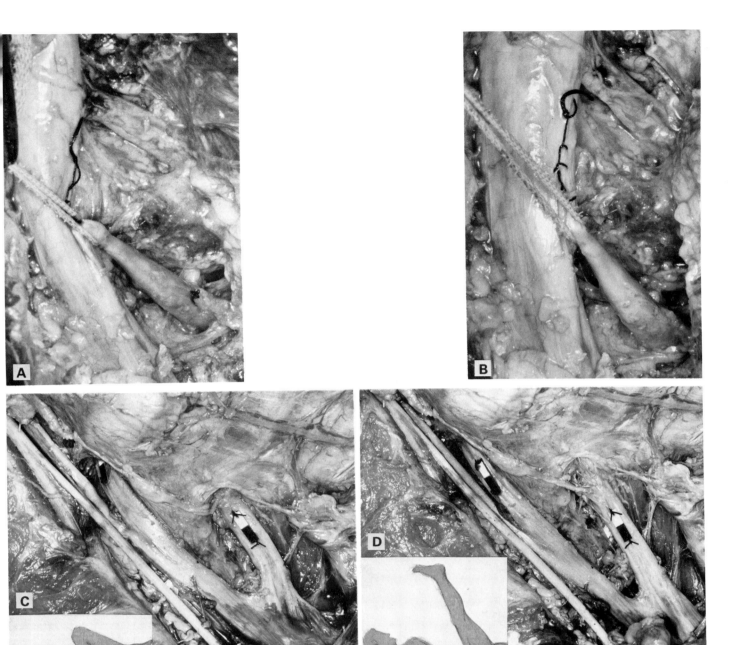

Fig. 133. The effect on the dura and the nerve-roots in the lumbar canal and on nerves of the lumbosacral trunk in the pelvis of (1) flexing the thigh and leg, and (2) straight leg raising as in performance of Lasègue's test (109, 258).

A, B. Dura and root-sheath at the intervertebral foramen. A gauze band round the root-sheath is pulling it cranially.

A. On flexion of the hip and knee with the spine extended there is relaxation of the dura, root-sheaths and nerve-roots and the nerves of the lumbosacral trunk. In its relaxed state the root-sheath (together with the anterior and posterior nerve-roots) is drawn further into the spinal canal by the cranially directed pull exerted by the gauze band. (The displacement is also evident from the fact that a black silk thread that had previously been concealed in the intervertebral foramen can now be seen.)

B. On straight leg raising with the spine flexed the root-sheath is drawn into the intervertebral foramen against the pull of the gauze band.

C, D. Sacral plexus and the exits of the spinal nerves from the intervertebral foramina. Paper markers are sutured to the perineurial sheaths.

C. Through the pull on the root-sheaths and nerve-roots, the nerves of the lumbosacral trunk have been drawn further into the intervertebral foramina, as the paper markers in this and the adjacent figure indicate.

D. Through the stretching of the great sciatic nerve produced on raising the extended leg, the nerves of the lumbosacral trunk are drawn further into the great sacrosciatic foramen, as is shown by the displacement of the paper markers.

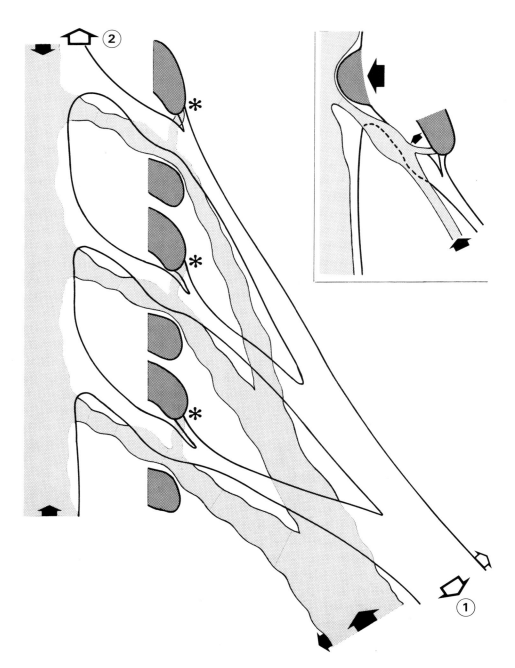

Fig. 134. Effect of the position of the leg on the sciatic nerve, sacral plexus, spinal ganglia, root-sheaths and dura.

Dark shading. Borders of intervertebral foramina. *Asterisks*. Ligamentous thickening of the transforaminal fascia between root-sheaths and bone at the exits of the foramina.

On raising the extended leg two mechanisms combine to produce stretching:

(1) The sciatic nerve is pulled towards the knee (238), resulting in stretching and caudalward movement of the root-sheaths and nerve-roots, the spinal ganglia with their suspensory apparatus and the sacral plexus.

(2) The column is flexed (35), the consequent elongation of the spinal canal further increasing the tension in the various structures.

Light shading. In flexion of the leg at the hip- and knee-joints the structures undergo relaxation, which is enhanced by extension of the lumbar spine.

Inset. The lumbar discal hernia 'borrows' relaxed tissue from the pelvis by drawing part of the dura, nerve-roots, and spinal ganglia further into the spinal canal and a small part of the plexus towards the intervertebral canal. This displacement only partly relieves the tension in the nerve-roots, and hence will not completely banish any neurological symptoms.

Fig. 135. The forces exerted on a nerve-root riding over a protrusion when the spine is flexed and by a clamping (pincer) action on the unloaded nerve-root.

P, pressure (geometrically determined); *T*, tension; σ_1, tension set up by transverse pressure; σ_2, tension set up by traction; ↔ direction of pressure (σ_1); ↔ direction of tension (σ_2); *white rectangles:* rigid surface supporting the nerve-root; *lower white rectangles:* firm bodies clamping a nerve-root.

A. In this system, representing a model of a nerve-root riding over a protrusion, there is a multi-directional state of tension. The main components are σ_1, acting perpendicular to the axis, and σ_2, acting axially. At each point the tension is determined by these two components and the angle α. σ_1 is a maximum at the surface of contact, and diminishes rapidly towards the diametrically opposite surface of the nerve-root, where it is zero; σ_2 increases towards this surface; σ_1 is practically negligible compared with σ_2.

B. In this system, representing a model of a clamping (pincer) action on a nerve-root, the bilateral compression sets up a uni-axial state of tension acting perpendicular to the axis. σ_2 is zero (53).

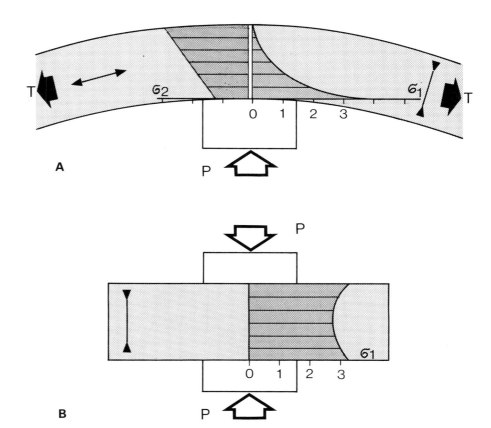

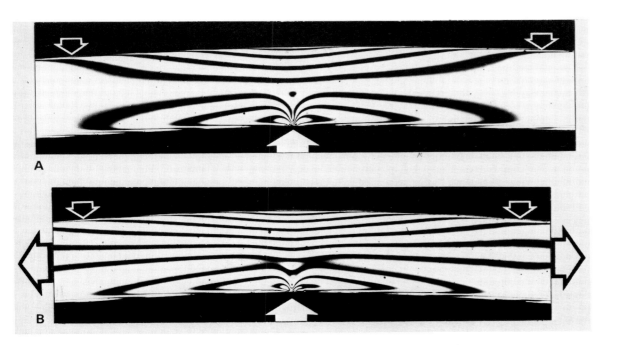

Fig. 136. Representation of the stress in a nerve-root that is stretched and simultaneously bent over an unyielding structure, as visualized in a photoelastic model.

An Araldite block was exposed to bending alone and to bending combined with stretching. The resulting stress field is indicated by the isochrome[1] pattern. The upper isochromes are due to tensile stress and the lower ones to unilateral pressure.

A. The block is bent over a support (*white arrow*) by application of downward forces (*black arrows*). The maximum tensile stress occurs along the upper edge (value 4.3).

B. The block is at the same time subjected to axial tension (*white, open arrows*). The tensile stress in the upper zone is then increased because the stress components due to the axial and bending tension are additive (value 6.5).

The model at the same time illustrates the production of a transverse bending tensile stress in a cross-section of the nerve-root or spinal cord when, on flexion of the spine, these structures are pressed against, and stretched over, an osteophyte or an internal firm lesion. This tension in the *cord* is accentuated by the lateral attachments of the dentate ligaments.

[1] *Isochrome.* A line joining points of equal stress.

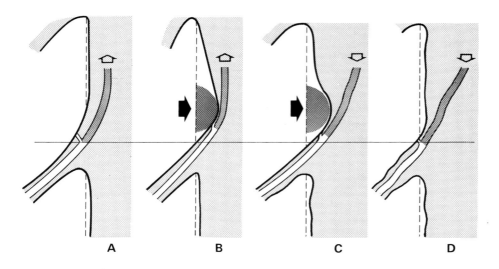

A   B   C   D

Fig. 137. Effect of the presence of a herniated disc on the tension in the dura and a nerve-root during changes in spinal posture.

A, D. The normal biomechanical events. B, C. Pathological events in the presence of a herniated lumbar disc.

A, B. Cervical spine flexed. C, D. Cervical spine extended.

White arrows. A, B. Direction of axial tension induced by flexion of the cervical spine. C, D. Direction of relaxation induced by extension of the cervical spine.

Black arrows. Direction of pressure resulting in increased axial tension from herniated disc.

A. The dura, root-sleeve and nerve-root are under normal tension.

B. Since the nerve-root is attached to the arachnoid membrane by gossamer fibres, it is drawn out to the same extent as the dura and membrane. The extent to which the root is stretched is indicated by the white segment above the reference line.

C. The dura, root-sleeve and nerve-root are slightly slackened but the protrusion of the herniated disc still sets up tension in the nerve-root.

D. The dura, root-sleeve and nerve-root are now greatly slackened.

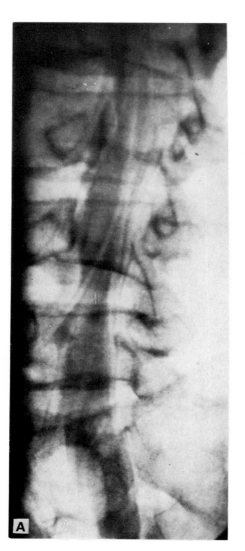

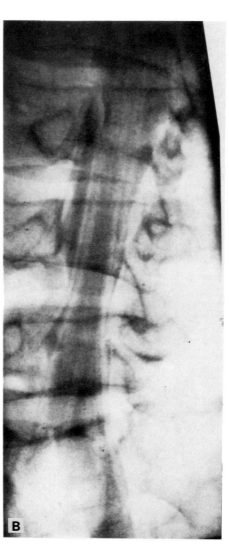

Fig. 138. Effect of a herniated disc on a nerve-root at the L_4/L_5 level shown during myelography in a patient (water-soluble contrast medium).

A. On extension of the cervical spine the involved lumbar nerve-root slackens and its upper portion loses contact with the disc.

B. On *flexion* the nerve-root is pressed against, and stretched over, the disc (53).

With kind permission of the Editor of Acta radiologica (Stockh.).

Fig. 139. Deformation of the dura and nerve-roots caused by a herniated disc shown during myelography in a patient (water-soluble contrast medium).

A. Since, in extension of the cervical spine, the dura together with the pons–cord tract is slack throughout its length, the dura is deflected by the pressure of the herniated disc at the L₅/S₁ level—visualized as a deep impression in the subarachnoid space.

B. Because, in flexion, the dura is stretched over the herniated disc its deflection is shallower and the nerve-root follows a straighter course (53).

With kind permission of the Editor of Acta radiologica (Stockh.).

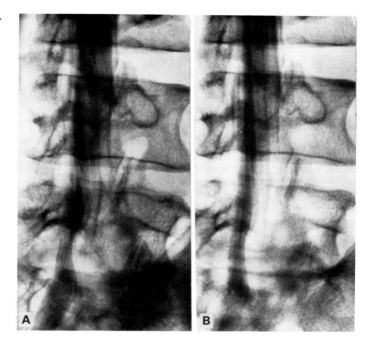

Fig. 140. Effect of lateral flexion of the spinal column on the lumbar spine, dura, nerve-roots and dentate ligaments.

A. Along the convex aspect of the lumbar spinal canal the pedicles move apart slightly and the dura is therefore stretched along the elongated side of the canal. The root-sheaths, also stretched, bear against the pedicles within the foramina. Because of the tension in their extraforaminal portion, however, this is pulled slightly towards the axis of curvature, which, for rightward flexion, is located on the right of the column. The nerve-roots are pulled even further towards the axis of curvature. The sacral nerves show only a very small tendency to straighten. Owing to approximation of the pedicles on the right side of the body, there is slackening of the dura, nerve-roots and dentate ligaments along the shortened side of the canal.

B. Herniated lumbar disc located on the inferomedial border of the right L₅ root-sheath (*arrow* points to outer, upper border). On flexing the trunk to the right both root-sheath and nerve-root slacken. If no part of the disc is located anterior to the root, neither stooping nor raising the extended leg will evoke neurological symptoms. If the trunk is flexed to the left, however, the involved root-sheath and nerve-root will be stretched over the disc and symptoms may be evoked.

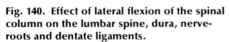
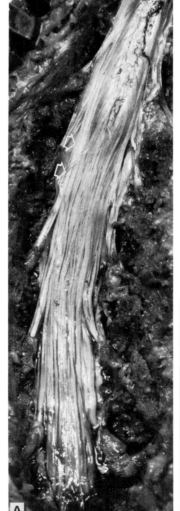
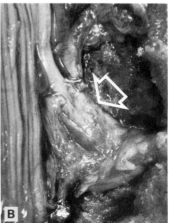

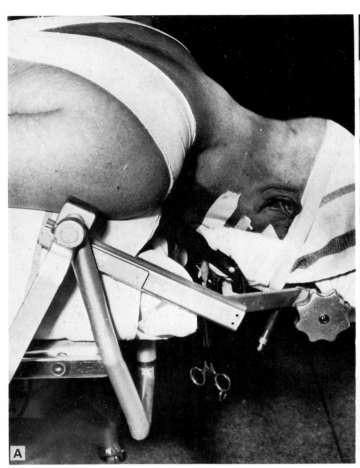

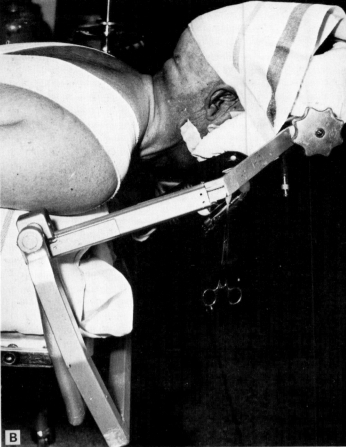

Fig. 141. Self-adjusting head support[1] for controlled spinal cord relaxation.

Attached to the operating table, the support can be adjusted by means of a crank. Its length is automatically adapted to that of the cervical spine. The photographs show the anaesthetized patient with the cervical spine (A) flexed and (B) extended.

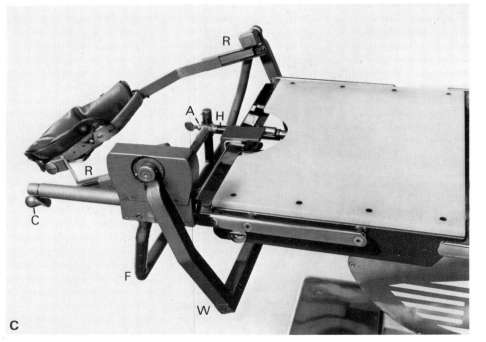

C. Construction of the head support.[2] *F*, Main transverse member; *C*, crank for vertical adjustment; *R*, ball-bearing track. On the right side, the entire length of the track is exposed, the head-frame having glided forwards and downwards under its own weight. *A*, Guide (with clamp) for vertical adjustment of the head support; *H*, guide for horizontal adjustment; *W*, counterbalance.

[1] Made by AB Stille-Werner, Stockholm, to author's design.
[2] Courtesy of Mr Arne Uggeldahl, Civ. Eng., Stockholm.

Fig. 142.

A. Deformation of the dura and cord in the anaesthetized patient during postural changes of the cervical spine.

a. Dura exposed after bilateral laminectomy at the C₄–C₇ levels. On *flexion* of the cervical spine the dura has stretched and its cross-sectional area diminished. A paper marker, attached to the dura by a suture at the cranial level, has moved in the cranial direction in relation to the reference point (*asterisk*).

b. On *extension* the marker has moved caudally, and the slackened dura is now clearly distended by the CSF pressure.[1] This distention ceased when the inelastic fibres of its transverse layer had been fully drawn out.

c. Dura opened and spine *extended*. The marker (still anchored to the cranial wall of the dura), now on the shortened cervical cord, has approached the silver clip. To visualize any slackening of the right dentate ligament a black silk thread has been wound round an attachment and loaded by a small weight hanging outside the neck. Since the cord is now slack the ligament can be drawn to the side.

d. On *flexion* the dura, dentate ligaments, cord and nerve-roots have been pulled taut, the black thread with the attached weight then being drawn medially. (The structural details are somewhat obscured by the arachnoid membrane, which was preserved during demonstration of the displacement of the marker.)

[1] The margins of a sagittal incision in the dura that are brought into close contact in the flexed position of the cervical spine, separate on extension to form an oval cavity (*cf.* the similar result of an incision in the cord on extension, Figs. 90 and 142 B).

B. Schematic representation of (1) the pathological axial and transverse tension in the dura and cord set up by a congenital gibbus of the cervical spine; and (2) the pathological pressure exerted on the cord by an epidural CSF-cyst following a decompressing operation during which a sagittal rift in the dura and arachnoid was inadvertently produced, with ensuing leakage of fluid.[2]

a. *Cervical spine flexed.* Pathologically increased axial and transverse tension in the dura and cord (cross- and sagittal sections).

b–e. *Cervical spine slightly extended* (in d and e the extended posture is secured permanently by a cervicolordodesis brake). The *axial* tension in the dura, cord and nerve-roots at the level of the gibbus has been practically eliminated, but the *transverse* tension has been only slightly diminished.

b. (*cylinder*). Shape and level of the accidental incision in the dura and arachnoid (indicated in the diagram by connecting lines - · - · -).

c. (*cross-section*). Pressure of the stretched dura exerted on the cord from behind.

d. (*frontal aspect*). Shaded band with large arrows. Zone within which the dura exerts pressure on the cord. The stress due to the CSF pressure and the widening of the dura as it shortens in extension have caused the

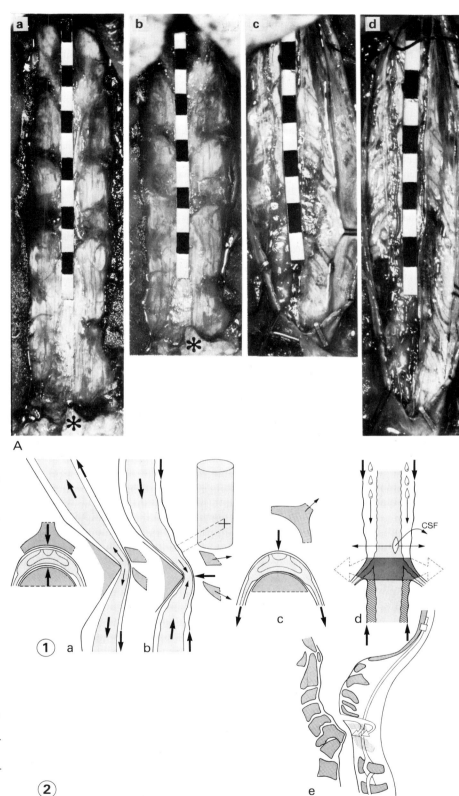

A

B

suture to rupture and a gap to open up in the dura (*small horizontal arrows*), through which cerebrospinal fluid has leaked into the epidural space (*curved arrow*). Below the site of transverse clamping of the cord by the dura due to the gibbus the CSF is trapped in the subarachnoid space (*hatching*).

e. (*bifurcated arrows*). Gap in the dura through which CSF has escaped to produce an epidural cyst. This has pressed on the dura and cord at the level of their maximum constriction.

[2] Case report see p. 192.

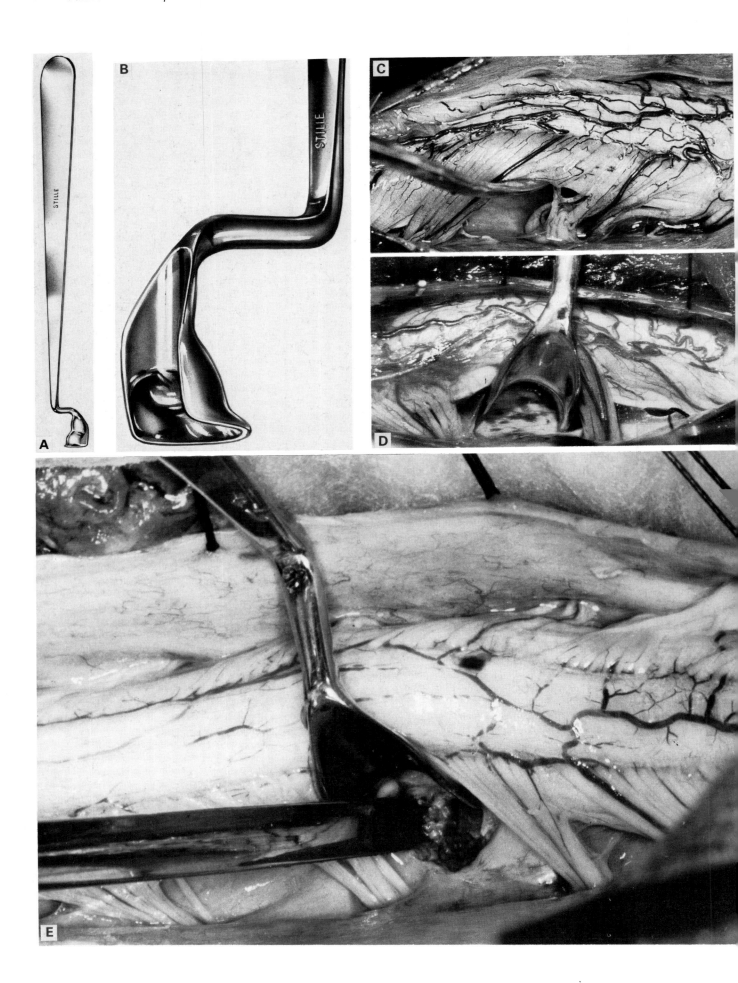

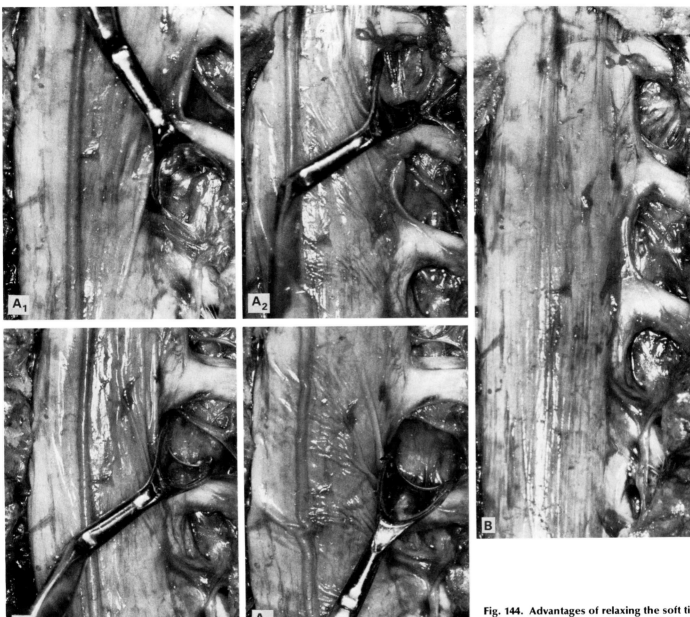

Fig. 143. Spatula for protecting the cord, with examples of its application in the cervical spinal canal.

A. The spatula; half scale.[1]

B. Lower end of the spatula.

C. Slack cord raised during the operation by a dissector for inspection of the anterior wall of the cervical canal before inserting the spatula.

D. The protecting spatula placed in front of the cord, which rides slack over it and thus reduces risk of damage during an operation. The nerve-roots are drawn out taut but not over-stretched.

E. Chiselling of an osteophyte (cadaver).

[1] Manufactured originally by Stille-Werner, Co., Ltd., Stockholm, to author's design. Production and distribution transferred to Aesculap-Werke, Tuttlingen, West Germany.

Fig. 144. Advantages of relaxing the soft tissues and using the protecting spatula in operations in the cervical spinal canal.

A. 1–4. With the cervical spine *extended,* the slackened tissues can be safely displaced with the protecting spatula. In the cadaver the reduced volume of cerebrospinal fluid and absence of bleeding facilitate exposure of the anterior aspect of the canal. In the living subject haemostasis is also rendered easier within the exposed area. Discal and osteophytic protrusions and discal herniations are then readily accessible from both the cranial and the caudal dural root-sheath angle. Not only is any extra- or intradural operation (on a disc, osteophyte, tumour, etc.) greatly facilitated, but the risk of damage to cord and nerve-roots is minimized.

B. On *flexion* of the cervical spine the dura and root-sheaths have been drawn taut and the nerve-roots resumed their caudalward course.

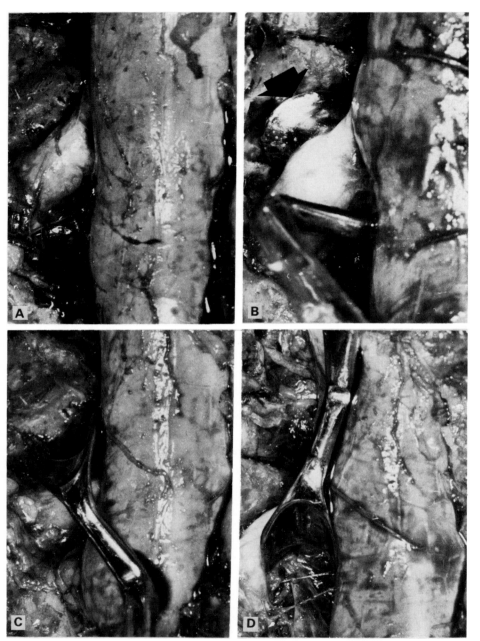

Fig. 145. The use of the protecting spatula in the lumbar canal with the neck extended to produce maximum relaxation of dura and roots —a measure for reducing the risk of injury to the nerve-roots.

A. Slackened lumbar dura and L_5 root-sheath.

B. The vault of the protecting spatula has been inserted under the sheath. The extent of the relaxation of the nerve-root is shown by the fact that the spatula could be pushed so far cranially that its edge is visible under the upper dural root-sheath junction (*black arrow*).

C, D. Spatula inserted at the upper and lower angles of the junction, respectively. The dura and nerve-roots in the lumbar region, too, can be displaced without risk of damage to the nerve-root tissue. In this region there is not infrequently pronounced discal herniation, through which the nerve-roots are subjected to both unilateral pressure and stretching. On instrumental deflection of the nerve-roots without previously induced slackening, this tension is invariably increased, possibly with harmful consequences.

Histodynamic factors in multiple sclerosis

At the New York Neurological Society in 1927 Lhermitte and Wechsler described the electrical discharge-like sensations in multiple sclerosis evoked on flexion of the cervical column. Lhermitte attributed them to lashing of demyelinized lengths of the cord against the bone of the spinal canal (177), a hypothetical phenomenon that is often referred to as 'concussion' of the spinal cord. At the Congrès Neurologique International de Berne held in 1931 Lhermitte referred to Borst's and Benda's supposition that the neurological symptoms were due to violent distortion and partial tearing of the axis of the medulla. This view, unconfirmed at that time by objective findings, was a good deal more consistent with the observed events. More recently it has been suggested that Lhermitte's sign might in some way be due to downward pulling of the cord (222). Postmortem histological examination of spinal cords of patients that, on bending the head forwards, had felt tingling sensations radiating down the back disclosed deformation of the blood-vessels with hyalinization, organized thrombi and partial or complete occlusion, leading to myelomalacia, gliosis and local shrinkage. As is clearly illustrated by one patient in particular (no. 4) (248), where multiple sclerosis had been diagnosed and where numerous small tortuous arteries extended from the C_4 to T_1, the neurological symptoms can be due to a wide variety of pathological alterations of the spinal cord (173, 235, 248).

More than a decade ago the author observed on the cadaver of a multiple sclerosis patient that flexion of the vertebral column produced a *pathological* increase in tension in the spinal cord (35). Since no case series was available for a close study of this phenomenon an attempt was made to produce the intramedullary scars experimentally so as to be able to examine their histodynamic effect. From observations confirming the presence of tension it was concluded that alleviation of the neurological symptoms might be obtained by relaxing the pons–cord tissue tract. These findings suggested a plausible explanation of the excessive tension in the cord tissue (Fig. 80).

It has been found that excitation and deficit symptoms in the multiple sclerosis patient may be accentuated on flexing the vertebral column so that the canal is elongated and the cord consequently stretched. This the author tentatively ascribed to pressure of the sclerotic changes in the spinal cord tissue on the neighbouring pathways, so that on flexion of the spine the nerve-fibres are over-stretched; the correctness of this view was confirmed in further biological experiments on the cadaveric spinal cord *in situ* (see Fig. 88). This opened up a new approach to the treatment of the symptoms, namely to render the cord slack by cervicolordodesis,

thus eliminating the pathologically high tension in the nervous tissue due to the oedematous or sclerotic foci.

When applied in a number of patients in the irreversible late stage of multiple sclerosis, surgical relaxation of the spinal cord has led in some cases to a rapid relief of symptoms (Cases 1–3, pp. 228–31). This improvement was probably due in some measure to the fact that the sclerotic foci no longer exerted a significant thrust on the slackened nerve fibres (Table 4; Figs. 80 and 88). If this beneficial effect can be confirmed, the cervicolordodesis operation in the late stage of the disease is clearly indicated.

What of the early stage, however? Since ACTH therapy frequently gives some alleviation of symptoms it might be held that surgical intervention is superfluous. The effect of relaxation in the early stage might be due to relief of pressure on, and hence tension in, the blood-vessels, the consequent widening of their lumen (Fig. 25) then leading to improved oxygenation of the nervous tissue, dispersal of oedema and harmful metabolites with consequent reduction of phagocytosis and myelin fragmentation. Since the relaxation of the tissue is permanent, so might be the improvement in the conditions so obtained. This would represent a clear advantage over the result obtainable with ACTH therapy. Moreover, spinal cord relaxation probably does not interfere with the patient's hormone and mineral balances. It is also conceivable that immobilization of the spinal cord promotes 'healing' of the multiple sclerosis lesions. (A superficial analogy is the effect of pneumothorax treatment—in which a lung is immobilized—on the healing of the tubercular lesions.) It would thus seem motivated to examine more closely the value of spinal cord relaxation also in the early stage of the disease, at least in patients with severe medullary symptoms. If the results should prove at least as good as in the late stage, it would be time to consider at what point there is no longer risk of relapse, so that the cervicolordodesis brake could be removed without disadvantage to the patient.

In a glimpse into the future of neurological surgery in 1949 Ernest Sachs expressed the opinion that "even some degenerative diseases of the nervous system, such as multiple sclerosis and the muscular dystrophies, may respond to surgical measures" (230). Today this goal seems to be nearer to realization. For, by applying spinal cord relaxation it is possible to alleviate not only the neurological symptoms produced by exogenous forces on the pons–cord tract, but also those evoked by intrinsic alterations of the cord tissue resulting from inflammation and reactive scar formation.

Histodynamic aspects of compressive spinal cord injury[1]

The suppression of biological and histochemical reactions following traumatic damage to the spinal cord is an interesting recent development of an idea first broached as long ago as 1914 (6). In experimental spinal cord trauma in the cat an increase in the amount of noradrenalin in the grey matter has been found at the level of impact (211). This discovery has aroused considerable interest following, as it does, the limited success of clinical attempts to utilize dehydrating hypertonic infusions, corticosteroids and local cooling of the damaged part of the cord (5, 26, 202). It was considered that if the production of noradrenalin is not arrested by a chemical antidote it might lead, some hours after the trauma, to further necrosis of the central spinal grey matter and paraplegia (212). It should be noted, however, that in both man and laboratory animals paraplegia and other severe functional disorders often occur suddenly at the very moment of trauma. This underlines the prime significance of mechanical trauma (241–4) vis-à-vis the secondary biological and biochemical reactions (145), and hence the importance of recognizing the hitherto neglected effects of compression, namely, momentary tearing of nerve-fibres and blood-vessels in the cord tissue. Logically, priority must then be accorded to surgical measures that may reduce the neurological effects of the lesion.

Some 20 years ago it was observed (60) that when an axis-cylinder is constricted circumferentially the incompressible cytoplasm is displaced towards the free ends of the cylinder. The greater the amount of plasma that collects here the more the plasma membrane protrudes. The nerve-cells in the spinal cord tissue behave in the same manner. The view that the brain and cord tissue is compacted on traumatic compression is thus incorrect (138).[2] Because nerve-cells cannot be compacted, an increase in the compressive force on spinal cord tissue will increase the axial tensile stress acting within the tissue; this will ultimately lead to tearing of axons and blood vessels (48)—a typical effect of any spinal cord trauma resulting from compression.

The mechanical events underlying spinal cord damage can be outlined in the following way. When an incompressible body is subjected to a pincer or clamping force a local tensile stress is set up; this will be greatest in a direction perpendicular to a plane through the points of contact of the pincer surfaces, and if it is great enough transverse fissuring of the body will result. In a comparison between the effects of a pincer action on a model elastic body (Fig. 77) and on the compressed cord

as observed in microscopic sections a close agreement was observed.

A brief diversion: Besides having the properties of a liquid and a cohesive gel, cytoplasm is elastic. When, on compression of an axis-cylinder, a certain volume of cytoplasm is displaced, its elasticity is increasingly drawn upon until it ultimately ruptures, together with its membrane. If such a rupture could be arrested just after it has occurred it would, of course, be possible to see only the above-mentioned transverse fissuring of the axon tissue, but this is probably never the case.

When after a compressive cord injury the spine is flexed and tension thus set up in the ruptured cord tissue, both the axoplasm and the small blood-vessels are displaced further in the cranial and caudal directions. This effect is amplified by retraction of the elastic elements, the ends of the torn axis-cylinders curling up into 'retraction balls' (Fig. 62). On close examination of greatly enlarged microangiograms (Fig. 59) it is seen that small torn capillaries belonging to the vertical lateral branches of the central arteries also coil in this way, though more loosely. This is probably a mechanism for arresting bleeding. (Under normal conditions the medial main trunks of the central arteries run largely transversely in the anteroposterior direction, but after rupture of the tissue and its consequent retraction they are deflected cranially and caudally; they thus approach the anterior aspect of the pia (Fig. 58). With this divergence of the central arteries their vertically coursing lateral branches are stretched in the axial direction, and they eventually rupture.

After infusion of radiopaque contrast medium into the spinal cord vessels in the cadaver there is no leakage from the torn arterioles so long as the cord is being compressed (this is probably also the case in the injured cord of a patient); only after the compressing dowel has been removed can the contrast medium leak out into the tissues, and then only provided that the infusion is continued (Fig. 65). If a perfusion pressure is maintained for a long time, pooling of medium in the lesion will increase.

Soon after a lesion has been inflicted in the spinal cord tissue of a living subject various reparative pro-

---

[1] High speed angular acceleration (and ensuing recoil) as a source of traumatic lesions of brain and spinal cord is disregarded in the present connection (114, 173, 195, 235, 257, 263).

[2] It is only blood-vessels that can collapse when all the blood has been displaced from the compressed zone.

cesses are initiated (65), which tend to localize the effects of the injury. After compression of the cerebral arterioles in the rabbit, release of catecholamine from adrenergic fibres in the vessel walls has been observed (214). If this is an essential feature of haemostasis (8, 145) it would seem that the effect of noradrenalin in spinal cord injury is not necessarily a detrimental one.

It has recently been established by the author that the surfaces of a traumatic rupture in the spinal cord tissue separate when the cervical spine is flexed (Fig. 67). At the present stage of our knowledge it is therefore important in such cases to immobilize the cord. To decide the best way of achieving this in the individual case is an urgent task for the surgeon.

Signs of excessive tension in the pons–cord tract; countermeasures

Histodynamic effects on nuclei and tracts at the cerebrospinal level

Respiratory failure due to tension in the medulla oblongata

Axial tension set up in the pons–cord tissue tract by firm extramedullary pathological structures or unyielding intramedullary lesions may be transmitted to the expiratory and inspiratory centres in the medulla oblongata. The responsible alterations include protruding tumours (Case 1, p. 207), myelopathic tissue lesions (p. 222), gliotic foci of multiple sclerosis (Case 1, p. 228) and traumatic tearing of medullary tissue (Cases 3–6, pp. 234–41). The compound histodynamic tension can obviously be great enough to deform the nerve-cells (including their supplying blood-vessels) in these centres by over-stretching, and thus to impair their function.[1] This is illustrated by the case reported by Maxwell & Kahn, where a thoracic kyphosis was the cause (187).

When skull traction is performed after a fresh spinal cord injury the excessive tension produced by the combination of oedema and traction (p. 55) is readily transmitted to the respiratory centres. The sequelae are familiar and well documented (17). Witness, for example, the 12 deaths among 70 injured patients due to respiratory failure soon after cervical spinal cord compression (129). The potentially deleterious result of intramedullary tension is exemplified by the following case. Twenty-four hours after compressive spinal cord injury, myelography disclosed eccentric swelling (enlargement of the medial and right paramidline portions) of the cord at the C_{3-4} levels. During skull traction diaphragmatic paralysis developed, and the patient, 64, died 4 days after the injury due to respiratory insufficiency (228). Local post-traumatic swelling of the cord was visualized by myelography in most of the patients in this series. Because the respiratory centres are obviously at risk in both acute (17) and chronic lesions of the cervical spinal cord, as well as in adverse situations where excessive tension is transmitted to the reticular substance of the medulla oblongata from pathological structures in other sections of the spine or the pons–cord tract, it is advisable to perform routine checks of respiration (17), pulmonary capacity, and P_{O_2}

and P_{CO_2} tension both on admission and at intervals thereafter.

Confusional state evoked by tension in cranial sections of the pons–cord tract

Five of the 6 patients with cervical spinal cord injury referred to suffered from confusion and delirium for between one day and a week. This condition is usually ascribed to the brain centres being deprived of informative sensory impulses; its ultimate cause might, however, be tension in cranial sections of the pons–cord tract, set up by a remote impinging extramedullary structure or by an unyielding intramedullary lesion in that section (see Case Reports, pp. 189, 233–40).

Tension set up in the various cord structures by osteophytes

Osteophytes frequently occur not only at points along the posteromedial margin of the vertebral body, but also in the region of the uncovertebral joints. There is thus a variety of sites at which pressure may be exerted on the dura and spinal cord, and so produce bending tensile stress in the nervous tissue. Thus, the tension set up in nerve-fibres, blood-vessels and supporting tissues will vary with the location of the responsible osteophyte(s). This explains why the uniform tension due to over-stretching of the pons–cord tissue tract can produce a variety of neurological symptoms. A greater prominence of symptoms on one side than the other may

---

[1] When the medulla oblongata is compressed by a cerebellar pressure cone the resulting axial tension in its tissue, which immediately produces dysfunction and respiratory failure, is usually so great that transverse fissures may occur, with resulting haemorrhage there and in the cerebellar tonsils (235); haemorrhage in the mid-brain or the pons in the case of uncal herniation has the same cause (152, 235) (*Frontispiece*).

indicate the site of the responsible structure in the spinal canal; confirmation may often be obtained by air myelography or at operation.

Predicting the biomechanical effects of surgical intervention

In planning surgical measures for the treatment of pathological lesions involving the pons and spinal cord it is important to understand their biomechanical background. In the case of a circumscribed pathological lesion (or several such lesions) that can be treated by a direct procedure it is a comparatively simple matter to analyse its (their) pre-operative biomechanical effects and to predict the biomechanical conditions resulting from an operation on the spine, dura, pons and spinal cord and the nerve-roots, and the biomechanical conditions that will obtain during and after healing.

As has been pointed out earlier by workers in this field, among the anatomical conditions that render the mechanical effects of space-occupying lesions almost unpredictable and that complicate the surgical approach (especially in the cervical region) are the mobility of the cervical spine and the constraining effect of the root-sheaths on the dura, nerve-roots and spinal cord (208). From the results of the above investigation it is evident that the effects of the pathological forces involving the pons and cervical cord are more complex than was previously believed; broadly speaking, as a result of pathological forces originating in this region potentially deleterious histodynamic stresses are invariably set up both in the nervous tissue and in its blood-vessels (central and peripheral arterial systems). If he is to be in a position to predict the effect of his therapeutic measures the neurosurgeon must be aware of their possible histodynamic consequences.

Estimation of stress in the spinal cord during surgery

Compression

The effects of neoplasms that compress the surrounding tissues are not dealt with.

Spinal cord. The detrimental effects of spondylosis and disc disease are usually ascribed to 'compression'. This is considered to be the mechanism underlying any form of mechanical damage of the spinal cord and nerve-roots, whether it is due to bony structures or lesions originating in the soft tissues—even that arising in spinal postures where compression of nervous tissue is hardly conceivable, such as flexion of the cervical spine or the whole column. The term 'compression' is still commonly used even when it must be obvious that there can be no true compression; for example, pressure on the anterior and posterior surfaces of the cord is referred to

as 'anterior' and 'posterior compression', respectively, although the cord is not in fact compressed against an opposing surface (the canal wall).

Compression can rarely be diagnosed directly during an operation; only in exceptional cases are there gross alterations of the dura, arachnoid and cord indicative of prolonged compression of these tissues; and it is unlikely that compression will still be acting after surgical exposure.

It is possible to define fairly precisely the mechanisms that result in compression of the cord in the spinal canal through alterations in the bone and, perhaps, other structures. Except when it is due to neoplasms and displaced bone fragments, compression occurs almost exclusively during *extension* of the vertebral column. This results in shortening of the spinal canal and folding of all the deformable soft tissues therein and in its vicinity; the cross-sectional area of the cord increases, its covering membranes fold and the bulging of the intervertebral discs and the ligamenta flava into the canal is accentuated. Other conditions that tend to favour transverse compression are a relatively narrow spinal canal, possibly of congenital origin (89, 159, 215, 258, 276), bony protrusions and spondylo-retrolisthesis (216).

Even in pathological situations were all the structures occupying the spinal canal have come in close contact with each other, actual compression may still not occur. Although he may be able to observe such contact with the naked eye, the surgeon is not in a position to predict the mechanical effects of a change in spinal posture. Since compression is a transient functional phenomenon it is rarely possible to recognize it by visual inspection during an operation.[2] Any impression gained during surgery that the cord is compressed by a thickened ligamentum is likely to be unreliable; an impression of close contact between the ligamentum flavum, dura and cord may often be due to widening of the dura by the cerebrospinal fluid after laminectomy, and the removal of part of the ligamentum flavum (Fig. 142). Moreover, laminectomy is usually performed with the spine flexed, a posture in which any compression of the cord will have been eliminated because of widening of the subarachnoid space.

The occurrence of compression of some section of the cord in the spinal canal can at present be reliably demonstrated only by gas myelography and tomography, which directly visualize the surfaces as they approach each other. The presence of compression can sometimes be established by measuring the cerebrospinal fluid pressure caudal to the site in question with the relevant portion of the spinal canal in neutral position or full extension, while Queckenstedt's test is being performed. If, however, the canal is wide the cerebrospinal fluid might pass lateral to the cord and the two surfaces between which the cord is com-

---

[2] Confirmation of true compression could be obtained only by cutting through the canal wall and its contents.

pressed. As has been demonstrated by preoperative to-mographic gas myelography, cord compression in the neutral posture is relatively uncommon. Positive contrast media are useless for this purpose, as they may give a misleading picture, if only because the gossamer arachnoid fibres, the vela and dentate ligaments in the subarachnoid space (35, 164, 178) may impede the flow of the medium at levels where the space is narrow (though still wide enough for the passage of gas). Any pooling of the contrast medium at such levels does not constitute proof of compression.

Nerve-roots. There is no objective method for demonstrating compression of *nerve-roots* in the intervertebral foramina. Even if the foramen is greatly narrowed by osteophytic spurs the only positive evidence of root compression is an increase in the intensity of pain resulting from involvement of the roots, and other sensory, and possibly also motor, symptoms evoked by extension of the spine. A reduction in the size of the foramina, within physiological limits, as seen in radiographs on extension of the column is usually unassociated with compression. (Because of the accompanying relaxation of the nerve-roots there is less risk of an anterior or anterolateral osteophyte exerting a thrust upon them.) A diagnosis of nerve-root or spinal cord compression is therefore justified only if the aforementioned conditions are present. The neurological manifestations ascribed to such compression are often due in fact to unilateral pressure on these components and their consequent over-stretching.

Choice of appropriate treatment. It is important to distinguish between the various sources of stress, since in principle the treatment for compression is protective bilateral laminectomy or facetectomy (p. 194), whereas in the case of over-stretching (bending tensile stress) due to unilateral pressure it is necessary to obtain relaxation of the pons–cord tract and its associated nerve-roots by shortening the cervical canal. It is true that not infrequently the same space-occupying structure, such as an anteriorly located osteophyte, can produce compression of the cord or nerve-root on spinal extension, and over-stretching of it on flexion; but the causes of the two kinds of stress cannot be removed by the same operative measure, because they have basically different origins.[3] Even when protective bilateral laminectomy or acro-cristectomy must be performed to remove the opposing structure for the pincer action, in cases where the anterior structure cannot be removed the cervical column must be fixed in slight extension to eliminate the thrust exerted by the offending structure when the column is flexed.

Tension

In an assessment of the causes of increased tension in the pons–cord tract there are various sources of error. An exact determination of the magnitude of the tension

and its site of origin is impossible. For example, a sharp snap when the dentate ligaments are divided (248) does not necessarily mean that the tension in them was increased to a pathological degree. When the dentate ligaments are severed with the column flexed, a physical phenomenon such as the snap may occur in the absence of any pathological alterations of the column, dura and dentate ligaments. When the cerebrospinal fluid has leaked from the subarachnoid space such a snap increases in loudness with the degree of flexion; thus, if the column is flexed this phenomenon is indicative of nothing more than a normal degree of elastic tension in the dura, cord and ligaments. Only when the spine is in the neutral position—in which the elastic tension has normally disappeared—do physical phenomena suggestive of residual, and thus pathologically increased, tension assume significance. For example, even if the cervical column is brought into this straight position a fairly large disc protrusion on the anterior aspect of the canal may well still generate a transverse tension between contralateral root-sheaths, and hence also in the dentate ligaments and the cord at this level. On dividing the ligaments in this posture they will then retract to a greater extent than normally. Incidentally, it is not entirely correct to maintain that Kahn's operation is worthless, as has been stated in recent papers. If the protrusion maintains some transverse tension in the relevant cord section even when the ligaments have been severed (160) this measure will still have produced some lowering of the transverse tension. (This is evident from the slight reduction in spasticity observed in most of the 21 patients that the author operated on with this method prior to 1960.) Because of the slackening of the dura obtained on extension of the cervical spine the division of the dentate ligaments is no longer of functional significance.

Incorrect estimates of the tension in the pons–cord tract have resulted from misinterpretation of the extent to which the two parts of the transected cord separate. For such an estimate it is necessary to take into account the exact position of the spine[4] (Fig. 26).

Surgical measures for reducing tension in the cord

During operations on several patients suffering from kyphoscoliosis who developed neurological symptoms

---

[3] The surgical measures intended to produce 'decompression' often have quite a different biomechanical effect. Only if the object is to alleviate established compression is the use of this term justified; it is inappropriate for alleviating unilateral thrust.

[4] After transverse transection of the cord in postmortem specimens the transected ends can, under certain conditions, separate at any level. So long as lordosis is maintained the tract will be slack and no separation will occur. Retraction starts in the neutral position of the spine, in which there is a change from the low tension phase to the high tension phase of the tract. The distance between the cut ends increases as the spine is flexed.

during adolescence it was observed that on transection of the filum terminale the ends moved apart (105). It was concluded that a tight filum terminale would exert traction on the spinal cord, pulling it against an angulated spine and tending to draw the hind-brain into the foramen magnum; it was inferred, moreover, that idiopathic scoliosis might have its origin in the tension in the filum terminale (105).

The pathological condition underlying the development of kyphosis and kyphoscoliosis may be associated with various malformations of the pons–cord tract and its encasing structures (Fig. 109). A relatively late event in the course of these disorders produced by the increasing curvature of the spine is over-stretching of the spinal cord, and this, too, may be traced to the filum terminale.[5]

Significance of spinal posture following compressive spinal cord injury

A spinal cord that has sustained traumatic injury should be protected from further, potentially harmful, tensile forces that would be produced by elongation of the spinal canal (50). It has been suggested that further damage might be avoided if the requirements for immediate management of the patient were better understood by first-aid personnel (123). That immobilization is necessary is usually realized; but one should also demonstrate the importance of ensuring that the spine is in an extended position during transportation, and *prescribe* that the head is never flexed forwards.[6]

In the hospital the night as well as the day staffs must realize the danger of aggravating the effects of spinal cord injury—whether acute or chronic—through flexion of the cervical spine. The need to avoid potentially harmful positions of the neck must be fully recognized by the anaesthetist, especially during intubation (17). The neurosurgeon who appreciates the dangers of stretching the traumatized cord through flexion, and thus separating the intramedullary wound surfaces, would take care to ensure that the spine is in the appropriate position of slight extension—when the patient is on a trolley, in bed, or being moved from, say, a trolley, to the operating table.

[5] At the Hospital for Sick Children, Toronto, 28 children with diastematomyelia and scoliosis underwent an operation in which a thickened and widened filum terminale was surgically severed. Most of the children displayed a postoperative improvement with disappearance of the neurological symptoms and signs. This would seem to indicate that the operation corrected a situation in which the cord had been pressed against, and stretched over, the bony or fibrous bar within the canal, or the otherwise deformed canal wall, during flexion of the spine.
Courtesy of Robin P. Humphreys (143).

[6] The immediate relaxation of the pons–cord tract that is required for adequate treatment of the patient with fresh compressive spinal cord injury may possibly be obtained most reliably by immobilizing his head and cervical spine *in slight extension* with an *adjustable* halo-pelvic splint; the use of this device (at present in course of construction) leaves the neck accessible from all directions for the reduction of any spinal fracture and dislocation by other surgical measures than traction.

Spinal and pons–cord tract surgery

Beneficial and adverse biomechanical effects

Neurosurgical operations are commonly performed with the object of alleviating local mechanical effects of certain lesions situated in the posterior cranial fossa or the spinal canal and involving the pons, medulla oblongata, spinal cord and nerve-roots. Rarely, however, is their purpose to correct biomechanical abnormalities by diminishing adverse tension throughout the pons–cord tract. The operation thus tends to consist mainly of local reparative measures, including elimination of pressure. This is the case whatever the type of procedure—whether laminectomy, partial or total removal of the uncinate processes, extirpation of a neoplasm, removal of an anterolateral disc or osteophyte, excision of displaced bone fragments after spinal injury, by a posterior, anterior or anterolateral approach (259, 261), or total removal of a disc with or without interbody substitution of bone, sagittal incision of the dura or severance of the dentate ligaments, etc. Where the lesion is restricted to a single major osteophyte or other structure these measures are usually adequate, bringing permanent or at least temporary relief.

Basis of beneficial effects

The beneficial effects of some surgical procedures are undoubtedly due to incidental improvements in biomechanical conditions.

Fusion

After the Cloward type of operation, performed to maintain the intervertebral space left on removal of a disc by inserting a bone dowel from the iliac crest, root symptoms can disappear at the level not only of the offending disc but also of protrusions or other structures located cranially or, especially, caudally on the anterior or anterolateral aspect of the spinal canal near the site of the intervertebral foramina (Fig. 94). The reason that the operation can be more effective than was originally expected (66, 68) is as follows. Usually the burr hole in the anterior aspect of the cervical spine, which is later to be plugged with a bone graft, is made while the neck is placed on a round bolster. In this position the head and neck are bent back to a greater or

lesser degree and the vertebral bodies separate at their anterior rims, while their posterior rims make intimate contact. Because of this separation, less bone is removed on the anterior part of the two vertebrae, and the cylindrical channel is then shallow on the anterior aspect and deep on the posterior. When the channel has been plugged with the cylindrical bone graft and there is consolidation in this position there will be a permanent backward tilt of the cervical spine at this level. Irrespective of its degree, any such tilt will result in some approximation of the arches, and this will shorten the canal more on its posterior than its anterior side. However slight the resulting slackening of the dura, root-sheaths, spinal cord and nerve-roots, it may still suffice either to relieve the tension resulting from pressure on, and stretching of, the cord or the nerve-roots passing over protrusions remote from the fused vertebrae, or to eliminate the tension produced in these tissues by other pathological firm structures. From these observations it would appear that a beneficial result of interbody fusion would be obtained more often if the spine was immobilized in an extended posture long enough to ensure osseous consolidation of the fusion.

When this tilt has not been exploited, the beneficial results of an interbody fusion may be ascribed to a reduction in height of the intervertebral space following the operation on the disc. By preventing the angulation of the two fused vertebrae the possible elongation of the canal has been reduced, and thus also the potential tension in the cord and nerve-roots (66, 68, 162).

Laminectomy

Bilateral laminectomy performed to secure decompression may result in backward tilting of the vertebrae, shortening of the posterior wall of the canal and hence slackening of the dura and cord. This situation will develop during healing of the muscle and fascia, through the traction exerted by the cicatrix on the spinous processes of the neighbouring vertebrae, thereby inducing a slight lordosis between two or more segments of the spine. This local extension is induced still more frequently after bilateral hemifacetectomy, and almost invariably develops after bilateral facetectomy (236).

Facetectomy

Bilateral facetectomy nearly always prevents elongation of the spinal canal at the level of the operation, owing to the removal of the joint facets and the subsequent consolidation with the two adjoining vertebrae tilting backwards, having been deprived of their supporting structures. Elongation will be prevented whether or not bilateral laminectomy has been performed. (During flexion of the spine the upper joint facets slide forwards and upwards on the lower ones and this upward component of the movement contributes to the elongation of the canal.)

Cervical region. Bilateral facetectomy combined with laminectomy has, however, still more far-reaching consequences. Under normal conditions adjacent vertebrae form an articular system comprised of the two intervertebral joints in question and one to three semi-joints. The latter consist in the first place of the syndesmosis of the intervertebral disc. Beside the two uncovertebral athroses (whose existence and functional significance are not generally accepted), the tesselated upper and lower surfaces of the arches between two adjacent cervical vertebrae resemble an articulation; however, the track between the two opposing surfaces is involved only at the end of the extension movement (Fig. 147 B). In full extension of the cervical spine the stabilizing effect of this track prevents excessive relative rotation of the two adjacent vertebrae. Moreover, when these surfaces are in close contact the range of extension is restricted and the load on the intervertebral joints is relieved through distribution of the axial compressive force. On full extension (backward flexion) of the neck the site of application of this force is displaced posteriorly to the surfaces of the track in the spinous processes.[1] If both bilateral laminectomy and bilateral facetectomy have been performed and the actual locking surfaces have thus been extirpated, only the restraining effect of the intervertebral disc and the annulus fibrosus will remain.

One object of bilateral facetectomy, just as bilateral laminectomy, is claimed to be the alleviation or elimination of the compression of the spinal cord and nerve-roots exerted by the joint pedicles (236). A widened dura after the operation is regarded as confirming that compression was present and that it was produced by the pedicles. But the widening of the dura can have another explanation. In the prone position with the head flexed, and thus below the level of the body, the cervical subarachnoid space and dura are dilated by the hydrostatic pressure of the cerebrospinal fluid in the thoracolumbar subarachnoid space. This widening occurs also when, with the body in the prone position, the head is raised during an operation; the cerebrospinal fluid in the intracranial subarachnoid space then causes bulging of the cervical arachnoid and dura. Thus, the widening of the dura does not in fact constitute proof that compression was present; nor does it indicate that

the tethering of the cord and nerve-roots to the anterior wall of the canal (208) has been released or that with the patient in the seated position the dura and cord separate from the anterior aspect of the canal (236). Only when the head and cervical spine are extended will the cord and the nerve-roots slacken; owing to gravity the bulging of the dura is then accompanied by sagging of the cord and nerve-roots towards the posterior surface of the arachnoid and dura, as far as the dentate ligaments and nerve-roots permit. Since, however, the anterior wall of the dura is still attached to Trolard's fascia, and by this to the periosteum and bone on the anterior aspect of the cervical canal, these bulging phenomena cannot be ascribed to a 'prolapse of the entire dural theca' (2).

The neurosurgical indications for bilateral facetectomy have been based on the view that protruding osteoarthritic spurs on the joint pedicles can clamp both the nerve-roots *and* the spinal cord against an anterior protrusion. However, from both topographical and biomechanical considerations it is unlikely that the cord itself can be compressed except in maximum extension of the spine in those rare cases where spurs located at the joint pedicles are exceptionally prominent and extend towards the midline. From the standpoint of the lumen of the canal the articular processes constitute part of its walls; but since the intervertebral joints are situated laterally and posteriorly, spurs protruding from them can hardly compress the dura and cord; since, however, the articular processes at the same time form the upper, lower and posterior margins of the intervertebral canals, any appreciably prominent pathological spurs of the superior or inferior articular processes of the intervertebral joints may readily compress the root-sheaths and nerve-roots during extension of the spine and exert a pincer action on them.

In fact, when the laminae of the vertebral arches and the articular processes with the joint facets have been removed, the vertebrae tilt backwards, thus resulting in slackening of the dura and the spinal cord and—if their compression in the interverteral canals is relieved—also of the root-sheaths and the associated nerve-roots.

Lumbar region. This biomechanical explanation of the frequently dramatic and far-reaching beneficial neurological effects of combined bilateral laminectomy and facetectomy in the cervical spine (236) applies also, with certain modifications, to the often beneficial effects of bilateral facetectomy in the lumbosacral region. The slackening of the sacral root-sheaths and nerve-roots (Fig. 138), which extends some distance into the sacral canal and towards the entrances of the sacral foramina—not easily accessible for surgery—accounts for

---

[1] Only when the cervical spine is forcibly hyperextended can the upper locking surfaces slide a short distance backwards on the lower ones; during this movement the intervertebral joints are subjected to a lever action, which can lead to rupture of their articular capsules.

relief of pain and recovery of function in the urogenital region. Slackening of the sacral roots will occur (i) if bilateral facetectomy of the articular processes of the L_5 vertebra has been performed, thereby resulting in backward tilting of this vertebra, (ii) if the intervertebral disc has been evacuated at this level or, still more reliably, (iii) if the vertebral body has been lowered. The greater the slackening, the less likely is it that a change of spinal posture will set up tension in these sheaths and roots, and hence subject them to pressure and tension.

Basis of adverse effects

Neurological impairment due to manipulation

In recent years the seated position of the patient with head and spine fully flexed has been increasingly used in surgical exposure of the posterior fossa and even sections of the spinal canal. When, in this position, pressure is exerted on the physiologically stretched tract by deflecting part of it with a spatula pathological tension is set up which can give rise to intramedullary and intraradicular damage, and hence neurological deficit. While symptoms evoked by pressure on sacral nerve-roots in the flexed posture of the spine (167) are usually only mild, damage to pathways in the pons and cord due to over-stretching of the nerve-fibres and supplying blood-vessels can have serious sequelae. This was the case in the following 2 female patients.[2] Both were operated on in the seated position for a left-sided acoustic tumour, which had been exposed with a self-retracting spatula and subjected to the pressure of it for several hours. After surgery one of the patients, 42, suffered from paraplegia of the legs and urinary incontinence, which regressed in about 2 months to slight paraspasticity. The other patient, 53, was unconscious for a week after the operation, during which time she needed respirator treatment; there was tetraplegia for some weeks and this regressed over 18 months to severe permanent left-sided spastic hemiparesis with some residual urinary incontinence and other symptoms.

The potentially deleterious effect exerted on the cord by protrusions located on the anterior aspect of the canal is to some extent offset by the narrowing of the intervertebral spaces, whereby the spinal canal is reduced in length, with consequent reduction of tension in the dura, ligaments, cord and nerve-roots caudal to the level at which the spine is shortened. Tension may be incidentally avoided, moreover, through the possible limitation of the range of spinal mobility resulting from spondylosis. The slackening of the soft tissues and restriction of the mobility of the spine that accompany disc degeneration prevent neurological symptoms developing in a large proportion of the aging population.

[2] Courtesy of L. Steiner, M.D., Dept. of Neurosurgery, Karolinska Hospital, Stockholm.

PART THREE

Measures of functional neurosurgery

Spinal cord relaxation as an aid in neurosurgery

Temporary relaxation

Preparatory to any operation involving the anterior aspect of the spinal canal temporary relaxation should be induced. This measure is also indicated in the removal of extramedullary and intramedullary tumours anywhere between the pons and the conus medullaris.

In extension of the cervical spine the slackened root-sheaths lose contact with the pedicles and move a short distance caudally; this is readily apparent to the naked eye (35). The slack cervical cord and the nerve-roots may now confidently be raised from the canal and drawn a little to one side with, say, a dissector. No resistance in either the caudal or cranial direction will be encountered, and the pressure and tension produced will be minimal. If the root-sheath is deflected by means of the protecting spatula (Fig. 143) the fields is clear for the removal of a herniated disc, tumour, etc;—any osteophytic protrusions in the exposed and protected area may then be resected with a high-speed drill burr.

If there are fibrous adhesions between the dura and the posterior longitudinal ligament (Trolard's fascia) on the posterior side of the cervical vertebral bodies, the dura in this region will also be slack when the cervical spine is extended. Though venous haemorrhage here can be most troublesome, the vessels will then be accessible for electro-coagulation. During these procedures it is advisable to use the above-mentioned special spatula to protect the nervous tissues.

Extirpation of tumours of posterior fossa and spinal canal

The relaxation technique made its début more than 16 years ago when it was used in the removal of ar extremely large clivus mengioma (25). Although the slack pons and medulla oblongata had been raised with a spatula and drawn to the side for more than 2 hours, the patient was able to breathe normally immediately the endotracheal tube had been removed (Case 2, p. 208).

If the pons and spinal cord have been slackened the pons can be moved laterally in the posterior cranial fossa, and the medulla oblongata and cervical (thoracic and lumbar) cord can be raised from the canal or drawn aside until the nerve-roots and the dentate ligaments are taut. If the ligaments are severed the mobility of the brain stem and the cord will be still greater; the tumour can then be better exposed, its vessels can be more readily examined, and there is more room for manipulation during its removal without risk of impairing the conductivity of the pons, cord or nerve-roots.[1] Here, too, the use of the protecting spatula is recommended. It may, for instance, be inserted anterior to and immediatley under the cord so that it bulges posteriorly (Fig. 143), a manipulation calling for great care. Just how much pressure and tension the cord will tolerate without risk of impairing its conductivity can be judged best from the resistance encountered on trying to stretch the nerve-roots. It is true that after somewhat prolonged and moderate traction of the cervical nerve-roots the patient may feel a radiating pain in the arms for a day or so, but in no case have any definite signs of deficit been observed.

Relaxation of the pons was originally conceived primarily as an aid in facilitating the extirpation of tumours beneath or lateral to the pons and medulla oblongata. This technique is obviously of value also in the extirpation of large tumours elsewhere in the posterior fossa, especially when the pressure exerted by such a tumour on the pons is great enough to depress it and hence to set up a tension high enough to be transmitted to the mid-brain.

This situation was found in the case of a 4-year-old child with a very large benign intracerebellar astrocytoma. After successful extirpation of the tumour in the *flexed* position of the head and cervical spine (during which the existing pressure on the pons and the resulting over-stretching were inevitably augmented) the child did not regain consciousness in the 5 postoperative weeks during which the author observed her. During the first 3 weeks the child needed continuous respirator treatment, after which this could be suspended periodically. A month or so after the operation slight reflex defence movements were occasionally noted. These observations are suggestive of a state of probably permanent decerebration.

Extirpation of paramedullary neurinoma (C_7–T_2)

Case. Man, aged 56 years.

Operation (author), July, 1971. Protective bilateral laminectomy by drilling sagittal grooves in arches C_7 to T_2 lateral to the dura and cord and raising the arches. The neurinoma was embedded in the left side of the cord at the cervico-

---

[1] By using the relaxation technique the surgery of vascular malformations is also greatly facilitated.

thoracic junction. After relaxing the cord by using the Breig–Stille-Werner self-adjusting head-rest the neurinoma was raised from the canal together with the adherent slack cord. Silver clips were placed on a large radicular artery entering the caudal pole of the neurinoma, and on arteries entering the middle of the tumour. The neurinoma removed, the cord was allowed to fall back into the canal.

This relaxation technique may also be used in patients with intramedullary neoplasms.

Extirpation of grade I–II intramedullary astrocytoma (C_2–C_3)

Case. Woman, aged 66 years.

Nuchal pain for 6 years, worse after traction therapy. For 3 months prior to admission sensation in right arm impaired; for 3 weeks sudden nuchal pain on turning head; right-sided hemiparesis and hemianaesthesia for 4 days, and faecal and urinary incontinence for 2 days.

Gas myelography, 20th August, 1971. Intramedullary tumour at C_1–C_3 level, completely obliterating the subarachnoid space.

Operation (author) same day. Protective bilateral laminectomy C_1 and C_2, ordinary bilateral laminectomy C_3. At level of arches of atlas and axis, local swelling of cervical cord. Cord relaxed by extending cervical spine by means of the self-adjusting head-rest. After dividing the left posterior root of C_3, a dentate ligament and a radicular artery, a 1 cm long incision was made laterally in pia mater. A reddish grey tumour, which had distended the surrounding tissue was removed with small forceps. When the tension in the cervical cord again increased as the cervical spine was allowed to recover its neutral position, more tumour tissue was extruded from the incision. The pulse and blood pressure were unaffected during the operation, and respiration was normal after extubation. Postoperative confusional state and anxiety. Improvement of sensibility and power in arms and legs, and pain reduced. Ten days later bladder control recovered.

Follow-up examination, 26th October, 1971. Slight paresis in right arm and hand, right leg dragged slightly (walked with aid). Slight numbness in buttocks and legs.

Comment. From the results of this operation it would appear that the risk of setting up potentially harmful tension in the surrounding nerve-fibres and blood-vessels during (partial) extirpation of intramedullary lesions is eliminated by inducing temporary relaxation of the cord.

Inspection of spinal canal

The relaxation technique makes division of the dentate ligaments both simpler and more reliable, as they can then be raised with a small blunt hook without subjecting the cord to tension, and divided without risk of cord damage. Access to the anterior aspect of the spinal canal is thus also facilitated. When this technique is used during open cordotomy the cord can be more easily and safely rotated, so that its anterior surface can be inspected, the site for the incision located, and damage to important blood-vessels avoided. The actual

incision in the spinothalamic tract must, however, be made with the cervical spine flexed so as to render the cord taut and thus to avoid damage to the pyramidal pathways.

Stereotaxic cordotomy. Flexion is also recommended in stereotaxic cordotomy. In certain commonly applied techniques this operation is usually performed with the cervical spine straight or slightly extended, but there is then a risk of missing the target area for the stereotaxic lesion (Fig. 102).

Protective technique for protruded thoracic disc

In view of the extreme sensitivity of the thoracic spinal cord to tension set up by a herniated thoracic disc (Fig. 118) it is especially important to apply the cord relaxation technique during removal of extra- or intradural expanding lesions located in this region. If there is a herniated disc or any other structure situated on the anterior aspect of this part of the canal slackening should be induced as a protective measure before the operation is started. As regards the thoracic region, in particular, it is necessary to bear in mind the risk of cord trauma from two different sources of tensile stress. One of these is a pincer action on the cord inflicted by error during laminectomy, for instance, through one of the jaws of the bone rongeur being pushed in under the laminae.[2] To eliminate this risk it is advisable to leave a good margin when sawing through the arches lateral to the dura and cord; the laminae can then be lifted out. The other source of tensile stress in the cord is that resulting from the unilateral pressure exerted by a protruding thoracic disc, or another anteriorly or anterolaterally located firm structure.

(A patient, who had had a herniated thoracic disc removed 8 years previously and suffered from postoperative paraparesis for several months, was digging in his garden when he suddenly had a recurrence of spastic paraparesis. Immobilization of the thoracic spine in the extended position on a Kifa back support (52) (fig. 104) led within a week to disappearance of the symptoms, and the patient volunteered that he felt

---

[2] During removal of the relevant vertebral arch in a patient with a calcified herniated intervertebral disc (Fig. 118) by 'conventional' bilateral laminectomy some 20 years ago the author's rongeur happened to press slightly for a short moment against the dura and the thoracic cord; after the operation paraparesis had developed. The histodynamic background is obvious: Pinching of the thoracic spinal cord between the jaw of the forceps and the calcified disc on the anterior wall of the canal produced local tension in the nervous tissue which probably resulted in immediate tearing of nerve-fibres especially in the centre of the cord, oedema and possibly haemorrhage. Such a mishap can now be avoided. To be able to remove the actual disc without risk of damage to the cord and ensuing neurological symptoms, the thoracic cord must be rendered slack immediately after exposing the vertebral arches; this can be effected by extending the cervical spine by means of the self-adjusting head rest (Fig. 141).

steadier on his legs than he had at any time for 8 years.[3]

Extirpation of herniated lumbar disc

In the lumbosacral region, too, the relaxation technique facilitates neurosurgical operations and reduces the risk of operative trauma (Fig. 145). Extension of the cervical spine produces no significant movement of the lumbosacral nerve-roots, though the root-sheaths may be seen to move slightly from the pedicles, and more fluid will enter the subarachnoid space. If the sheaths are thin and translucent, evidence of the slackening of the roots can sometimes be clearly seen; the floating roots then move to and fro over a short distance in time with the pulse. Even if the sheaths are not translucent, their distention by cerebrospinal fluid when the spine is extended indicates that the roots are slack. As a rule, however, it is only during manipulation that the slackening produced by extension of the spine will be apparent; for example, the usual resistance to deflection or elevation of the roots will be found to be appreciably reduced. Thus, both to touch and to the naked eye it is now obvious that the nerve-roots can be moved more freely and for a greater distance without increasing their tension.

Thus, also in the lumbar section of the spinal canal relaxation of the root-sheaths and nerve-roots will afford better exposure of a herniated disc, osteophytes, tumours, etc. Although the nerve-roots tolerate pressure and tension better than the spinal cord, the relaxation technique may also be useful in this region of the canal. This is especially pertinent in the case of paresis of the dorsiflexor muscles due to tension in the L_5 motor nerve-root. Because of the sensitivity of this root and the fact that any motor paresis resulting from damage to it may be irreversible, an immediate operation is usually recommended. In this situation much would be gained by using the relaxation technique to minimize surgical trauma. Another advantage of the procedure is that the quite common postoperative bladder dysfunction is avoided. There is evidence that discal hernia operations can result in permanent reduction of bladder capacity and similar dysfunctions to a greater extent than is usually realized (90, 165, 227).

As has been mentioned above, if it is intended to use the relaxation technique at operation it is necessary to perform a preoperative radiological examination of the anteroposterior width of the cervical canal with the neck bent back. The small effort involved may be amply rewarded by the confidence derived from knowing that the cervical cord cannot be compressed during extension of the cervical column.

Since 1958 the author has induced temporary relaxation of the cord and nerve-roots in a large number of operations for a variety of lesions in the posterior fossa and the spinal canal. The beneficial results in most of these patients have been achieved thanks to this method (Case Reports, pp. 207–10). In a number of patients the relaxation technique has been used in the removal of what would otherwise have been almost inaccessible tumours at the anterior border of the foramen magnum and the upper cervical canal.

---

[3] R. Frykholm: Personal communication, 1963.

Long-term or permanent relaxation
—Cervicolordodesis

Definition

Cervicolordodesis is the operation whereby a 'brake' is introduced between the back of head and the spinous processes of the thoracic vertebrae T_1–T_3. Its purpose is to maintain slight extension of the head and cervical spine.

Technique

See Figs. 150 and 153

Object

The object of this measure is to relax the whole pons–cord tract so as to diminish, if not eliminate, the symptom-producing pathological tension in its tissue set up by various firm extra- or intramedullary lesions or structures. When the tract is stretched elastically on flexing the spinal column the extramedullary lesions or structures exert a unilateral thrust on the adjacent portion of the cord, and the intramedullary ones a multilateral thrust on the cord tissue.

Indications

The histodynamic causes of cord disorders range from purely mechanical lesions (such as rupture of the cord in acute spinal cord injury) to extra- or intramedullary alterations. The latter include local oedema and reactive sclerosis as in multiple sclerosis, and cysts as in syringomyelia; the former include bony spurs, as in cervical myelopathy.

The recognition of the source of tension responsible for the neurological symptoms has implications for the choice of therapy. In myelopathy patients, however, where the moderate extension of the cervical column necessary to eliminate the thrust threatens to result in a pincer action on the cord, the first step is to avoid this possibility by protective arco-cristectomy or protective bilateral laminectomy at the appropriate level. The second step is to inhibit the flexion of the cervical spine by cervicolordodesis.

Materials used; foreign body reaction

In the search for a suitable implant material strong enough to withstand the forces generated during everyday activity and passive—though possibly forceful—flexion of the neck, the fascia lata strips originally used were replaced by Marlex and Mersilene mesh and, more recently, by a 2 cm wide Teflon ribbon.[4] It was, of course, some time before it was possible to assess the

mechanical suitability and histocompatibility of these materials. Probably owing to stretching, the fascia lata could not be relied on to maintain the degree of extension of the cervical spine originally applied at the operation. On inspection at re-operation after some months (Case 2, p. 224 and Case 3, p. 230) the rather loosely woven Marlex and Mersilene meshes had torn at their anchorages in the occipital bone and at the spinous processes. There was a good deal of reactive connective tissue, often indistinguishable from the mesh itself.

Trevira ribbon appeared at first to be mechanically suitable.[5] One patient (Case 1, p. 225) fell twice and struck her neck on the edge of the bath; as there was no immediate relapse of neurological manifestations from the long pathways it was concluded that the brake had withstood the impact.[5] Furthermore, at 3 re-operations no evidence of any visible deterioration of the material of the ribbon was found. Only round the places where the ribbon was affixed to the bone was there adhesion by connective tissue fibres. In the channel through the neck muscles the ribbon was for the most part only loosely attached to the tissue, and it could easily be withdrawn. In no case was there evidence of a foreign-body reaction around the clamp and the cement (61). There has so far been no reason to check for any reaction to the Trevira ribbon in the bone of the spinous processes. In those cases where the ribbon had to be removed owing to infection it was severed just cranial to the uppermost process, and the caudal part of the ribbon was left in place with no manifest untoward effects. The surgical wounds healed well, but antibiotics were administered in 3 cases because of infection that prompted removal of the ribbon (see below).

Infection occurred immediately after implantation of the fascia lata in one patient (Case 2, p. 234) and after implantation of Mersilene mesh in another 2 patients (Case 3, p. 230 and Case 9, p. 220). The cause of the infection in the first 2 cases is not known; in the third, the surgical wound had not healed properly when the patient was transferred to another hospital. In the second of these patients, where there had twice been infection after implanting Mersilene meshes, it was decided to try a Trevira ribbon. The feared relapse of the previous infection occurred, and after several months the ribbon was removed. An interesting development in

---

[4] Later identified as Trevira polyester fibre material, see 'Recent advances and conclusions' (p. 193).
[5] This assumption has proved to have been in error; see 'Recent advances and conclusions' (p. 193).

this patient, and in the 2 others whose Trevira brake had to be removed, is the formation of a relatively firm tube of connective tissue around the tunnel through the neck muscles, and this seemed to restrict flexion of the neck to some extent.

The Trevira ribbon had to be removed in 2 more patients owing to infection unassociated with the operation. In one of them (Case 5, p. 238) there was infection of a tracheostomy, which eventually spread to the site of the ribbon. The patient's neurological condition ruled out discarding the cervicolordodesis, and antibiotic therapy was introduced. The ribbon was left in place for several months before it was cut off just above the uppermost anchoring spinous process; the wound then healed uneventfully. In the second patient (Case 2, p. 224), who was living in the country, the Trevira ribbon had to be removed several months after the operation because of a superficial infection, which could have been avoided had the patient been under supervision.

In view of the vital importance of the implant remaining sterile, clean air systems in the theatre are mandatory (63)—as in any other implant operation (62).

Possible drawbacks

The number of patients submitted to the cervicolordodesis operation is at present too small to permit of any general appraisal of the associated risks.[6,7]

Duration of the treatment

In the case of any severe traumatic injury to the spinal cord it is necessary, in view of the probable presence of transverse fissures in the cord, to relax it without delay so as to avoid the risk of increasing the damage by over-stretching unaffected nerve-fibres and blood-vessels, as well as any already placed under tension by the lesion. After administration of dexamethasone to avoid oedema, one of the available surgical measures for establishing a slight degree of extension of the cervical spine must be chosen—on the basis of a thorough X-ray analysis. The choice lies at present between a bone graft and cervicolordodesis. (Another device for maintaining long-term extension of the cervical spine is a halo-pelvic splint that has been adjusted to this purpose.) The graft fuses all the cervical vertebrae and permanently immobilizes the cervical column. Cervicolordodesis, in which forward flexion of the head and cervical spine is prevented by a brake has the advantage that the patients retain some mobility of the cervical spine and that there is always the possibility of removing the brake and recovering full mobility. Because of the small number of patients receiving this form of treatment and the relatively short follow-up periods it is not known how long after the operation the spinal cord relaxation must be maintained. In any case, it might be justifiable to lengthen the ribbon 6 months or so after the cervicolordodesis operation so as to allow the neck to be bent through approximately

one-half of its ordinary range of movement. Since the ribbon is clamped at a distance from its end (the excess being folded back over the clamp and buried in the canal) it is an easy matter to provide this range of mobility by opening the transverse incision in the neck under local anaesthesia, unscrewing the clamp and letting out the ribbon the required amount.

If a substantial intramedullary scar has formed after the cord injury, on bending the neck it might exert a multilateral thrust on the fibres in the adjacent intact pathways and impair their conductivity. Aggravation of the neurological symptoms after the ribbon has been

[6] When meningeal irritation is suspected after a cervicolordodesis operation it is, of course, no longer possible to rely on bending of the neck as a diagnostic aid. Equally informative examinations are available, however—for example, Kernig's and Lasègue's tests.

[7] When, after protective laminectomy in which a sagittal incision has been inflicted inadvertently in the dura and arachnoid, the cervical spine is kept extended by a cervicolordodesis operation, the mechanism described in Figs. 142 A and B invariably results in a gap in the dura and liquorrhoea when the arachnoid opens.

Case report (condensed). Woman, 35, suffering from severe cervical myelopathy arising from congenital malformation of the vertebral bodies and arches, especially in the lower part of the cervical spine. The neurological condition of the patient, which included extensive atrophy of the muscles of the hands and right leg, had deteriorated at an accelerating rate over the previous 4–5 years and the patient was ultimately confined to a wheel-chair. During tentative skull traction at another hospital the patient's neurological condition had deteriorated rapidly (Fig. 97[9]). The main radiographic features were severe kyphosis of the lower cervical spine with marked narrowing of the canal at the C_6 and C_7 levels (anteroposterior diameter 0.5 cm, enlargement factor subtracted) (see Fig. 142 B).

Operation (author & Håkansson), May 1975. Bilateral protective laminectomy C_6 and C_7 and cervicolordodesis (with improved Trevira ribbon). When the arch of the C_6 was raised and the ligamentum flavum was divided, a *ca.* 5 mm long sagittal incision in the adherent dura was accidently produced; the edges of this rift were approximated by a transverse suture.

Postoperative course. Uneventful during the first week after the operation; then a fairly sudden and copious secretion of fluid through the channels of the upper skin sutures; this ceased after placing some secondary sutures and applying a compression pack.

After the formation of the fistula and probably of an epidural cyst (that had exerted pressure on the dura and cervical cord) there was a reversal of the trend towards a general neurological improvement; this improvement had been reflected in the perception of heat in the legs the day after the operation, steady recovery of sensibility in the lower body during the next few days (amounting to practically normal sensation) and an increasing range of movement of the toes and left leg. (*cf.* p. 218).

Surgical closure of the rupture in the dura and a shunt operation were also considered. For organizational reasons the indicated operation was not performed; the patient's condition deteriorated, with the development of paraplegia.

Practical conclusions. When some form of protective laminectomy has been performed prior to a cervicolordodesis operation the surgeon should check that this procedure has not resulted in a rift in the dura; any such rift should be reliably closed and, especially one in the sagittal direction, stitched far enough from its edges so that the sutures can withstand the transverse tension in the dura invariably set up in the extended posture.

lengthened would probably indicate the presence of such a scar, and the ribbon would then have to be shortened again.

Isometric training of the neck muscles after cervicolordodesis

In particular during the time when the cord injured patient is confined to bed or a wheel-chair it is important to exercise the neck muscles at least daily by contraction against resistance, so as to maintain an adequate circulation and thus to avoid atrophy. This is most effectively accomplished by isometric training. As the head can be rotated and extended after the cervicolordodesis operation, there are enough initial positions for the training contraction. If there is a risk of the intramedullary wound surfaces separating, however, it is inadvisable to choose lateral flexion of the head as the initial position. Also rotation of the head should be avoided since this movement might well give rise to shearing forces across a cord rupture.

Results and reliability of the cervicolordodesis operation

For the results obtained by permanent spinal cord relaxation the conventional five-point scale 'excellent', 'good', 'fairly good', 'no change', and 'worse', was originally applied; fortunately, however, the last two classes have proved to be superfluous, since all the patients operated on have displayed a distinct improvement. In all of them the regression of the individual neurological symptoms followed approximately the described pattern (p. 231). The time varied from case to case, however, as is seen from Table 5. In all patients, where the effective degree of extension of the spine was not maintained, for example, because the ribbon loosened from its anchorage, the initial improvements was followed by some relapse. In one patient there was a rapid and almost complete neurological relapse after only 5 days (Case 3, p. 230), and in another patient as much as 4 years later (caused by skull traction!, Case 2, p. 216). As the improvement was permanent in only about one half of the patients, there is clearly room for improving the technique—for instance, by ensuring a more reliable anchorage of the ribbon.

Experience has consistently shown that the more reclined the head and the more lordosed the neck, the slacker is the cord and the greater the chance of neurological improvement. Moreover, the more strictly the reclined head position is maintained the more reliable will be the long-term neurological recovery. It is therefore of the utmost importance to use a reliable braking device to restrain flexion of the head, and one that is histocompatible as well as mechanically sound.

Recent advances and conclusions

The 2-cm wide Teflon ribbon, which superseded the fascia lata graft, Marlex and Mersilene mesh as the material for the cervicolordodesis brake, at first promised to be eminently suitable for the purpose. The ribbon was claimed to possess the desired strength by a large margin. However, doubts as to the material's properties were aroused when steadily progressing neurological deterioration was observed in several patients in whom this ribbon was used; it was noticed, moreover, that they were able to bend the head forwards much further than just after the operation.

An analysis of the old Teflon ribbon[8] carried out by the manufacturers showed that an increase in its total length may well have occurred. Such an increase in length would have permitted a considerable increase in the flexion angle. (This is consistent with the observations in the Case Reports.)

The elasticity of the material was accordingly reduced and the yield introduced in the weaving process was eliminated.

As the polyethylene material recovers its stretchability under dry or moist heat, sterilization must be performed either with gamma radiation (2.5 Mrad cobalt-60) or high-energy electrons; ethylene oxide may also be used.

The improvement in the properties of the new Trevira ribbon[9] over those of the old one are evident from the graph in the figure given below, where the tensile force is expressed in Newtons (1 Newton=0.120 kgf).

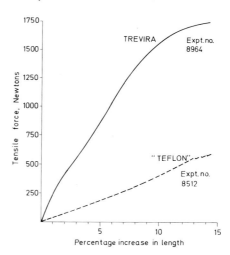

The new Trevira ribbon was first used on 29th May, 1975.[10]

[8] Courtesy of L. C. Lammers, M.D., Hoechst Company, Ltd., Frankfurt am Main, West Germany.
[9] Manufactured and distributed by Hoechst Company, Ltd., Frankfurt am Main, West Germany.
[10] See also Footnote 2, Fig. 153 C.

Functional neurosurgery for eliminating a pincer or clamping action

Protective arco-cristectomy and protective bilateral laminectomy

Definitions

Protective arco-cristectomy consists in sawing out only the upper part of each lamina of the vertebral arch. In protective bilateral laminectomy the whole of each lamina is sawn out.

Technique

See below (p. 195) and Figs. 147 and 148.

Object

The object of protective arco-cristectomy is to remove the crest of the vertebral arch; that of protective bilateral laminectomy, to remove both laminae. The surgical methods outlined below are used in both operations.

Anatomical background

In extension of the cervical spine the posterior wall of the cervical canal shortens and forms a curve that is convex towards the canal. This wall consists of the dura mater and the ligamenta flava, and, just below these, the anterosuperior rims of the arches, which in sagittal section are wedge-shaped. As the arches approach each other in full extension the ligaments flava are pressed both forwards and backwards between them. (If, after stripping the cervical dura from the periosteum of the vertebrae of the cadaver, a finger is passed over the posterior surface of the cervical canal, the resilient ligaments are found to form a somewhat corrugated surface (52). If the finger-pressure is increased the rims of the arches will be felt.)

Besides the obvious protection of the cord in general from the wedge action of the crista arci afforded by the ligamenta flava there is the protection of the cervical cord provided by the greater rigidity of the rhomboid network of the medullary tissue in its posterior than in its anterior zone. When the cervical cord is compressed axially and hence widened in its transverse plane on extending the cervical column, the network stiffens and

expands towards the posterior contour of the canal, thereby protecting the conducting nerve elements from mechanical damage.

Traumatic mechanisms responsible for pincer or clamping action. The potential pincer effect of the crista arci on the cervical cord will not be exerted until this protective system has broken down; this can occur in the following pathological situations (fractures are disregarded here):

(a) In spondylo-retrolisthesis after tearing of the anterior longitudinal ligament in a so-called hyperextension or whip-lash injury (with or without fracture of the involved articular processes). The crista arci then protrudes more prominently beneath the ligamentum flavum because its protective fold is eliminated through posterior displacement of the neighbouring arch; at the same time the lower border of the suprajacent vertebral body moves towards the now unprotected crista arci, causing a marked narrowing of the cervical canal, and hence pinching of the cord. In this case the indications for selective decompression by means of protective arco-cristectomy (black in the diagram, p. 198) are of secondary importance (Fig. 147).

(b) Another pathological situation in which the protective system is broken down is that in which, on extension of the spine, the cord is pinched between an osteophyte and the crista arci. The level at which the constriction of the cord and the resulting axial tension are greatest is at the line connecting the tip of the anterior protrusion and the crista arci (Fig. 148, *Inset*). Protective arco-cristectomy or protective bilateral laminectomy is now indicated to obtain selective decompression.

Diagnostic requirements for functional neurosurgery. Plain lateral tomographic films of the cervical spine in the neutral or slightly extended posture. Measurement of the distance between the lower border of the dislocated vertebra (or osteophytic protrusion) and the crista arci of the subjacent vertebra. Oxygen myelographic and tomographic films, where possible. Note should be taken of the magnification factor.

Indications. To relieve the local axial tension in the cervical cord in the above pathological situations (in spondylo-retrolisthesis only if reduction is impossible) it is necessary either to remove just the upper rims of the vertebral arch (protective arco-cristectomy) or to perform bilateral protective laminectomy (see below). Through the support the arch rims give to the protruding ligamenta flava they form a relatively broad pincer or clamping surface, which, together with the anterior such surface, is responsible for the compression and hence the tension. Protective arco-cristectomy at one or more levels will suffice so long as the canal is wide enough. Otherwise it is necessary to resort to protective bilateral laminectomy (see below).

These two operations dispense with the need for immediate extirpation of the protrusion located on the anterior surface of the canal by removing the bony structure that constitutes the opposing pincer surface. In order to eliminate the unilateral thrust of this protrusion on the cord it will then be necessary to prevent flexion of the head and cervical spine by means of a brake (cervicolordodesis; Fig. 153). When the structure forming the anterior pincer or clamping surface is still protruding far into the canal it should be extirpated by anterior access (p. 250) (259).

Surgical techniques. In the case of a pincer action due to the presence of osteophytes the operation for removing the opposing laminae or their upper rims should be performed in the neutral position of the spine.

In the case of a pincer or clamping action due to spondylo-retrolisthesis, where there is always instability, laminectomy must also be carried out in the neutral position but with adequate stabilization of the cervical spine—for instance, by applying gentle traction with Crutchfield's forceps (load 500 g) under television monitor control. If a permanent stabilizing measure is indicated (for example, spondylodesis by an intracorporal bone graft or the steel-frame prosthesis [Fig. 154 A], procedures during which renewed or increased retrolisthesis can occur before stabilization has been achieved), protective arco-cristectomy or protective bilateral laminectomy should be performed in advance in order to eliminate the risk of damage to the cord during these operations.

Protective arco-cristectomy and protective bilateral laminectomy. Since the cord is under high local tension due to the fracture or dislocation, under no circumstances should any instrument be inserted between the vertebral arch and the dura; for in arco-cristectomy and

bilateral laminectomy any constriction of the cord by the laminae will increase the total intramedullary tension and possibly cause tearing of the nervous tissue (or extend a tear already present), and hence result in irreversible neurological deficits.[1] Protective resection of the crista arci (arco-cristectomy) should therefore be performed. This is done by making two sagittal grooves in the vertebral arch just medial to the intervertebral joint, using a high-speed drill burr; a transverse groove is then sawn in the arch—at right-angles to its surface—about 4–6 mm below the upper border of the crista, depending on the extent of the constriction (Fig. 147). When the crista arci has been sawn out in this way it must always be raised carefully. When the ligamentum flavum has been lifted up from the dura together with the laminae it is advisable to cut off its stretched lateral parts with a small sickle-shaped blade, the cutting edge of which is directed upwards. The remaining parts of the ligamentum flavum need not be removed since owing to their elasticity, they will probably not exert compression. In protective bilateral laminectomy, the whole vertebral arch is sawn out. The cuts are made at right angles just behind the pedicles (Figs. 147, 148); the same precautions are then observed as in arco-cristectomy.

Arco-cristectomy is usually indicated at the C_5/C_6 level. Exposure should be restricted to the arch responsible for the pincer action, together with part of its spinous process. To gain access to the crista in the narrow space available it may be necessary to resect the upper border of the process, but to ensure stability its lower part should always be left intact. Although technically more demanding this operation offers definite advantages.[2] If an anterior protrusion reaches the anterior aspect of the intervertebral foramen and thus compresses the nerve-root arco-cristectomy may be combined with hemifacetectomy.

---

[1] In the part of the cord subjected to compression the nerve-fibres are over-stretched, or nearly so. Since the cytoplasm of the axis-cylinders is incompressible, any instrument that happens to be pressed against the cord in an attempt to obtain decompression by removing bone or other tissue will displace a further volume of cohesive cytoplasm, and thus increase the potentially harmful tension in the axis-cylinders. If they have not already been torn in the spinal injury, this can occur when an instrument is inserted between the bone and the dura; for this reason the slightest pressure on the section of the cord already under tension must be avoided.

[2] In spinal trauma that has led to anterolisthesis (through the catapult mechanism) the perhaps bilaterally fractured arch usually does not follow the anteriorly displaced vertebral body (171). The cord will thus be exposed only to the unilateral thrust of the lower border of the body, which remains in place. This produces tension in the fibres in the medullary tissue network which, compared with the pincer action, is relatively harmless, as is evident from the fact that the resulting neurological symptoms are mostly reversible (28, 91, 171, 190).

TABLE 4. Survery of lesions where the symptom-producing tension in the pons–cord tract can be diminished by methods of functional spinal cord surgery.

	Mechanical effects			
	External thrust of firm structures impinging on anterior or anterolateral surfaces of the pons—cord tract[a]	Outward thrust	Pincer action due to firm structures pressing on anterior or posterior surfaces of the pons–cord tract[b]	Rupture of nerve-fibres as effect of pincer/clamping action
Foramen magnum tumour	+	–	?	(+)
Cervical myelopathy	+	–	+ (at level of narrowing)	(+)
Kyphosis	+	–	? (posterior aspect of dural theca)	?
Kyphoscoliosis	+	–	? (posterior aspect of dural theca)	?
Anterolateral osteophytes and discal herniation	(extraforaminal)	–	+ (intraforaminal ?)	(+)
Multiple sclerosis	–	+ (due to localized oedema or glial scar)	–	?
Intramedullary cyst	–	+	–	?
Spinal cord injury: Partial cross-sectional lesions	+ (in impinging structures, bone fragment, herniated disc etc.)	+ (in oedema, astroglial or collagenous scar etc.)	+ (protracted if responsible structures are not removed; temporary in case of 'hyper-extension trauma')	+
Total cross-sectional lesions	+ (in impinging structures on cranial intact cord section and nerve-roots; at caudal level on the completely isolated cord section)	(at caudal level on completely isolated cord)	+ (pincer action is invariably the cause of the lesion)	+

Note. Even transient (possibly incapacitating) neurological symptoms can be elicited on a histodynamic basis (outward thrust on, or tension round fissures in, the nervous tissue) by cytologic changes; for example, in multiple sclerosis, by perivascular oedema and infiltration, haemorrhagic infarction, myelin fragmentation and demyelinization, reactive gliosis and secondary degeneration of fibre tracts (Fig. 100).

[a] In the case of a thrust on the cord from within and a thrust from without, the tension throughout the cord increases in proportion to the degree of *flexion* of the head and spine and elongation of the spinal canal.

[b] The local axial tension in the cord due to compression increases in proportion to the narrowing of the spinal canal, the degree of *extension* of the spine and the accompanying widening of the cross-section of the cord.

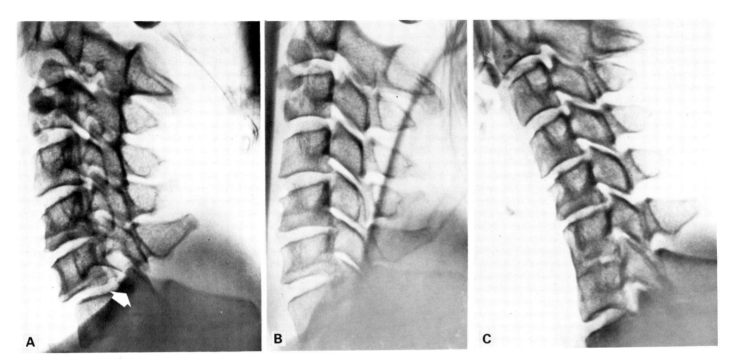

Fig. 146. Mobile anterolisthesis at the C_6/C_7 level caused by a whip-lash injury and treated by postural reduction and interbody fusion.

A. Slight anterolisthesis with rupture of the interspinous ligament and probable damage to the posterior longitudinal ligament. Relatively wide cervical spinal canal. The radiograph disclosed no fracture of the vertebral arch. (*White arrow.* Upper, inner edge of the C_7 body.)

B. Complete reduction a few hours after placing the neck on a round bolster so that the head was slightly extended. In order to mobilize the patient as early as possible interbody fusion was performed and a supporting collar provided.

C. Complete fusion of the C_6 and C_7 bodies after one month. The vertebral interspace is still visible. Slight compensatory forward angulation at the C_5/C_6 level in full flexion.

Comment. Since experience has shown that the bone graft may not be perfectly stable, immobilization should always be applied in interbody fusion, just as in the reduction of any other fracture.

Histodynamics. If the dislocation of the cervical column is not reduced, the upper, inner edge of the C_7 body (*white arrow*) presses on the spinal cord and sets up a bending tensile stress in it (Fig. 136). Any resulting neurological symptoms due to transverse stretching of the cord tissue have proved to be largely reversible. A pincer action on the cervical spinal cord in anterolisthesis seems to be a relatively rare event, since, when the pedicles are fractured, the arch of the vertebra is frequently left behind.

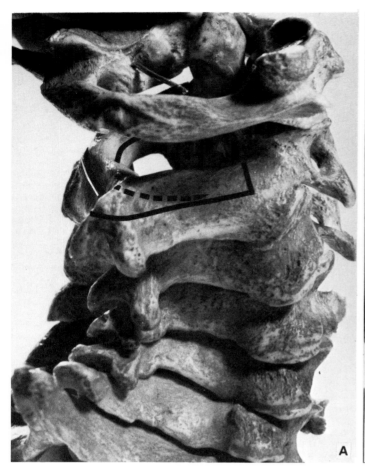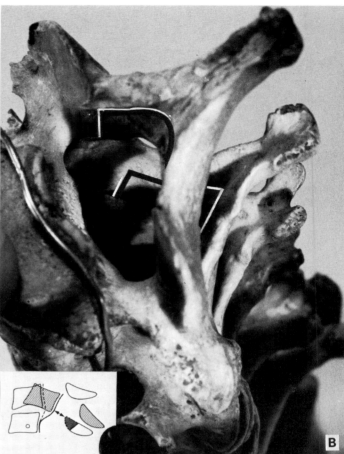

Fig. 147. Arco-cristectomy. A protective surgical method of relieving the compression of the cervical spinal cord, but retaining the supporting functions of the neural arch by resecting its anterosuperior rim, thus guaranteeing the stability of the cervical spine—the apophyseal joints being preserved.

A. Line of resection marked on the bone from behind and above to afford a better view of the arch of the second cervical vertebra. *Broken line.* Line of resection of the upper part of the spinous process.

B. Line of resection marked from below on the C_6 and C_7 arches and the spinous processes, the levels where these structures are usually involved in a pincer action on the cord, together with the C_5 and C_6 bodies.

Inset. The lower border of a posteriorly displaced vertebra (*shaded*) approaches the anterosuperior rim of the neural arch of the lower vertebral body (216). On performing arco-cristectomy the rim of this arch is resected (*black zone*).

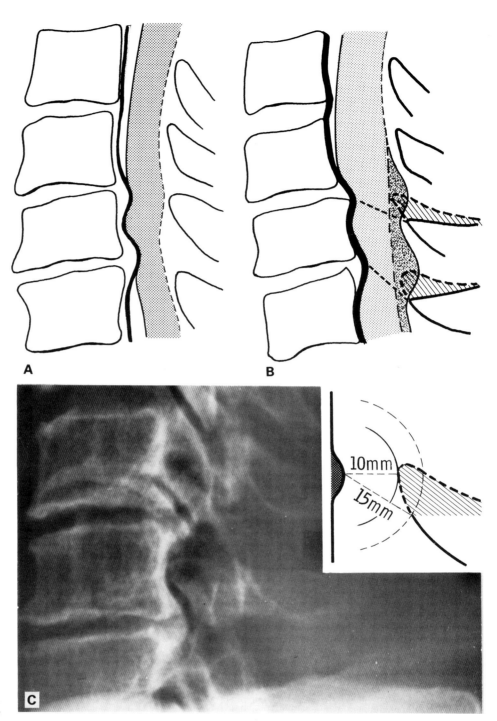

A   **B**

C

Fig. 148. Arco-cristectomy at the C_6 and C_7 levels (combined with cervicolordodesis).

The patient, a man aged 61 with cervical myelopathy (Case 4, p. 218), was troubled mainly with migraine cervicale, spastic gait that had increased over 5–10 years and disturbed balance.

A. Drawing from a gas myelogram before operation. Only the anterior contour of the cervical cord was visualized. (Stippled line indicates defective visibility of posterior contour.)

B. Drawing from superimposed radiographs of the cervical spine before and after arco-cristectomy. Before the operation (author, November, 1970) the lumen of the canal between the large osteophytes at C_6 and C_7 and the corresponding vertebral arches had been reduced to 10 mm; after the operation it was

enlarged to 14 mm at C_6 and 15 mm at C_7. Removal of the respective ligamenta flava together with the cristae arcorum, and slackening of the dura by cervicolordodesis provided room for the cervical cord to ride tensionless over the osteophytic humps. The shaded area shows the space available for the cord after arco-cristectomy.

C. Radiograph taken after arco-cristectomy and cervicolordodesis (Mersilene mesh).

After the operation the headache vanished, the spasticity and loss of power in the arms and legs diminished slowly, and the ankle clonus disappeared, but Babinski's sign remained positive.

Inset. To determine on the plain radiograph the amount of bone to be excised from the vertebral arch in arco-cristectomy draw a circle of 15–18 mm radius, with the most prominent point of the anterior wall of the cervical canal (often an osteophyte) as its centre. The maximum anteroposterior width of the cervical canal that, after the operation, will be available to accommodate the spinal cord, the nerve-roots and their investing soft tissues is indicated by the intersection of the circle with the vertebral arch. To obtain the true value it is necessary to subtract the enlargement factor for the radiograph.

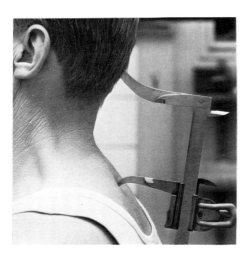

Fig. 149. Calipers for determining the degree of extension of the cervical spine required to secure relaxation of the cord prior to and during the cervicolordodesis operation.

An alternative, and often more exact, measure is the distance between the (lowermost) tip of the mandible and the jugular notch; however, during the operation this region is usually not accessible for measurement.

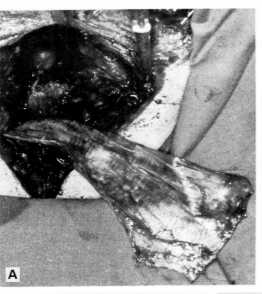
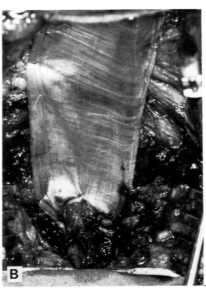
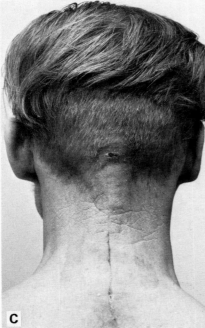
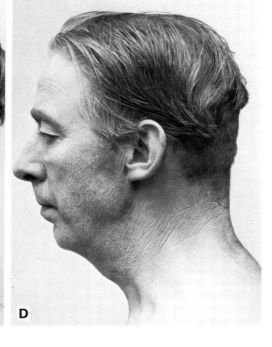

Fig. 150. The cervicolordodesis procedure. Transplantation of fascia lata to the neck to serve as a brake to prevent flexion and thus to avoid setting up tension in the pons–cord tract.

Photographed at operation (Bengt Nylén, author, March, 1970) on a 45 year-old patient with cervical myelopathy (central hemiparesis of the right leg, paraspasticity, reduced sensibility from the iliac crest to the anus, with Brown-Séquard's syndrome (Case no. 5, p. 218)).

A. After protective bilateral laminectomy C_6 and selective protective resection of about one-fifth of the upper border of the arch of C_7 (arco-cristectomy), a fascia lata autograft about 13 cm long and 4 cm wide was anchored around the spinous process of the T_1 by means of polyester sutures.

B. The head and cervical spine have been extended enough to ensure effective slackening of the spinal cord, the required degree of which must be ascertained in advance radiographically; then using image-intensifier control at operation. Along its whole width the upper part of the fascia is sutured to the fascia colli transversa and the periosteum of the external occipital protuberance.

C. The area 10 days after the operation showing the scar after a T-shaped incision. The cervical spine could be turned and bent freely in all directions except forwards.

D. The cervical spine on attempting to flex the neck to its maximum.

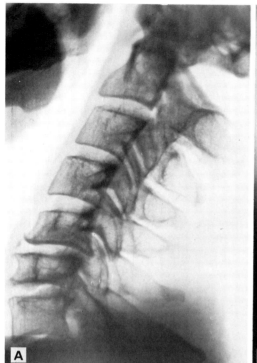
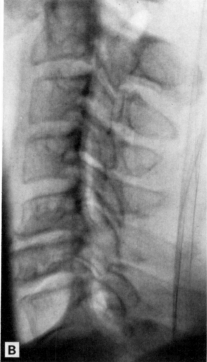
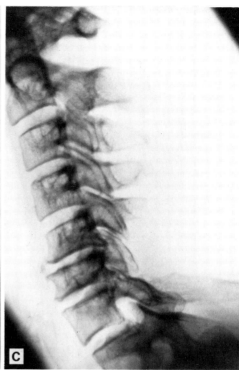

Fig. 151. Pre- and postoperative radiographs of the cervical spinal cord and spine before and after cervicolordodesis (same patient as in Fig. 150).

A. Marked reduction of the C_5/C_6 and C_6/C_7 intervertebral spaces with large osteophytes on all three vertebrae. The C_5 body is slightly, and the C_6 body greatly, reduced in height with calcification of the anterior longitudinal ligament. There is considerable narrowing of the cervical canal between the osteophytes on the C_5 body and the C_6 arch,

and slightly less between the osteophytes on the C_6 and C_7 bodies and the upper part of the C_7 arch.

B. Gas myelogram of the cervical cord (supine position). The gas (*light strip*) can be followed to the upper and lower contour of the large protrusion at the C_5/C_6 level, and is found again below C_6.

C. Full flexion of the head and cervical spine 10 days after the operation. (Because of the myelopathy no preoperative radiographs were taken in full flexion.)

By protective bilateral laminectomy C_6 and protective arco-cristectomy C_7 the possibility of a pincer action developing at these levels on extension of the cervical spine has been removed. A tangential line along the posterior surface of the C_4 body to the superior posterior border of the T_1 body shows that the osteophyte at the C_5/C_6 level together with the associated soft tissues can still exert unilateral pressure on the cord; at the C_6/C_7 level, too, the conditions for such pressure remain, but it has been prevented by the cervicolordodesis.

Fig. 152. Relief of compression by protective arco-cristectomy and relaxation of over-stretched nervous tissue (approximation of possible intramedullary wound surfaces) by cervicolordodesis in the treatment of cervical spinal cord injury.

Radiograph after arco-cristectomy at the C_7 level combined with cervicolordodesis showing the marked osteophytic spurs at the C_6/C_7 intervertebral level and the bone defect after the operation.

Fourteen weeks after surgery the patient, a man aged 67, who had sustained a central cervical spinal cord injury when he fell on his face from a bicycle, had regained fairly good power in his totally paralysed hands and severely paretic arms; the complete urinary incontinence had disappeared (Case 1, p. 232).

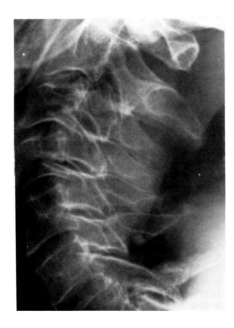

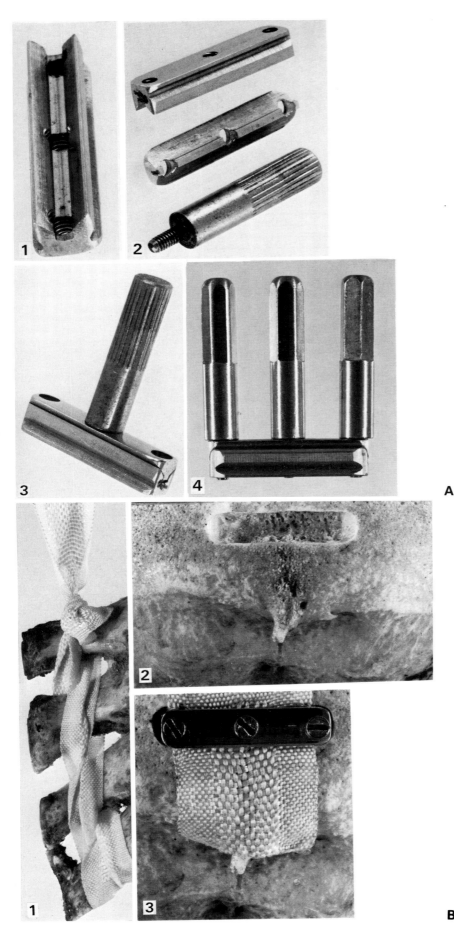

Fig. 153. Apparatus and technique for the cervicolordodesis operation.

A. *Prosthesis clamp*. Dimensions 26 by 6 by 4.5 mm.[1]

1. Lower part of the clamp, seen from above. Each side of the baseplate contains a groove for anchoring it in the cement.

2. *Top.* The baseplate of the clamp seen from below. *Middle.* The V-shaped upper component of the clamp. *Bottom.* One of the 3 clamp grips with knurled shaft and screw for temporary assembly of the 3 clamp components (see below).

3. Clamp with one of the 3 grips in place. During cementing in the channel in the bone all 3 grips must be screwed in so that the clamp can be pressed down evenly into the cement and none can enter the screw-holes.

4. The most recent version of the prosthesis clamp grips.

[1] Manufactured and distributed by Hans Malmgren, Medical Prosthesis Co., Ltd., Harpsundsvägen 152, 124 40 Stockholm–Bandhagen, Sweden. (Patent pending.)

A

B. *Cervicolordodesis ribbon and its anchorage.*

1. Trevira ribbon, 2 cm wide, laced round the T_3, T_2, T_1 and C_7 spinous processes and tied over the C_7 (no longer done).[2]

2. Channel cut in the occipital bone to take the clamp; it is placed 2 cm cranial to the tip of the external occipital process.

3. The clamp in place in the channel, its 3 screws tightened to secure the Trevira ribbon. (The channel in the figure is too large. A templet and a special drill—see below—are now used to ensure that the channel is cut exactly to size.)

[2] It may soon be possible to replace the synthetic fibre material by denatured fascia lata from the human or bovine cadaver. If this should prove to be as strong as the synthetic product and otherwise suitable, it could be stored in a fascia lata bank, just as denatured tendon tissue for tendon sutures.

B

C. *The surgical technique.*

A transverse incision about 5 cm long is made about 1.5 cm above the external occipital protuberance. With the aid of the templet and special drill, a transverse channel is cut in the bone to accommodate the clamp. With its 3 grips in place the clamp is cemented (61, 139). A vertical, slightly curved, incision in the skin (convex to the left) is made from C_6 or C_7 to T_3/T_4. The fascia of the trapezius muscle is exposed on each side of the C_7 or T_1 to T_3 spinous processes. Approximately 2 cm long sagittal incisions are made in the fascia and muscles about 1.5–2 cm from the sagittal line on each side of the supra- and interspinous ligaments C_7/T_1, T_1/T_2, T_3/T_4. From one lowermost parasagittal incision to the other a large Deschamp's needle is inserted transversely below the T_3/T_4 supraspinous ligament. The Trevira ribbon is threaded and drawn under the ligament. From the next higher incision a large less curved Deschamp's needle is inserted diagonally below the T_2/T_3 supraspinous ligament until its eye emerges on the opposite side in the incision at the lower level. When the ribbon has been threaded the needle is withdrawn back. When the manipulation has been repeated on the opposite side and the 2 ends have been pulled as tight as possible the ribbon is drawn down out of sight between the muscle and the spinous process. This shoe-lacing technique is repeated at the higher levels.

Through a channel cut in the muscles just above the spinous processes by means of a long curved debriding forceps with external cutting edges the two ends of the ribbon are drawn to the prosthesis clamp (they usually lie flat one on the other). When the cervical spine has been extended to the predetermined degree with the aid of the self-adjusting head-rest, the 2 ends of the ribbon are screwed tight in the clamp.

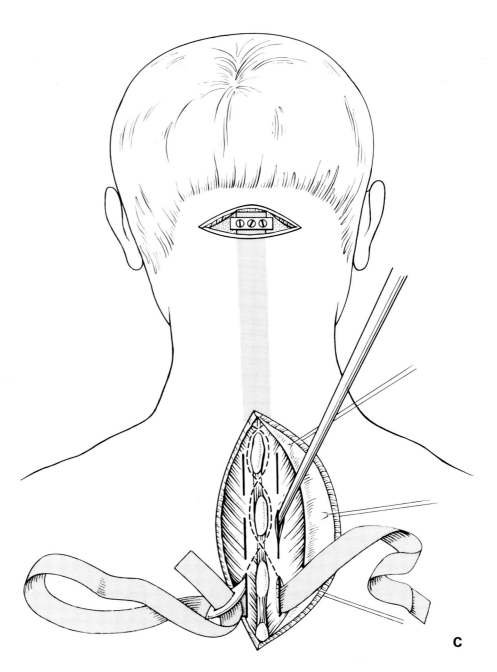

C

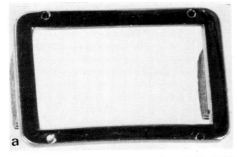

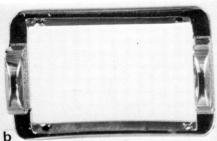

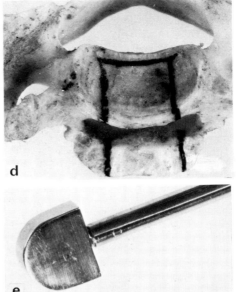

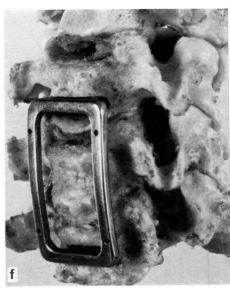

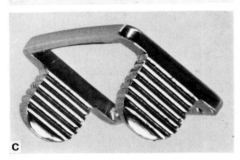

Fig. 154.
A. Steel-frame prosthesis for immobilization of vertebral fracture in spinal cord injury by means of a bridging spondylodesis on the extended cervical spine.

Before cementing the lugs of the frame in the intact vertebral bodies cranial and caudal to the damaged vertebra the cervical canal is lordosed by extending the cervical spine over a firm round bolster (X-ray check). The shape of the frame permits subsequent adjustment of the damaged vertebra and, if necessary, its extirpation if the fracture is found to be inadequately reduced.

a. The prosthesis, front view; dimensions 3.3 by 2.3 cm.[1] The slightly curved frame fits the anterior convexity of the cervical spine; its edges are rounded to avoid damage to the soft tissues. The holes in the frame provide anchorage for fragments or transplanted bone.

b. The prosthesis, rear view. The inner surfaces of the long sides slope backward and outward; the resulting widening prevents the frame from pressing on the longus colli muscle when cemented in place.

c. The lugs, with corrugated surfaces.

d. Cervical vertebra with channel drilled to take the lug. The channel occupies about one-half the width of the vertebra (*black lines*). The width of the lines includes the thickness of cement.

e. Gauge for checking the width and depth of the channel. (This instrument has been superseded by a drill guide.)

f. Steel-frame prosthesis in place in a cadaveric specimen of the cervical spine; it bridges the C_5 vertebral body.

g. Lateral view of the cervical spine with forward displacement of the C_4 over the C_5 (Case 6, p. 240).

h. The prosthesis anchored in the vertebral bodies C_4 and C_6; wedge-shaped tibial graft; dislocation reduced. As the intended extension at the level of the fracture could not be achieved solely with the guidance of the television monitor, a normal X-ray check was necessary before the frame was cemented in place.

i. Radiograph showing the prosthesis cemented in the vertebral bodies C_4 and C_6; a tibial bone graft has been secured with fine steel wires through the holes in the frame (same patient as under g, h).

[1] Manufactured and distributed by Hans Malmgren, Medical Prosthesis Co. Ltd., Harpsundsvägen 152, 124 40 Stockholm–Bandhagen, Sweden. (Patent pending.)

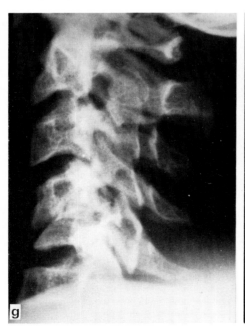

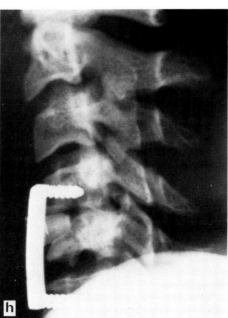

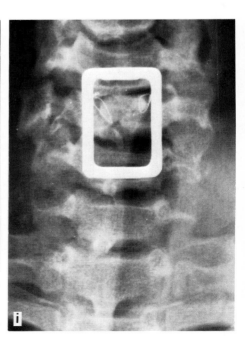

B. Supplementary instruments for cervicolordodesis *(upper row)* and bridging spondylodesis *(lower rows)*.

a. Templet for drilling the groove in the occipital bone, special drill and hexagonal key (about 45 per cent of actual size).[2]

The *templet*, which is of aluminium, consists essentially of two wings connected by a bar of rectangular section. The wings of 6 mm plate are curved slightly upward and outward. The connecting bar forms a socle 1 mm high and directed downward. In this a jig is fastened with 2 screws; it consists of a steel plate with three holes 7 mm wide, from each of which extends a steel tube 16 mm long. Four pins projecting from the plate pass far enough into the base of the socle to provide an anchorage for the templet in the occipital bone.

The *drill* is used for cutting the holes for the groove in the occipital bone. It is provided with an adjustable stop; when the drill projects far enough from the jig to cut a hole of the required length the stop is locked by tightening 2 hexagonal-headed screws with the *key*.

b, c. Debriding scissors for cutting the cervicolordodesis channel through the muscle (about 45 per cent of actual size).[3] b, slightly curved model; c, strongly curved model.

The outer edges of the scissors are blunt; the blades taper 2 cm from their tips. When cutting the channel in the muscles the scissors need not be opened more than 2 cm, in which position their outer edges retain taper, thereby preventing the tips of the scissors from fastening inadvertently and causing unnecessary damage to the tissue.

d. Deschamps's needle, screwdriver for prosthesis clamp,[2] and ribbon pull-through[4] (about 45 per cent of actual size).

The *pull-through* can be bent into a suitable shape for drawing the Trevira ribbon from the incision in the upper thoracic region, through the tunnel in the neck muscles, to the prosthesis clamp.

The *Deschamps' needle* is used for lacing the Trevira ribbon around the spinous processes.

e. Guide for drilling the channel in the vertebral body to accommodate the steel-frame prosthesis; special drill and hexagonal key (about 55 per cent of actual size).[2]

Three long, round parallel channels running the length of the drill guide serve as a jig for the drills. Two drills are supplied; in one of these the adjustable stop is set to cut a hole just deep enough to accommodate the most prominent convex point of the lug of the prosthesis, with a small margin for the cement; in the other drill the stop is set for cutting a hole long enough to take the lateral part of the prosthesis lug. The remaining bone partitions between the 3 holes are then removed with an ordinary burr.

f. Lower end of the drill guide (enlarged).

From the lower edge of the drill guide project 4 sharp points for anchoring the guide to the anterior surface of the vertebral body; the inner two points are shorter than the

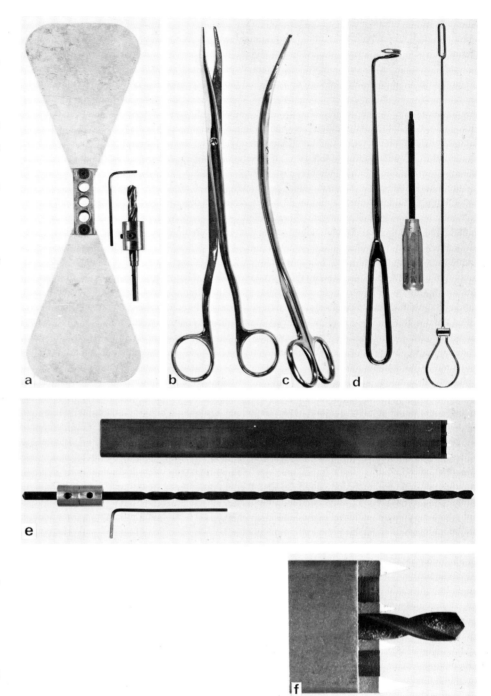

outer ones, so that the guide fits the convex surface of the vertebral body. (Before the transverse groove is cut in the vertebral body it is advisable to insert a needle into each of the adjacent intervertebral discs, as close as possible to the upper and lower surfaces of the vertebral body, so that the needles will indicate the slope of these surfaces. From the direction of the needles it is possible to estimate the angle that the guide must make with the vertebral body, and thus the position in which it must be held throughout the drilling procedure—which takes about 2–3

minutes—to ensure that the groove is placed in the middle of the vertebra.)

[1,2] Manufactured and distributed by Hans Malmgren, Medical Prosthesis Co., Ltd., Harpsundsvägen 152, 124 40 Stockholm–Bandhagen, Sweden. (Patent pending.)
[3] Manufactured and distributed by Aesculap-Werke, Tuttlingen, West Germany.
[4] Manufactured and distributed by Stille-Werner Co., Stockholm, Sweden.

The effects of tension on neural conductivity

The alleviation of signs and symptoms through the surgical elimination of tension in the pons–cord tract has occasionally been unpredictably good. The fact that sensory deficit, pain, paresis and sometimes also spasticity of months' or even years' duration can be relieved transforms the prognosis for this group of patients (47, 49) and confirms that several neurological disorders are caused by excessive intramedullary tension. It is not possible to say whether these manifestations have their origin in loss of elasticity of the affected tissue, stiffness due to scarring, tensile ischaemia or other causes.

Axonal conductivity appears to be independant of physiological changes in tension in the axon that occur between the normal extremes of spinal posture (35). The conduction velocity of the action potentials varies with the diameter of the axis-cylinder, and a 20 per cent increase in fibre length would theoretically be accompanied by a 10 per cent decrease in the diameter. Yet there is no evidence that the amplitude of the action potential decreases as the fibre is lengthened. One possible reason for this is that a change in the length of the cylinder results in a change in impedance across the cell membrane. It would be rewarding to investigate the phenomenon in flexed and extended postures, possibly with the use of evoked cortical responses (75). When an isolated nerve-fibre from a peripheral nerve is stretched at a constant rate, its conductivity is not blocked until near the point of actual rupture (78, 117, 232, 240). The conductivity of the myelinated fibre in the spinal cord probably behaves in a similar way.

It is thus unlikely that the neurological manifestations are due simply to changes in the physical properties of the axis-cylinders—especially if it can be demonstrated that neural function can recover even after fibres have been stretched beyond their elastic limit. Nonetheless, local sclerotic lesions in a myelopathic cord may well lead to excessive tension in the zone between scarred and normal tissue, where nerve-fibres may be over-stretched over short lengths. A further possible cause of over-stretching is local oedema. Both sclerotic foci and sites of oedema are surrounded by an ischaemic zone, the extent of which may vary with the tension in the cord during changes in posture. The venous pressure will therefore also fluctuate and with it the concentration of the by-products of 'stagnation'. Anoxia in over-stretched nervous tissue, if prolonged, is bound to lead to irreversible loss of conductivity and cell death.

It would thus seem that the nervous tissue which dramatically recovers its function—with relief of pain, sensory deficit, bladder dysfunction and spasticity—will have been subjected to excessive tension and recurrent spells of ischaemia and hypoxia, though not of long enough duration to lead to cell death; and when the cause of the over-stretching and hypoxia is eliminated, signs of recovery are observed—usually after a few weeks or days, but perhaps even in a matter of hours.

Results of surgically induced slackening of the pons–cord tissue tract

Case Reports[1]

In the operations reported in the following section spinal cord relaxation has been applied:

(a) as a temporary measure, designed to obtain and facilitate access to the basal aspect of the posterior cranial fossa, the anterior border of the foramen magnum and the anterior aspect of the spinal canal at the appropriate level; and

(b) as a permanent measure.

(a) With the exception of some operations for foramen magnum tumours none of the surgical results reported here have been achieved by temporary relaxation of the spinal cord. The value of this technique in facilitating the operation, and reducing the risk of damage to the nervous tissue is self-evident. Since 1958 the author has applied the method in scores of operations on patients with a wide variety of extra- and intradural lesions. Its technical advantages are described in the chapter entitled 'Pons–Cord Tract Surgery, Beneficial and Adverse Biomechanical Effects', in connection with the presentation of a number of cases.

(b) As will be evident from the following accounts of the operations and their discussion, the surgical technique for the permanent relaxation of the spinal cord has been improved in various respects over the years, and this process is continuing. With the accumulation of experience of the biomechanical effects of the method at the microscopic level, the range of indications is also being extended.

Foramen magnum tumours

Case 1. Man, aged 55.

Neurological history. February, 1962. Sensation of warmth radiating from the neck to both arms; numbness and weakness in the hands; fine movements difficult to perform. Forward bending of the head evoked electric shock-like sensations, radiating towards the diaphragm area. Difficulty in keeping balance; left leg weaker and could be moved forwards only with an effort. *June.* Respiratory, bladder and rectal function impaired.

Admitted to Department of Neurosurgery, South Stockholm Hospital, 5 July, 1962.

Neurological findings. Unsteady gait. Reduced sensibility for all qualities below C_4 to umbilical plane. Severe atrophy of small muscles of both hands. Unable to raise arms more than about 20 cm, and in supine position unable to raise legs more than about 30° from the couch. Bilateral extensor plantar reflexes.

Gas myelogram. Expanding process at level of atlas and anterior aspect of foramen magnum (Fig. 156).

Operation (author), 23 July, 1962. Removal of extradural neurinoma 3.8 cm across, situated on anterior right aspect of cervical canal, extending from the axis several centimetres upwards and into the posterior fossa. Part of the squama occipitalis on the right side removed to obtain access to the upper dome of the tumour. Atlas and axis arches on right side totally destroyed. Tumour, with rubbery consistency, enclosed in thick capsule, adherent to C_2 root-sheath. Right vertebral artery stretched to a thin strand over tumour. Some time after division of the obliterated arterial strand, severe haemorrhage from the cranial stump in the posterior fossa and caudal stump near the transverse foramen; arrested with silver clips.

Operation performed with the cervical spine in extension and with aid of self-adjusting head-rest (Fig. 141). Relaxation of dura mater and the upper section of the pons–cord tract permitted leftward displacement of medulla oblongata, so that tumour could easily be freed from all adhesions. Wide view of the whole field of operation and ample room for manipulation facilitated application of silver clips to stumps of vertebral artery, greatly retracted at moment of haemorrhage.

Histological diagnosis. Schwannoma.

Postoperative course. Uneventful. Sciatic pains of several years standing disappeared completely and had not recurred

---

[1] For extraneous reasons the intended follow-up examinations could not be continued after July, 1975.

by 1965. Discharged 8th August with marked regression of all above-mentioned neurological symptoms.

Case 2. Woman, aged 57.[1]

Neurological history. Nuchal pains for the past 8 years. In 1958, paraesthesia, reduced power and clumsiness in both hands; paraesthesia in both legs.

Admitted to Department of Neurosurgery, South Stockholm Hospital, October, 1960.

Neurological findings. Feeling of pressure in neck, radiating to both shoulders. Marked paraesthesia and clumsiness in hands, especially the left. Unsteady gait. Periodic difficulty in swallowing. Difficulty in micturition (retention of urine). Atrophy of neck and shoulder muscles; slightly increased tension in neck muscles on right. Marked loss of power in both hands (dynamometer: zero). Joint kinaesthesia and vibratory sensation in all fingers reduced. Dys-stereognosis and dys-diadochokinesis in left hand. Tendon reflexes in the arms increased; some spasticity (Trömner's sign positive bilaterally), increasing distinctly on bending head forward and flexing the cervical spine. Vibratoty sensation reduced in legs. Deep sensibility reduced in toes. Spastic tendon reflexes in both legs; cloni. Bilateral extensor plantar responses. Gait unsteady; spastic and atactic.

Gas myelogram. Uppermost section of cervical cord displaced posteriorly in an arc. Distance between aquaeductus cerebri and clivus plane strikingly large. Cisterna pontis widened (films taken in neutral posture). Scarcely any difference in contrast visible at posterior border of foramen magnum (Fig. 157).

Arteriography (vertebral artery). Basilar artery displaced 1.5–2.0 cm in occipital direction from posterior clinoid processes (sella turcica).

Operation (Frykholm), October, 1960. Meningioma issuing from caudal part of clivus and anterior aspect of foramen magnum. After exposure of upper section of cervical spinal canal and posterior fossa, upper part of the cervical cord found to be displaced far posteriorly and slightly to the left. Pons, oblongata and cord slackened by bending head and neck backwards; the pons could then be raised from the clivus, and upper part of the cord easily moved to right, thus giving better access to the large tumour which could then be radically removed.

Histological diagnosis. Meningioma with psammoma granules.

Postoperative course uneventful except for slight paresis of left facial and glossopharyngeal nerves. Within a week the spasticity in the arms and legs had disappeared and extensor plantar reflexes could no longer be elicited.

Case 3. Woman, aged 32.

Neurological history. For previous 2 years, nuchal pain radiating to the back of the head; worse at night; increasing greatly on bending head and neck forwards. Six months after onset of symptoms, paraesthesia in both hands; difficulty in grasping small objects. Gradually increasing heaviness in shoulders, arms and legs. After cisternal puncture (Cairo), (severe flexion?, haemorrhage?) sudden paraplegia of legs, progressing in 2 days to tetraplegia. Slow regression over 6

weeks; 2 months later, able to take a few steps when supported. Capable of feeble arm movements. Six months later, sudden relapse of tetraplegia. Since March, 1962, difficulty in micturition and defaecation (urinary incontinence and constipation).

Admitted to Centre for Neurosurgery, Cairo, March, 1962.

Neurological findings. Hypaesthesia on right side of body. Vibratory sensation abolished in arms and legs; spastic reflexes. Bilateral extensor plantar responses.

Gas myelogram (Ahmed Fouad El-Nadi). Obliteration of subarachnoid space below anterior border of foramen magnum at level of C_1 and C_2, with thickening of soft tissues by more than 1 cm. Extramedullary expanding process (Fig. 158).

Operation 1 (Tauwfik), 7 April, 1962. Bilateral laminectomy C_1 and C_2. Opening of dura mater disclosed arachnitic adhesions; no further exploration; dura left open. Neurological condition unchanged.

Operation 2 (author), 1 November, 1962. Large dumbbell-shaped neurinoma with large extradural portion on anterior and left aspect of dura, extending from inferior border of clivus caudally to just below arch of axis. On flexion of cervical spine, displacement of dura and cervical cord posteriorly and to right. Extension of cervical column slackened dura, root-sheaths, cervical cord and nerve-roots. First, complete removal of extradural part of the tumour—greatly facilitated by easy access through slackening of dura; second, extirpation of intradural pea-sized part of the tumour, adherent to and issuing from rootlet of posterior second cervical nerve-root.

Histological examination. Neurofibroma.

Postoperative course uneventful; rapid recovery. After a week the patient could move her arms, and after 10 days stand on her legs; began to walk with support. Her state had further improved considerably when, 3 weeks later, there was sudden coffee-ground-like vomiting, shock and coma. Abdomen distended and silent. Pulse imperceptible. Died during transfusion. No autopsy.

Case 4. Man, aged 53.

Neurological history. In 1959, after lifting heavy logs, numbness and burning sensation in the neck, radiating to right shoulder, and 6 months later to radial aspect of the lower arm. Burning pains increased on turning the head to the left. In 1960, reduced power in right arm and hand; about 6 months later paresis in right leg, which began to drag. Occasional sensation of warmth on right side of body, hyperaesthesia to cold in right foot and to warmth in right leg.

Admitted to Department of Neurosurgery, South Stockholm Hospital, June 1961.

Neurological findings. Muscles of shoulder girdle on right side severely atrophied, those of right arm, hand, thigh and lower leg less so. Thermaesthesia abolished in C_2–C_5 dermatomes on right side of neck. Tendon reflexes in right arm and leg exaggerated. Foot clonus and extensor plantar response on right side.

Radiographic examination. Fairly marked scoliosis of spinal column at level of cervicothoracic junction.

---

[1] Patient identical with Case 1, J Neurosurg *19:* 661, 1962.

Gas myelogram (combined with encephalography). Soft tissue shadow with lower curved border at level of atlas; tumour in posterior fossa? cerebellar tonsil?

Operation (author), June, 1961. Syringomyelia. After laminectomy of the upper cervical vertebrae and making a sagittal incision in the median line of the dura, the cervical spine was extended. The lower part of the left cerebellar tonsil extended below the upper rim of the arch of the atlas. After 2nd and 3rd dentate ligaments had been divided, the cord— slackened by extension of cervical spine—was raised from the canal and rotated slightly to the side. On the anterior aspect of the cord at C_2 level the pia mater bulged and moved to and fro synchronously with respiration, disclosing a syringomyelic cyst extending from C_1 to C_5. This cyst was completely concealed when the cord was in place in canal. C_1–C_5 anterior and posterior nerve-roots were grey and atrophied. Cyst punctured; content slightly yellow.

Postoperative course uneventful. At examination next day, spasticity greatly reduced, sensibility slightly improved.

Comments and discussion (Cases 1–4)

Surgical technique. Cases 1–3 illustrate well the extent to which relaxation of the dura and pons–cord tract by extension of the cervical spinal canal facilitates the removal of extremely large tumours in otherwise almost inaccessible regions along the clivus, anterior border of the foramen magnum and the anterior aspect of the upper cervical canal. Surgical operations in this region have hitherto presented great technical difficulties. Slackening the tract not only facilitates the technical procedure, but minimizes the risk of surgical trauma to the pons, oblongata, cord and nerve-roots.

The advantages of the relaxation method are best illustrated against the background of the circumstances for both surgeon and patient that prevailed only a few years ago. The tumour in Case 2 may be compared in size and location with that in Case 2 of Smolik & Sachs, 1954 (239): "The spinal cord bulged markedly . . . pushed back by tumor . . . lying anterior to the spinal cord . . . the tumor was retracted gently . . . even this slight manipulation affected the patient's respiration." Again, Dodge writes (Mayo Clinic, 1956): "It should be realized that complete removal of tumors in this anterior (basilar groove) or anterolateral position despite their benignity may yield only a Pyrrhic victory gained at the cost of great damage to the cord or medulla or ultimate demise of the patient" (81). To achieve a better mobility of the cord Dodge recommended bilateral division of the dentate ligaments and of the superior (anterior and posterior) cervical nerve-roots.

Case 2 was the first one in which relaxation of the pons–cord tract was utilized in removal of a tumour in the foramen magnum region. Since it was necessary to draw the pons and oblongata quite forcibly to one side, an unavoidable manipulation entailing the application of considerable pressure of the spatula on the medulla oblongata, it would not have been surprising if some

damage had been caused to the respiratory centre; but in fact, immediately after disconnecting the respirator, spontaneous respiration was observed and no respiratory assistance was required.

In Case 4 the relaxation of the tract enabled an examination to be made of the anterior aspect of the cervical spinal cord leading to the discovery of a syringomyelic cyst which otherwise might well have been overlooked. Its exact extent could not have been established in any case, and percutaneous puncture, which is now applied in the diagnosis of, and to some extent also the treatment for, spinal cord cysts would hardly have been utilized.

Radiographic examination. In the gas myelograms the upper section of the cervical cord in Cases 1 and 3 and the pons in Case 2 were displaced a considerable distance posteriorly, as was confirmed at the operation. In both supine and prone positions the relevant films were taken with the cervical spine approximately neutral. As seen from Figs. 156–8, the head and the cervical spinal column were bent slightly forwards or backwards. At the time these films were taken no study had been made of the influence of the spinal posture on the pons–cord tract, and therefore no films had been taken in extreme functional positions; the posterior contour of the posteriorly displaced cord is consitent with earlier descriptions of such tumours; "arising in an anterior position (basilar groove) the upper cervical part of the cord and the medulla were pushed posteriorly, rotated and stretched over the tumor . . . the first and second cervical roots and the rootlets of the eleventh nerve were often stretched over the tumor" (81), (Fig. 155).

Neurological findings. In the presence of such tumours forward bending of the head and spine increases the over-stretching of, and pressure on, the pons–cord tract. In Cases 1 and 3 the bending of the cervical spine resulted in a clear increase in spasticity in the extremities through an increase in the already exaggerated tendon reflexes. This has been confirmed indirectly by the above surgeons: "flexion of the neck is hazardous in positioning patients with benign tumors at the foramen magnum".

The sudden tetraplegia in Case 3 illustrates the latent dangers of bending the head and cervical spine forwards. Here, the tension in the cervical cord tissue may have been produced by over-stretching of the tract and the associated increase in pressure on the cord and, at the same time, puncture of the cord or an artery, with consequent haemorrhage. Not only does the posterior displacement of the pons–cord tract by the tumour shift the oblongata towards the posterior boundary of the cisterna cerebellomedullaris so that it is readily accessible for any puncture (which in such cases is, of course, inadmissible), but through increased axial tension it is retained in this position.

In Case 3 in which the tumour (neurinoma) was

located at the spinocranial junction the pseudoathetotic movements of the fingers were observed that have been regarded as an early sign of meningioma in the foramen magnum region (25) (Fig. 159).

Case 1 with an extradural neurinoma at the level of the foramen magnum had been suffering for several years from sciatic pain on the left side. This completely disappeared immediately after removal of the tumour, and the patient was still well 3 years after the operation (see also 'brachialgic sciatica' p. 111). A positive relationship between foramen magnum tumours and sciatic pain—has been observed by Dodge, 1956: "the initial symptom was low back pain and sciatic pain. This reminds one of the not infrequent occurrence of sciatic pain associated with tumors of the cervical portion of the cord" . . . "The blood supply may progressively be compromised and may give peculiar unrelated and distant bizarre symptoms" (81). A more likely explanation of the symptoms, however, is that they are due to the stress in the nervous tissue set up by an unyielding structure on bending of the cervical cord with the consequent traction in the dura, pons–cord tract and lumbosacral nerve-roots (Fig. 29 G).

Of still greater practical and theoretical importance is the fact that in Cases 1–3 the bladder and rectal control were recovered on removal of the tumour. Since the sciatic pain in Case 1 and the above cases reported by Dodge would seem to have been due to the effect of stress in the nervous tissue set up by pressure on, and over-stretching of, the lumbar or sacral nerve-roots, and transmitted *via* the over-stretched pons–cord tract, it is reasonable to wonder whether the urinary incontinence and difficulty in defaecation in Cases 1–3 might have been due to the same transmitted forces. The situation is complicated, however, by the fact that the tumour produces a similar pressure on, and bending tensile stress in, the relevant section of the pons–cord tract (and hence the centrifugal pathways for micturi-

tion within the tract (200) which is stretched over the actual tumour (Fig. 157), and that extirpation of the tumour produces relaxation both of the cranial section of the tract and of the sacral nerve-roots.

This question bears on the main clinical theme of the present study. It is notable that the urinary incontinence almost invariably occurs in the case of changes of the pons–cord tract that result in either chronic or chronically intermittent over-stretching of it. A search for the causes of this tension brings to light pathological processes of varying nature and origin that ultimately lead to distortion of adjacent nerve-fibres and blood-vessels (106, 180). This is the common denominator of all these chronically invalidizing disorders of the spinal cord, whether they have an allergic inflammatory basis—as multiple sclerosis—a chronic mechanical (cervical myelopathy) or acute traumatic basis, such as spinal cord injury; foramen magnum and high cervical cord lesions can, in fact, simulate, or be associated with, degenerative disease of the nervous system (1, 30). If this nonspecific histodynamic stress in the nerve-fibres is eliminated by procuring relaxation of the pons–cord tract by functional surgery (36), the relevant neurological symptoms usually decrease or disappear—so long as there has been no irreversible break in conductivity. After the relaxation of the tract the conductivity of the motor, sensory and urinary pathways not infrequently displays a remarkably rapid recovery.

The reduction of the neurological symptoms (Case 4) obtained by puncture of a spinal cord cyst is due to the elimination of its outward thrust on the nerve-fibres in the adjacent pathways.[2]

---

[2] It is known that the forces set up in the intact nerve-fibres around a lesion—for instance, an intramedullary cyst—on flexion of the cervical spine may be about three times greater than normal (Figs. 76 A and A').

Fig. 155. Typical deformation of the medulla oblongata produced by a foramen magnum tumour.

The tumour is located in front and slightly to the right of the oblongata, at the junction between the posterior fossa (clivus) and the upper cervical canal. It bears against quite a long section of the pons–cord tract, stretching and deflecting it. The cervical nerve-roots riding over the tumour are pressed posteriorly and thus also stretched. As a result of the backward and leftward displacement of the cord, tension is set up in the cranial nerves located in the right ponto-cerebellar angle. The nerve-roots and cranial nerves along the left aspect of the involved part of the tract are slackened. The tension produced in the nervous tissue by the tumour will give rise to a bending tensile stress, with both transverse and axial components.

On slackening of the cord obtained on extension of the cervical spine in a case such as the present one, the stress in the nervous tissue will be slightly reduced but, because of the size of the tumour, it cannot be entirely eliminated. Better access to the tumour during surgery without risk of damage to the cord can only be provided by resorting to spinal cord relaxation, which eliminates pressure of the tumour on the blood-vessels and nerve-fibres in the involved pathways.

Courtesy of H. W. Dodge, M. D., The Mayo Clinic (81). With kind permission of the Executive Assistant of the Mayo Foundation.

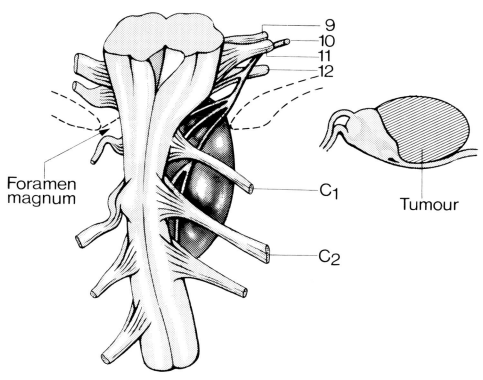

Fig. 156.

Extradural neurinoma situated on the anterior and right walls of the cervical canal. The upper section of the cervical cord is displaced posteriorly and to the left, and hence over-stretched (Case 1, p. 207).

Arrows. Denote the tumour's border-line visualized in the gas myelogram.

Courtesy of Torgny Greitz, M.D. and Arne Grepe, M.D., Karolinska Hospital, Stockholm.

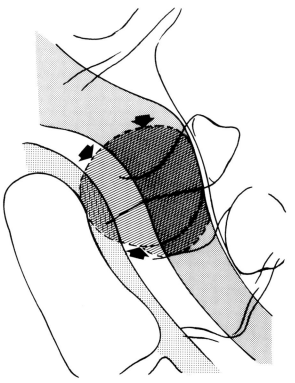

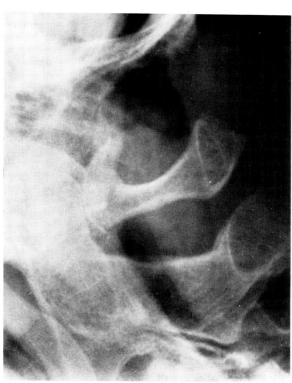

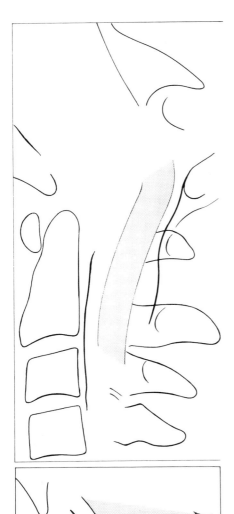

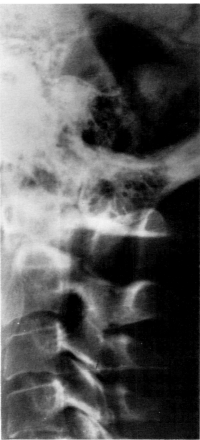

Fig. 157.

Meningioma issuing from the dura on the clivus and the anterior aspect of the foramen magnum. The uppermost section of the cord (*shaded* in the diagram) is deflected posteriorly in a wide arc, resulting in over-stretching of and bending tensile stress in the nervous tissue (Case 2, p. 208).

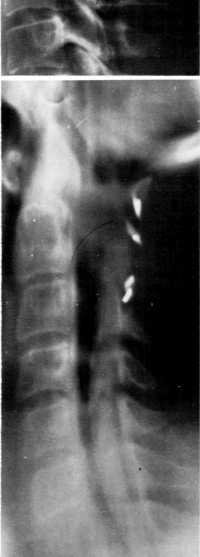

Fig. 158.

Extra- and intradural neurinoma, the extradural part of which was situated on the anterior and left surfaces of the dura, while the intradural part issued from the posterior second cervical nerve-root.

The dura and upper cervical cord are displaced posteriorly and to the right, thereby over-stretching the cord tissue (Case 3, p. 208).

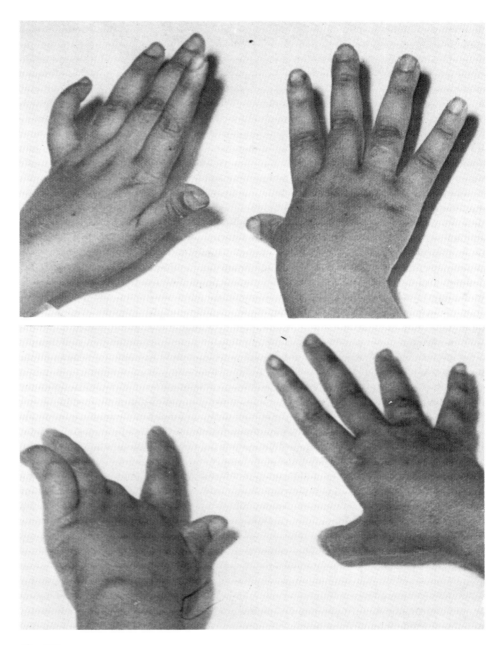

Fig. 159.

Pseudoathetosis in a patient with a neurinoma near the foramen magnum (Fig. 158)
(125). (Photographed in Cairo, 1962.)

TABLE 5. Regression of motor and sensory deficit and urinary incontinence in 18 patients with spinal cord lesions of various origins after relaxation of the pons–cord tract by cervicolordodesis.

Diagnosis	Case no.	Age	Sex	Year of operation	Preoperative state	Increase warmth in legs	Sensibility on trunk improved below level of hypaesthesia	largely recovered
Spinal cord injury (Partial transverse lesions)	1	67	♂	1970	Tetraparetic; paraplegic hands; total urinary incontinence	no annotation	not collab.	2 w
	2	18	♂	1971	Tetraparetic; paraplegic hands; total urinary incontinence	no annotation	1 d	1 w
	3	58	♂	1972	Tetraparetic; hemiplegia rt.; paraplegic hands; total urinary incontinence	no annotation	1 d	2 d
Multiple sclerosis (Spinal cord manifestations)	1	38	♂	1961	Bedridden; paraplegic spastic legs; total urinary incontinence	no annotation	1 w	3 d rt. arm
	2	29	♀	1962	Paraparetic spastic legs; total urinary incontinence	no annotation	4 d	?
	3	51	♂	1972 April 4	Tetraspasticity; impaired gait; subtotal urinary incontinence; paretic rt. arm and hand	?	–	–
				May 17	Condition unchanged except for improved power rt. arm		?	14 d
Cervical myelopathy	1	51	♀	1963	Bedridden; paraparetic spastic legs; total urinary incontinence	no annotation	14 h	?
	2	49	♀	1966	Paraparetic legs; needs cane support; subtotal urinary incontinence	no annotation	2 d	1 w
	3	59	♂	1967	Bedridden; spastic tetraparesis; total urinary incontinence	no annotation	?	?
	4	61	♂	1970	Paraparetic, spastic legs; impaired gait	+	?	?
	5	45	♂	1970	Paretic rt. leg; thermoanaesthetic rt. buttock; paraspasticity; poor rectal control	no annotation	1 d	2 w–3 mo
	6	55	♂	1971	Muscle atrophy, paresis, hypaesthesia in forearms and hands; acrocyanosis	6 h	–	–
	7	62	♂	1971	Bedridden; spastic tetraparesis; Lhermitte's sign; total urinary incontinence	6 h	2 d	1 w
	8	51	♂	1971	Muscle atrophy, paresis lt. hand; paraparetic spastic legs; Lhermitte's sign; urinary incontinence	1 d	1 d	1 d
	9	52	♂	1971	Spastic tetraparesis; Lhermitte's sign; impaired gait; urinary incontinence	4 h	1 d	1 mo
	10	52	♂	1971	Spastic tetraparesis; impaired gait; slight urinary incontinence	6 h	1 d	1 d
	11	45	♂	1972	Spastic paraparesis; impaired gait; Romberg's sign and dysarthria; slight voiding difficulty	?	–	–
	12	61	♂	1972	Spastic paraparesis; needs sticks support; severe pain in arms, increasing on flexion; slight voiding difficulty	3h	3h	2d

Cervical myelopathy

Case 1. Woman, aged 51.

Neurological history. December, 1960: paraesthesia and a feeling of heaviness in the legs, progressing in a few weeks to paraparesis. Radiating paraesthesia to the arms; on flexion of the neck, electric shock-like sensations in arms, trunk and legs.

Admitted to Karolinska Hospital, Stockholm, March, 1961.

Neurological findings. Greatly reduced power on flexing the legs, unable to extend the feet. Spastic reflexes in both legs. Bilateral extensor plantar responses. Reduced sensibility for all qualities from the iliac crest to the toes on both sides.

Radiographic and gas myelographic examination. Spondylosis with extremely large protrusions, especially on a level with the intervertebral discs C_5/C_6 and C_6/C_7.

Operation 1 (X.X.), March, 1961. Conventional bilateral

Bladder/bowel		Recovery of mobility in arms (A), legs (L)		Able to walk with support (S), unsupported (U)	Spasticity of legs clearly reduced	Factors bearing on efficiency of spinal cord relaxation; degree of restriction
Sensation largely improved	control recovered	Slight	Marked			
w	?	(A) 4 d–2 w	(A) rt., 4 w	(U) 4 w	6.5 mo	Prostatectomy some years earlier; indwelling catheter not removed for 3 mo
w	1 w	1 w	(L) lt., 2.5 mo	(S) 2.5 mo	2.5 mo	
d	4 d	(L) rt. 2 d +(hand) lt. 10 d	able to sit	6 d		10 d postop., urinary infection and epididymitis; 10 d later, haematemesis and melaena (X-ray exam. some weeks later disclosed gastric carcinoma)
w	4 w	(L) 3 w	–	–	–	Movements in legs and toes transient and feeble; micturition urgency after 3 h
w	1 w	(L) 2 w	(A) 2 w	(S) 2 w	?	Urinary retention (4 d)
–		(A) rt., 1 d		–	–	5 d postop., wound infection. Graft loosened and range of flexion of head increased
	1 d	3 h	8 d	(U) 8 d	14 d	After reoperation head kept firmly in slight extension
d	2 d (transient)	(L) 3 d (transient)	–	to sit	3 d (transient)	Relapse after recovery of neck mobility due to slipping of bone graft
w	1 w	(L) 2 d	(L) 1 w	(U) 1 w	–	Tendon reflexes absent (congenital lues). Symptom-free 4 years. Relapse after spinal traction
w	1 w	1 w	(L) 1 w	(U) 1 w	1 w	Burning sensation in rt. leg returned at nights. Motor power normalized. Spastic & atactic gait
–		(A) 3 w	(L) 3 mo	+	?	20-yr left-sided headache relieved. Unsatisfactory operative technique
	3 mo	(L) 3 d	(L) 3 w	+	3 w	3 mo: sphincter ani function
–		(A) 3 w +hands		+		Raynaud-like acrocyanosis and power recovered in hands
d	4 d	1 w	(A) 1 w (L) 2 w	to sit	+	Urinary retention after operation. Neurological signs after 6 800 rad for laryngeal cancer
d	4 d	(A) 1 d	(A) 1 d (L) 1 d	4 d	4 d–4 w	Paraesthesia in fingers for 1 w after operation
d	1 d	(A) 1 d	(A) 1 mo (L) 1 mo	(U) 1 mo	(U) 1 mo	3 d after operation urinary retention lasting some days
d	2 d	(A) 1 w (L) 2 w	(A) 2 w (L) 2 w	(U) 2 w	?	8 h after op. urinary retention; tapped once; thereafter normal function
	3 d	(L) 1 d	(L) 2 w	2 w gait improved	3 w	Low back pain vanished; Romberg's sign relieved
	3 d	(A) 3 d (L) 3 d	(L) 1 w (A) 3 w	1 w gait nearly normalized	1 w	Postoperative urinary infection, controlled by antibiotics

laminectomy C_5 to C_7. Cervical spinal cord made closest contact with the protrusions at C_7 level (effect of maximum functional positions not checked). Borders of the dura, opened in the midline, sutured up to the neck muscles on both sides.

Postoperative course. A cerebrospinal fluid fistula had to be closed by secondary suture. Neurological condition deteriorated, with moderate urinary and bowel incontinence. Unable to rise from the supine position or to stand or walk. Superficial sensibility slightly improved, deep sensibility worse. Admitted to hospital for the disabled.

Neurological findings. August, 1962, condition unchanged. Paraparesis, almost amounting to paraplegia. Bilateral foot clonus and extensor plantar responses. Sensibility reduced below umbilical level. No vibratory sensation on either side. Paraesthesia in both arms, power not appreciably reduced. Biceps and triceps reflexes spastic. Bladder automatism: spontaneous emptying every second hour or so; could start but not stop urination.

Gas myelogram (July, 1963). The largest protrusions at C_4/C_5 level.

Operation 2 (author) at Red Cross Hospital, Stockholm, July 1963. Extirpation of C_4/C_5 protrusion by anterior access and Cloward's instruments. On the anterior side of vertebral bodies of C_4 to C_7 a diagonal groove was drilled to take a tibia

bone graft about 8–9 mm wide. With the patient's neck reclined over a firm round bolster the graft was hammered into
this groove so as to achieve osseous healing of the spine in
extension.

Postoperative course uneventful apart from mild, transient
adynamic ileus. Neck placed on round bolster to keep the cervical spine in extension. Day after the operation paraesthesia
diminished appreciably in the arms and below umbilical level.
Increased sensibility in the sacral and perineovaginal region
and better control over bladder and bowels.

On second and third postoperative days spasticity in the legs
diminished markedly and power in foot extensor muscles and
gluteal muscles increased. For the first time for many years
could perform small abduction and adduction movements of
legs. From the 4th postoperative day no further improvements.

Radiographic examination, August and October, 1963. Lower
section of cervical spine straight. In lateral view, bone transplant projects 1–2 mm on anterior aspect of vertebrae. Stabilization of whole cervical column in straight position.

Two or three weeks after operation spasticity returned, with
difficulty in controlling bladder. After energetic rehabilitatory
training patient since 1964 able to stand with support and other
aids and to manage household work. Compared with former
bedridden existence at a hospital for chronic invalids, present
state represents progress for her, despite persisting difficulties.

Case 2. Woman, aged 49.

Admitted to Department of Neurology, Karolinska Hospital,
Stockholm, November, 1966.

Neurological history. Hutchinson teeth from congenital
syphilis. Several specific forms of treatment received. Since
1940 sporadic temporal lobe attacks. No mental defect, rather
intelligent and quick-witted. Dragged left leg for last 9 years.
1962, began to feel a cushion-like paraesthesia under right
foot, spreading gradually through whole leg to thigh and but-
tock; numbness appeared in left foot and leg and in both
palms. For 1 year, 1965, heaviness in legs. Since 1960 irregular
bowels; since 1964 urgency and incontinence of urine. For
some months, girdle pains around abdomen; almost daily
radiating pain in occipital region. Unable to walk without a
stick.

Neurological findings. Gait unsteady. Romberg's sign positive. Vibratory sensation reduced below both iliac crests and
abolished in both legs; perception for touch and temperature
and pain slightly diminished below umbilical level. Tendon
reflexes abolished in legs.

Radiographic examination of cervical spine. Large bony protrusions at C_5/C_6 level with great reduction in height of disc.

Gas myelogram. (No examination in extreme functional positions.) Cervical canal quite narrow, with soft tissue borders
3 mm wide on anterior and posterior contours. In the neutral
position cord was in contact with the protrusion present at the
level of the degenerated C_5/C_6 disc.

Cerebrospinal fluid pressure. Complete block on extension
of cervical spine.

Operation (author), 8 November, 1966. Protective bilateral
laminectomy C_2–C_7; immobilization of cervical spine in
moderate extension by fascia lata graft (same procedure as in
Case 3).

Postoperative course uneventful. Considerable improvement according to neurologist who took over the check of
postoperative state. Paresis of central type in right leg disappeared, sensibility in legs much recovered. Regained normal
control of bladder. Gait steady; no longer reliant on support.

Radiographic examination of cervical spine. Lordosis remained even when the patient tried to bend head forwards
as much as possible.

Follow-up check (author), February, 1967. On bending neck
forwards from neutral position strain encountered; hence difficulty in descending stairs; lateral movements of head and extension unrestricted. Extremely satisfied with the results of the
operation. Gait normal on flat ground; stick no longer required. No occipital pain. Vibratory sensation normalized in
legs. Deep sensibility slightly impaired in toes of right foot.

The strength of the fascia lata graft was evidenced in a dras-
tic manner. A physician unaware of the purpose of the operation was unable to bend the head forward a fortnight after the
operation.

Follow-up-check at Visby Hospital, November, 1970. Postoperative improvement largely retained; arm and leg reflexes
normal, no spasticity. Babinski's sign absent. Sensibility decreased in right hand, power slightly decreased in right hand
and leg. Sensibility for all qualities, including vibratory sensation, normal below umbilical plane with the exception of slight
paraesthesia in the sole of the right foot. After spinal traction
by a physiotherapist for pain in the lower back (*sic*) pain
developed in the neck, with periodic slight difficulty in controlling the bladder. Cervicolordodesis properly retained (X-
ray check) with no impediment to the movements of head or
spine other than flexion.

Case 3. Man, aged 59.

Neurological history. Severe cervical myelopathy and cervical rhizopathy.

In May, 1966, there was paraesthesia and numbness in the
legs and spasmodic pain in the calves; legs unsteady. Loss of
power and numbness in the arms followed, especially the right
one, which it was difficult to raise to the neck. Fingers stiff
and fumbling. Pain between the shoulder blades on coughing
and sneezing. Headache resembling migraine cervicale.

Neurological findings. Spastic tetraparesis. Babinski's sign
positive bilaterally. Sensibility reduced below the C_4 level.

Admitted to Department of Neurosurgery, Karolinska Hospital, January, 1967. Bedridden. Total urinary incontinence;
catheter *à demeure*. Frozen right shoulder; severe pain.
Oedema in right hand involving all fingers. Able to move the
right hand only slightly; unable to raise arms through more
than 45°. Constant pain in right lower leg.

Severe spasticity in both legs with inexhaustible patellar and
Achilles tendon clonus. Bilateral extensor plantar reflexes.
Below iliac crest vibratory sensation abolished in legs and pain
sensibility reduced. Below middle of lower legs pin-prick perceived only as pressure.

Radiographic examination of cervical spine. Prominent
protrusions at C_6/C_7 and C_7/T_1. On flexion, anterolisthesis between C_5 and C_6.

Operation (author), January, 1967. Protective bilateral laminectomy C_2 to C_7. Cervical column immobilized in moderate

extension by means of a 5–6 cm wide fascia lata graft sutured to periosteum of lower border of occipital bone and spinous process of T_1. Between these points, fascia folded double to form, between neck muscles, a sagittal band whose posterior border was sutured to transverse cervical fascia. Day after operation, wound rupture (neck muscles unusually voluminous).

Postoperative course after resuturing uneventful. In next few days spasticity in arms and legs diminished. No patellar clonus, no Achilles tendon clonus on left side any longer (right Achilles tendon reflex absent since earlier discal hernia). After intensive physiotherapy right arm could be abducted again to 90° in shoulder joint. Now able to bend the fingers to about 3–4 cm from palm of right hand. Burning sensation in the right leg disappeared during daytime but returned at nights. Normal strength in the legs recovered except for an old extensor paresis in right foot (defect after discal hernia). Vibratory sensation recovered in both legs except on inside of right tibia. Able to walk without support, but gait definitely spastic and atactic. Recovered practically normal 24-hour bladder control. Able to urinate even in supine position.

Radiographic examination of cervical column in extreme functional positions. Kyphosis still marked in lower cervical column. On slight flexion of cervical spine, a pulling sensation in the neck; full flexion no longer possible because of the graft.

Follow-up check. One year later the patient complained of increased, barely tolerable brachialgia (telephone conversation) but none of the previous neurological symptoms had recurred. Patient did not appear for follow-up examination.

Comments and discussion (Cases 1–3)

Only some 24 hours after surgical slackening of the pons–cord tract, all 3 patients found an increase in sensibility in the lower part of the body, including the legs. The paraesthesia in arms and hands also disappeared almost completely after a time. The vibratory sensation returned in Cases 2 and 3. Urinary incontinence, which had been slight in Cases 1 and 2 and total in no. 3, completely disappeared in Cases 2 and 3. These two patients recovered complete bladder control; the patient presented as Case 1 recovered good control of the bladder and bowels only temporarily—probably only so long as the cervical spine was in extension (see below).

In Cases 1 and 3 the severe spasticity diminished significantly in 2–3 days. In Case 2 there was also an increase in the mobility of the paretic leg; the nature of the paresis, probably spastic, was difficult to assess, because the ankle reflexes were absent as a consequence of tabes in connection with the congenital syphilis. In any case this paresis ultimately also disappeared almost completely after the operation; the patient was again able to walk without a stick. If the paresis was not connected with the myelopathy due to the protrusion but with the sequelae of the congenital syphilis, the improvement might throw light on the value of using slackening of the pons–cord tract to diminish symptom-producing histodynamic effects of other parenchymal

processes than those considered here. The cause of the paresis of the leg in the present case is, however, so obscure that there is little to be gained by discussing the circumstances surrounding its occurrence and disappearance.

There are, on the other hand, some other aspects of this case that are of particular interest. To obtain a reliable basis for analysing the mechanism of origin of the cervical myelopathy, it is necessary to perform tomographic air myelography and to check the mechanical effect of the protrusion on the cervical cord in extreme functional positions (43). Since this examination was not performed for some reason, reliance was placed on measurement of CSF pressure during Queckenstedt's test in extension of the cervical spine; a block being recorded in this position, the myelopathy was ascribed to compression of the cervical cord. It is true that the cervical canal was fairly shallow (no preoperative measurements of its diameter or that of the cord were available) and the soft tissues were so thick that, to judge from the block, they interfered with the normal passage of fluid. However, since full extension of the cervical spine obviously did not result in any increase in the neurological symptoms, this mechanical constellation cannot have resulted in more than extremely slight and intermittent compression. If there had in fact been compression and it was not simply a question of contact between the intraspinal soft tissues the degree of this compression will therefore have been so small as hardly to justify use of the term compression. This conclusion is justified in the light of the results of the present investigation into the nature of the compressive stress and the outcome for the present and similar cases. Furthermore, the mere fact that the neurological symptoms disappeared completely almost immediately after relaxation of the pons–cord tract indicates the absence of appreciable compression; for such compression always leads to persistent symptoms, as it invariably produces permanent damage to the nervous tissues (p. 55). The gas myelographic evidence that, even in the neutral posture, the cord was in contact with the large protrusion on the anterior aspect of the cervical canal suggests that the symptoms must have had their origin in the familiar tension produced by the spondylotic protrusions (52, 216). If the neurological symptoms had been produced by compression they would have been of a different nature, namely of the type associated with central cervical spinal cord injury. However, in spite of the fact that marked compression had thus not yet supervened, there were well-founded grounds for performing laminectomy, since there was a risk that in forced extension of the cervical spine—for instance, in a whip-lash movement—the cervical cord might ultimately have been subjected to a deleterious pincer action (91, 216).

Postoperative radiographic checks of the cervical spine provided an acceptable explanation of the positive effects of the operation in Case 2 (permanent extension position of the cervical spine), the not entirely adequate effect in Case 3 (the lower cervical vertebrae still kyphosed with increasing kyphosis in full flexion) and failure in Case 1. If in this case it had been possible to obtain permanent extension with the bone graft, this patient would have constituted an example *par excellence* where the clearly unsatisfactory result of the earlier 'classic' method—laminectomy, division of the dentate ligaments and suturing of the dura to the neck muscles (which in the present case was followed by definite deterioration)—could be compared with the otherwise irrefutable advantages of the relaxation method.

As is evident from the radiographs in Case 1, which were not taken until some weeks after the operation, the tibia bone graft, which had initially been adapted to the extended posture of the cervical column, healed firmly in the *neutral* posture. The first few days after the operation a careful watch had been kept to ensure that the extended position of the cervical spine was retained. Since no Crutchfield's forceps had been applied to guarantee this position, a single flexion movement—for instance, while the bed was being made—might have sufficed to disturb the position of the graft. There can be little doubt at all today that the patient's neurological deterioration after the initial improvement was due to a change in position of the cervical column. On the other hand, the reason why the neurological symptoms were not so definite and therefore as incapacitating as before the reoperation is most probably that immobilization of the cervical spine occurred in the neutral position. In any case, in this position the lowermost and otherwise most mobile part of the cervical spine could no longer be flexed. That the neutral position of the cervical column was not more effective may be due to the fact that the protrusions could not be completely removed and a thrust on the cord thus persisted; furthermore, the vertebrae may have been forced into an extended (elongated) position by the bone graft when it was pressed into its groove. It is also possible that the suturing of the dura to the muscles performed at the first operation may have accounted in part for the fact that the relaxation effect on the dura, and hence on the remaining dentate ligaments and the pons–cord tract, was smaller than would otherwise have been the case.

In Case 3 a slightly better result was achieved after the fascia lata graft. The reason why a laminectomy was performed in this patient despite the spacious cervical canal is that there was a spondylolisthesis between C_5 and C_6 that in extension may have been converted into a retrolisthesis, thus resulting in a pincer action on the cord. In transplantation of the fascia lata strip it was intended to fix it in a stretched position corresponding to the slight extension of the head, but this was not entirely successful, as the postoperative radiographs showed (wound rupture may have been one reason). The residual kyphosis of the lower section of the cervical spine prompted the idea of inserting wedge-shaped bone grafts in the intervertebral spaces by an-

terolateral access *ad modum* Verbiest at any reoperation (260). In Case 2 with a positive postoperative result there was a clear relationship between the total disappearance of the neurological symptoms and the perfectly stable extension position of the cervical spine. The negative experience in Case 1 means that a pair of Crutchfield's forceps inserted in the frontal bone and loaded with a weight of 500 grams (rather than a plaster cast) are to be recommended as a means of ensuring and safely retaining the reclined position over a round bolster—even at night. The requisite degree of extension should be determined by means of a radiograph of the cervical spine. This picture can then be compared with lateral films taken on the operating-table before and after application of the fascia or bone graft. This has proved an indispensable measure for guaranteeing an adequate degree of extension of the cervical column.

Cases 1 and 2 had slight and Case 3 extremely marked cervical rhizopathy. In the latter case the relaxation of the tract was followed by reduction both of the radicular symptoms such as the nerve-root pains, the weakness and fibrillations in the arm muscles and hands and of the funicular symptoms such as the spastic arm reflexes. In this way confirmation was obtained of the polyvalent effects of the functional spinal cord surgery.

Because of the traction on the dura, dentate ligaments, cord and nerve-roots in the caudal part of the spinal canal, with undesirable neurological symptoms as a possible consequence, the suturing of the cervical dura to the muscle has no place as a standard neurosurgical method.

Case 4. Fig. 148.

Case 5. Figs. 149 and 150.

Case 6. Man aged 55.

Neurological history, 1958. Reduced power in right hand, atrophy of small hand muscles and hypersensitivity to cold. Steady loss of power. Troubled by stiffness and fumbling of hands and fingers and reduced sensation in tips of fingers and toes. *1961:* Sciatica on right side.

1959: Radiographic examination of cervical spine showed spondylosis deformans with osteophytes, especially at the C_5/C_6 and C_6/C_7 levels.

1962: Electromyogram. Damage to peripheral motor neurones with partial denervation. *Operation.* Right ulnar nerve transposition. No improvement.

1967: Neurological findings. Power in left hand diminished. Mobility reduced in thumb, followed by the whole hand and the forearm. Aching at the back of the neck in the mornings.

1968: Gas myelogram. Marked protrusion of soft tissues corresponding to C_5/C_6 disc, mostly on left side. *Cerebrospinal fluid pressure.* Partial block on bending cervical spine backwards. *Neurological findings.* Marked atrophy of interossei muscles (and short abductor muscle of thumb) of right hand, slight atrophy of interossei muscles and abductor muscle of little finger of left hand and left triceps muscle. Squeeze dynamometer right 15, left 30.

1970: Neurological findings. Rapid progress of symptoms in left arm and hand, increasing fasciculations in both arms up to shoulders. No pain. Marked reduction in power of left triceps muscle and wrist-drop. Reduction in sensibility in both hands, especially thumb and index finger of left hand. Slight hypoaesthesia on the radial aspect of left upper arm, more markedly so on radial aspect of forearm.

Radiographic examination. Greatly reduced height of C_5/C_6 and C_6/C_7 intervertebral spaces with osteophytes on borders of vertebral bodies, especially at the C_5/C_6 level. These protruded far into the intervertebral foramina, especially at the C_5/C_6 level.

Fairly marked cyanosis of the arms and especially hands, which were cold and sweaty. Likewise marked acrocyanosis of feet (reminiscent of Raynaud's disease). Fasciculations in left thumb, especially on waking. No definite neurological manifestations from the long spinal pathways.

Neurophysiological examination. Signs of injury to the peripheral motor neurones in left extensor muscle of fingers, abductor muscle of little finger and left dorsal interossei muscles with partial denervation of the last of these muscles. The reason for the ulnar nerve neuropathy could not be detected by ENG.

Neurological findings, 1971. Both arms atrophied, especially left triceps muscle. Extensor muscles of forearm also paretic, with wrist-drop and greatly diminished extensor power in all fingers. Fourth and fifth fingers slightly flexed, suggesting paresis of ulnar nerve. Sense of touch, pain and temperature reduced from elbow, increasing in distal direction, especially marked in finger and toe pads. Reflexes brisk in arms and legs, absent in triceps and brachioradialis muscles on left side. Plantar response normal bilaterally. *ENG:* Left ulnar nerve lesion at level of elbow; peripheral radial nerve paresis. *Synchronous oscillography.* No sign of obstruction of larger arm arteries.

Operation (author), February, 1971. Bilateral hemifacetectomy C_5/C_6 and exposure of C_6 root-sheaths to the ganglia; bilateral minor hemifacetectomy C_6/C_7 and protective bilateral laminectomy C_5; cervicolordodesis with fascia lata graft. To relieve load on graft neck was placed on a round bolster and bent backwards. Schantz collar.

Postoperative course and neurological findings. Postoperative course uneventful. Some hours after operation a sensation of warmth in both hands and feet was experienced for first time for several years. A fortnight later sensation in the arms and hands was restored almost to normal. Increased motor power in left arm and both hands. Acrocyanosis no longer apparent. Subjective and objective improvement in general condition; sleep satisfactory and balance recovered.

Follow-up examinations (3 May, 1971). Left thumb could be opposed and fingers could be separated and approximated; power in hand and forearm (extension) increased. No longer wrist-drop or fibrillations in left forearm.

15 February and 3 May, 1972. The postoperative improvement lasted some months. Then, after stretching in bed (no further details available, but presumably forced flexion of the cervical spine on changing his position) the patient had radiating pains in left shoulder. Power in left arm and hand diminished again;

now some fumbling; slight reduction in sensibility of ulnar aspect of left hand. *Objective findings.* Head could be bent forwards much more than during the first months just after the operation, and it is obvious that the graft was no longer fully effective. The patient associated the deterioration with an increased range of flexion of the cervical spine; reoperation desired. Promised graft of stronger material.

Case 7. Man aged 62.

Neurological history, 1952; Low back pain treated with corset. *1968:* Carcinoma of the larynx, confirmed by extirpation in June, 1970, and treated by high voltage X-rays with the cervical glands as the target (altogether 6 800 rad); three months later weakness of left leg, and soon thereafter of right leg and left arm. Paralysis progressed rapidly, ultimately to affect all four extremities; the patient could no longer walk. Towards the end of January, cushion-sensation in both feet, with increasing spread cranialwards. On slight bending of the neck electric shock-like sensation radiating into both legs and, on further bending, also to arms and hands (Lhermitte's sign). Permanent paraesthesia in both hands especially the left. On admission to the Department of Neurosurgery total urinary and bowel incontinence (indwelling catheter); no sensation when bladder filled or stool passed.

Neurological findings. Spastic tetraparesis, more marked on left. Unable to extend left foot; able to extend knee slightly but not flex it. Greatly reduced power for same movements in right leg. Paresis of right arm and especially of right hand; left arm weak, fingers could not be extended, and bent only feebly. Much reduced sensitivity to touch below umbilical plane, on left more than right. Anaesthesia to warm and cold from costal arch to groin on right side; greatly reduced below this level, less so in left leg; anaesthesia for pain in same region as for temperature; greatly reduced in the rest of the right leg, except for foot; sensitivity to pain also greatly reduced from middle of left tibia peripherally.

Radiographic examination. Height of intervertebral spaces greatly reduced at C_3/C_4, C_4/C_5 and C_5/C_6 with big osteophytes reducing the anteroposterior diameter of *canal* to about 10 mm. Anterolisthesis of C_3 vertebral body. Cervical spine displayed marked kyphosis through the section in question.

Gas myelogram. Space visible only above the C_4 and below the C_7 vertebrae. Anteroposterior diameter of thoracic *cord* reduced to about 6 mm.

Operation (author), 12 March, 1971. Protective bilateral laminectomy C_4–C_6, protective arco-cristectomy C_7 and cervicolordodesis with Marlex mesh.[1]

Postoperative course and neurological findings. About 6 hours after surgery patient had a sensation of warmth in arms and feet. Gradual regression of anaesthesia and hypoaesthesia during next 2 days; sensitivity to pain and temperature stimuli recovered soon on right side of abdomen and lower part of left leg and foot. Sensitivity to distention of bladder and bowels returned 3–4 days after surgery. After a fortnight, power in right arm, hand, leg and foot much improved. Persistent tenderness in left wrist; fingers remained semiflexed but looser;

---

[1] C. R. Bard Davol, Murley Hills, New Jersey, USA.

grasp slightly more powerful but still feeble. Spasticity regressed slowly bilaterally.

On 2nd day after surgery slight fluid discharge from lower part of neck wound, which ruptured 12 days after operation (discharge so copious that CSF discharge suspected). Resuturing of all layers.

Comment. Spinal cord relaxation was regarded as especially urgent in view of the probable X-ray damage to the cord besides that due to the marked narrowing and kyphosis of the cervical spine. A sensitive cord is probably still more susceptible to mechanical stress (local over-stretching due to sub-critical compression, and bending tensile stress).

Case 8. Man, aged 51 (no. 8, Table 5).

Case 9. Man, aged 52.

Neurological history. In summer of 1969 the cervical spine had been forced sharply backwards when the patient dived into shallow water. He felt an electric shock-like sensation radiating to both arms. Persistent numbness in arms and hands together with a sensation of cold. Pain in arms elicited by coughing. Sensation in arms and hands deteriorated after December, 1969. Since then also slowly progressing weakness of arms, hands and legs.

Neurological findings, January, *1970.* Flaccid paresis in arms and hands; spastic paraparesis in legs. Babinski's sign positive bilaterally.

Admitted to Department of Neurosurgery, Karolinska Hospital, March 1971.

Neurological findings. Greatly reduced power in arms and hands, especially on right. Fingers of right hand crooked and could not be extended. Could not manage buttons or wind up the clock. Reduced power in legs. Spastic and atactic gait. Could walk only slowly, with aid of a stick. Spastic tremor in legs when seated; unable to rise from this position. Able to walk downstairs only with difficulty. Reduced sensation in arms, greatly so in hands. Proprioception and vibratory sensation normal. On flexing of the head and coughing, paraesthesia radiated to ulnar aspect of forearms and hands, and to knee region. Reduced sensibility below nipple level; reduced perception for all qualities in the legs; abolished vibratory sensation. Urinary incontinence; perception of defaecation; able to void only small portions after delay. Paresis of anal sphincter; much reduced perception on evacuating bowels; urgency of defaecation. Reflexes in arms slightly increased, in legs still more so; Babinski's sign positive bilaterally.

Radiographic examination. Reduced height of the C_5/C_6 and C_6/C_7 intervertebral spaces. Shallow cervical canal with large osteophytes on margins of vertebral bodies protruding into the intervertebral foramina at these levels.

Gas myelogram. From C_3 to C_7, soft tissues on anterior aspect of canal thickened. Between C_6 and C_7, large protrusion impinging slightly on the narrowed but not atrophied cervical cord in the supine position.

Operation (author), September, 1971. Protective bilateral laminectomy C_4–C_6, protective arco-cristectomy C_7, bilateral hemifacetectomy C_5/C_6 and cervicolordodesis (Mersilene mesh).

Postoperative course and neurological findings. The healing of the surgical wound was poor; there was bleeding and, later, an accumulation of serous fluid around the mesh. Local administration of penicillin.

Four hours after the operation the hands and feet were warm, subjectively warmer than for several years. According to bedside test there was no longer any loss of sensibility in the arms, trunk or legs. Twenty-four hours after operation, voiding was satisfactory and there was no longer urinary incontinence; could pass urine even in the supine position. On the 3rd postoperative day, urinary retention 950 ml; after that, micturition was normal. Normal sensation over whole body, including sacral dermatomes, except for slight residual reduction in sensibility below the knees. Proprioception slightly reduced. Able to move arms and legs freely in supine position. Improved power and mobility in hands; right hand was still weaker than normal but previously crooked fingers now extended without difficulty. On day after operation he could sit on the edge of the bed; thereafter mobilized increasingly; 4 weeks later persistent (possibly increased) disturbance of sensibility on volar aspect of finger-tips where a pin-prick could just be perceived. Improved power in arms and hands on both flexion and extension but still difficulty in managing buttons. Walking considerably improved; able to go up 7 flights without resting, and 3 without holding the banister, but still some difficulty in balancing. Required support of banister when going downstairs to avoid swaying to the side. No bladder problems; normal sensation of filling and emptying; no retention. Power in arms and legs fully recovered (right only slightly weaker); reflexes on right slightly increased. Patellar reflexes normal, slightly increased reflexogenic zone. Achilles reflexes: clonus of short duration on right, one beat on left. Babinski's sign ambiguous bilaterally. Flexion of head braked in neutral position; unable to tie his shoe-laces. He was most pleased with the results of the operation, and no longer felt any Lhermitte's paraesthesia. Surgical wound not completely healed when discharged.

Case 10. Man, aged 52.

Neurological history. Since spring of 1970 aching pain in lumbar region, radiating to right leg. Increasing weakness in both legs especially the right. Some months later, pain and fumbling, first in right hand and then in the left, associated with numbness in the ulnar fingers. Difficulty in controlling bladder.

Neurological findings, January, *1971.* Reduced gross power in all extremities, especially the legs. Muscular atrophy and contracture in right hand. Slight tremor in right hand, reduced vibratory sensation in left leg. Increased tendon reflexes in arms and legs with patellar and Achilles clonus.

Admitted to Department of Neurosurgery, Karolinska Hospital, 26 October, 1971.

Radiographic examination. C_5/C_6 disc lowered. Osteophytes on borders of adjacent vertebral bodies decrease the lumen of a slightly shallow cervical canal.

Gas myelogram. Protrusions of soft tissues along anterior aspect of cervical canal. Cord at C_5–C_6 level flattened; practically no gas visible.

Neurological findings. Gross power reduced in arms and

hands, especially the right hand, where there was contracture of thenar and atrophy of hypothenar. Gross power reduced in legs, especially the right. Difficulty in raising right leg from couch and in standing on toes; unable to stand on right heel. Increased tendon reflexes in arms and legs. Bilateral patellar clonus, inexhaustible Achilles clonus. Babinski's sign positive bilaterally.

Operation (author), 4 November, 1971. Protective bilateral laminectomy C_5 and C_6, protective arco-cristectomy C_7 and cervicolordodesis (Mersilene mesh). The mesh was anchored in the periosteum around the external occipital protuberance and in the T_1/T_2 interspinous ligament with Tycron sutures.

Postoperative course and neurological findings. Wound healing delayed. About 6 hours after operation there was a sensation of warmth in the hands and feet; after 8 hours, urinary retention, 500 ml drained; catheter *à demeure* in place for about 24 hours. Temperature 38.8°. On postoperative day 2 able to sit up in bed, and on day 3 in a chair. Power in arms and hands increasingly improved. Transferred to Red Cross Hospital for exercise of arms, legs and right hand. Gradual improvement. Gait still uncertain, with tendency to limp on right side; tires easily. Mobility and power good in right leg, somewhat weaker in left. Right arm weaker than left in all functions. On discharge after 3 months, reflexes lively, Babinski's sign positive bilaterally.

Follow-up, 15 March, 1972. Managed daily walks of at least 1 hour before tiring. Gait still unsteady. Right arm and hand stronger, fumbling unchanged. Flexion of cervical spine evokes radiating paraesthesia in ulnar fingers of left hand.

15 May. Less marked fumbling with right hand. Greater steadiness in walking. Able to stand on the heels and raise both feet equally well; could stand on either leg and keep balance with the other leg raised high. Babinski's sign positive; clonus disappeared. Working 4 hours a day in former occupation as car enameller. Graft came into action as a brake only when the head was bent forwards almost halfway from the erect posture.

26 March, 1973. Power normalized in both arms and hands. Has resumed his former work. Walks 6–7 hours daily. Slightly atactic gait.

Case 11. Man, aged 45.

Neurological history. Over previous 3 years increasing fatigue and loss of control of right leg, followed a year later by same symptoms in left leg. Limped; fell easily, then difficult to get on legs again. Difficulty in starting micturition. Effort followed by pain on right side above iliac crest and in lumbar region. Felt invalidized through his inability to walk properly.

Admitted to Department of Neurosurgery, Karolinska Hospital, 23 February, 1972.

Neurological findings. Suspected pallor of the optic disc; sometimes dysarthria; slight facial palsy on right side. Paraspasticity especially on right side, stiff dragging spastic gait. Drop-foot on right, occasional overextension of right knee (*genu recurvatum*). Some evidence of atrophy of right thigh and extensor muscles of lower leg. Unable to stand on heels, or raise right foot. Vibratory sensation reduced, especially on the right, increasing distally from thorax; on left, distally from iliac crest. Proprioception reduced, especially on left. Reflexes: patellar reflex raised on right, inexhaustible foot clonus on

right, 3 or 4 beats on left. Babinski's sign positive on right, less marked on left side. Romberg's sign: marked swaying in all directions.

Radiographic examination. Cervical canal normal in width. All intervertebral spaces below C_4 lowered; C_5/C_6 lowered to less than one half. Large osteophytes on adjacent vertebral bodies, protruding into the canal and slightly into the intervertebral foramina.

Gas myelogram. Protrusions of soft tissues from C_3 to C_7. Protrusion C_5/C_6 narrowed canal lumen by 6 mm, and in supine position made contact with the cervical cord.

CSF pressure normal.

Other examinations. Electrophoresis on CSF: no definite evidence of a demyelinizing process. Tecnetium scintigram (suspected parasagittal meningioma) July, 1970, normal.

Operation, (author) 24 February, 1972. Protective bilateral laminectomy C_5 and C_6; protective arco-cristectomy C_4 and cervicolordodesis (Mersilene mesh).

Postoperative course and neurological findings. Uneventful. The wound healed normally (drain removed on the second, and the last sutures on tenth postoperative day.) The patient sat on the edge of the bed the day after the operation, and was thereafter increasingly mobilized. The bladder symptoms disappeared completely, as did the pains in the hip and back. Gait slowly improved. A fortnight after the operation the patient walked from the second to the tenth floor under the supervision of a physiotherapist, taking 2 steps at a time; longer paces were now possible, but the gait was still slightly spastic and atactic, with a tendency for a slight limp on the right. Now able to lift the leg and foot more easily and higher; there was hardly any difference between the right and left limbs. The feeling of unsteadiness was less marked although it was still experienced after rapid turns. The brake took effect just when the cervical spine was in the neutral position. The patient warmly recommended the operation to others with similar symptoms.

Objective findings. Vibratory sensation still slightly worse on right. Patellar reflexes lively (had been walking just before the check), but no increase in reflexogenic zone. Achilles reflexes lively, left 2 slight beats, right none. Babinski's sign weakly positive on right side, indeterminate or normal on left.

Discharged to Rehabilitation Department for further exercise.

Follow-up examination 14 August, 1972. Range of foward bending movement of head greater than intended. Walking capacity slightly poorer than during first months after operation; able to manage stairs and to lift feet well; gait slightly unsteady. Troubled by poor balance, especially during warm summer days; tended to stumble, especially over right leg. Occasional tenderness along right trapezius muscle. Recovery of normal sensibility and bladder control maintained. Habitually held head bent forwards and slightly to right.

Case 12. Man, aged 61.

Neurological history. Since 1965 constant dull pain in back of neck and shoulder region. Mid-1970, radiating pain and paraesthesia in both arms, spreading from little fingers to involve hands, forearms and upper arms. Since early 1971 tingling sensation in both legs, which felt cold and dead, especially the backs; periodic reduction in sensation over the whole body. Simultaneously weakness and reduced power in the legs and feet, most noticeable when standing. Unable to raise toes from ground. In summer of 1971 power reduced in hands. Sometimes unable to hold a fork or manage buttons. In both forward and backward bending of the head, radiating electric shock-like sensation in arms, hands and all fingers (Lhermitte's sign).

Unsteady on legs; obliged to use a stick or crutch to feel safe. After walking a few hundred metres, increasing numbness, stiffness and fatigue in legs. Dragging gait increasingly marked, it being necessary to swing the feet forwards. Fell frequently, especially when turning. Six months previously urinary incontinence; now better, though unable to control flow.

Neurological findings. General atrophy of muscles of shoulder, upper arm, forearm and hands, especially of thumbs. Lively arm reflexes bilaterally. Reduced sense of touch on the volar and dorsal aspects of the hands; could not feel pin-prick in thumbs. Vibratory sensation in arms and hands normal. Sensibility to touch reduced below costal arch; sensation of cold on anterior and posterior surfaces of body. Lower extremities: no definite atrophy. Reduced power in raising legs and extending knees, especially on left; unable to stand on heels. Increased reflexes, spasticity in left leg. Babinski's sign uncertain on right, positive on left, withdrawal reflex. Proprioception more or less normal. Vibratory sensation reduced below knees, absent in right foot. Gait spastic-atactic, left leg less well controlled. Need to raise legs unusually high because the feet dropped. Romberg's sign: inclined to fall forwards. Knee–heel test: slight ataxia and dysdiadochokinesia.

Radiographic examination and gas myelogram. All cervical discs lowered, especially C_4/C_5, C_5/C_6 and C_6/C_7. Large osteophytes on borders of adjacent vertebral bodies, with narrowing of intervertebral foramina, same on right and left sides. Narrow spinal canal. Anterolisthesis C_4/C_5, C_4 displaced 3–4 mm anterior to C_5. Soft tissues from C_4–C_7, inclusive, thickened on the anterior aspect of canal. At levels C_5/C_6 and C_6/C_7 large protrusions, narrowing sagittal diameter to 7–8 mm.

Other laboratory tests. CSF electrophoresis: Total protein 71 mg/100 ml; increased permeability of blood–CSF barrier.

Operation (author), 7 March, 1972. Protective bilateral laminectomy C_5/C_6, protective arco-cristectomy C_7, hemifacetectomy C_6/C_7 right, C_5/C_6 and C_6/C_7 left, and cervicolordodesis (Mersilene mesh). Intervertebral foramina greatly narrowed by sclerotic osteophytic protrusions. Mesh anchored cranially in periosteum around occipital protuberance, and caudally with sutures through C_7 spinous process and in fascia around T_1.

Postoperative course and neurological findings. Drain at lower end of wound removed after 2 days. Postoperative course uneventful. An hour or so after waking, improvement in sensibility in left leg; only slight reduction to touch, pin-pricks and cold below the knee on each side. Sensitivity to all qualities normalized in arms and legs within 24 hours, paraesthesia and Lhermitte's sign no longer present. Within 14 days power in the arms, hands, legs and feet considerably improved. Two days after operation residual urine 150 ml; after the fourth day

bladder control normal. Romberg's sign no longer positive. Could now walk straight and steady, though slightly unresilient. Withdrawal tendency remained on stimulating the soles of the feet. Wound was not completely healed on discharge.

Case 13. Man, aged 50.[2]

Neurological history. Abuse of alcohol over many years. In the 4 years prior to operation, legs weak and difficulty in walking, occasionally needing two sticks. Peripheral neuropathy due to alcoholism diagnosed some years earlier. In April, 1972, condition worse. Atrophy and weakness of arm and leg muscles. Able to take only a few steps with support. Sensibility reduced on dorsal aspect of arms and absent in hands; loss of sensibility to touch below navel level, reduction of sensibility to pain and vibration increasing distally in both legs. Periodic severe pain in back of neck.

Neurological findings, 10 August, 1972. Practically total tetraparesis (only very slight movements of shoulder muscles, especially the right, of right brachioradialis muscle and left quadriceps femoris). Complete bilateral wrist-drop. Arm and leg reflexes absent, Babinski's sign positive bilaterally. Total urinary incontinence. Lumbar puncture: CSF protein level 825 mg/100 ml.

Radiographic examination, 10 August. Kyphotic and shallow cervical spinal canal. Large osteophytic protrusions at C_4–C_6 levels.

Gas myelogram. No contrast visible from C_3 to C_7.

Admitted to Department of Neurosurgery, Karolinska Hospital on 16 August.

Operation (author) 17 August, 1972. Protective bilateral laminectomy C_4–C_7 and cervicolordodesis (Mersilene mesh). Dura highly vascularized; on opening xanthochromic fluid escaped. Cervical spine placed in predetermined extension posture by means of self-adjusting head support. In its relaxed state, cervical cord still slightly stretched over anterior protrusions. Adhesions between cord on anterior aspect of dura severed with dissector. Dura sutured.

A fourfold layer of Mersilene mesh then attached with Tycron sutures in small holes drilled in a transverse groove in the occipital bone and in holes through the spinous processes T_1–T_3.

Postoperative course and neurological findings. Course uneventful. Neck pains diminished 24 hours after operation. On second day sensibility level had fallen to the inguinal region on both sides. One week later, sensibility to touch over whole of lower left leg, and one hand width below inguinal fold on right side. Now able to extend and flex left arm several times, though with greatly reduced power. Small but distinct movements of left fingers. Able to flex right arm once or twice but not to extend it. Finger movements better than on left side. Able to approximate and separate thumb and forefinger though without power. Catheter à *demeure* still used; no sensation of bladder filling.

31 August. Further improvement, including respiration. Now able to extend and flex right arm with increased power and also fingers, with all movements of right thumb. Grip still

---

[2] Not included in Table 5.

weak. Left arm and hand similarly improved, though to a lesser extent. Able to flex and extend both legs and feet, range of movement increasing daily. Perceived painful stimuli in sacral dermatomes. Still no sensation of bladder filling. Referred to another hospital. No follow-up examination possible.

Comments. In this patient the neurological symptoms and signs were identical with those seen after central spinal cord injury. The total bilateral wrist-drop, with very slight move-

ments in left quadriceps, might equally well have been due to an acute trauma of the cord; in either case the symptoms are a result of the short-range axial tension in the cord tissue produced on compression. The only difference between the two causations is that in spinal cord injury the compression is momentary, whereas in myelopathy it is repeated and usually somewhat weaker.

Cervical nerve-root lesions

Case 1. Woman, aged 59.[1]

Neurological history. For more than 15 years there had been pain in the cervical region radiating towards both shoulders. Resection of the C_5, C_6 and C_7 discs in 1964 led to an improvement. A traumatic injury in the spring of 1969 was followed by a deterioration, with pain in the neck radiating to the right shoulder and arm.

Radiographic examination, October, 1970. Marked degenerative changes C_3/C_4; the C_4 and C_5 were fused.

Operation (at another hospital), October, 1970. Intercorporal spondylodesis C_5/C_6 by Cloward's method. After operation pain even worse, affecting right shoulder and back of head. A collar and physiotheraphy, etc., provided no permanent relief.

Neurological findings, February, 1972. Rhizopathy symptoms C_5–C_7 right side. Severe migraine cervicale type of headache, mostly on right side, radiating over vertex to temples; troubled by persistent buzzing and ringing in one ear.

Radiographic examination. Fused C_4–C_6 vertebrae. Intervertebral disc C_3/C_4 lowered, with osteophytes on borders of adjacent vertebral bodies. In flexion of head, the C_3 body slipped about 3 mm forwards over C_4 leading to local kyphosis (about 25°). This disappeared on extension, and axis of cervical canal from a tangential plane through upper contour of atlas arch to a plane through lower contour of C_3 vertebral body was shortened by about 1 cm (enlargement factor not subtracted). The changed angle between C_6 and C_7 contributed a further 0.5 cm. Headache and pain in right arm worse on head flexion and diminished on extension and on abducting right arm.

Deliberations before re-operation. It was considered that if the maximum shortening of the cervical canal could be obtained in the cervcolordodesis operation and, moreover, if the osteophytes in the narrowed intervertebral spaces could be removed, it would be possible to slacken the nerve-roots involved so that the bending tensile stresses in them that were responsible for the symptoms could be eliminated.

Operation (author), February, 1972. Protective hemifacetectomy C_4/C_5, C_5/C_6, C_6/C_7 right side and cervicolordodesis (Mersilene mesh). Sclerotic osteophytes narrowing the intervertebral foramina removed with Stryker burr.

Postoperative course and neurological findings. About a week after the operation, the symptoms and signs had practically disappeared. The improvement lasted about 5

weeks. Then the pains and occasional buzzing and ringing in the ear returned; 15 May. Wound healed, no irritation. On bending the head the Mersilene mesh could be felt to tighten beneath the skin; however, the range of forward bending of the head had greatly increased.

Radiographic examination (cervical column in extreme functional postures) 15 May, 1972. Able to flex the cervical spine more than had been calculated. If the cervical canal had in fact been shortened as intended, the symptoms would probably not have reappeared.

Immediate reoperation was considered inappropriate because a few weeks previously the patient had had heart failure, with myocardial affections and pulmonary stasis, and exudation into the left pleural cavity.

Case 2. Woman, aged 59.[2]

Neurological history. A 10-year history of persistent severe neck pain and bilateral brachialgia, more pronounced on left, sometimes lasting for several hours. Migraine cervicale with pain in back of neck, radiating to left temple and left ear lobe. Tendency for left eye to lacrimate. Resection of 6th and 5th discs and anterior interbody fusions in 1963 and 1959.

From July, 1969, fairly severe pains radiating to occipital region and left arm and hand. Grip weaker in left than right hand. Fusion of the now degenerated 4th disc contemplated. In recent years also radiating pain and tremor in legs; fell occasionally when there was no opportunity to sit down; frequency of attacks ranged from once a fortnight to several times a week.

Admitted to Department of Orthopaedics, Karolinska Hospital, in March, 1972. Neurological manifestations accentuated on flexion of the neck.

Radiographic assessement (author). Diagrams of cervical spine in full flexion and extension superimposed. Axis of cervical canal from a tangential plane through upper contour of atlas arch to a plane through lower contour of C_3 vertebral body shortened in extended position by about 1.5 cm (enlargement factor unknown). Caudal of C_3 plane, axis of canal not shortened in normal way owing to postoperative kyphosis and spondylotic rigidity between C_4 and C_5. (Although the canal shortened only slightly on extending the cervical spine,

---

[1] Not included in Table 5.
[2] Not included in Table 5.

cervicolordodesis was decided on with a view to eliminating tension in cervical nerve-roots and hence the symtoms.)

Operation (author) March, 1972. Protective hemifacetectomy C_4/C_5, C_5/C_6, C_6/C_7, C_7/T_1 left side and cervicolordodesis (Mersilene mesh). Just above external occipital protuberance a transverse groove 3.5 cm long and 4 mm deep was cut in the squama occipitalis, and in lower edge of the groove 5 holes were drilled. After extending the cervical spine by means of self-adjusting head-rest, Mersilene mesh was affixed to occipital bone and fascia colli at levels of T_1 and T_2 with Tycron sutures.

Postoperative course and neurological findings. After the operation the brachialgia disappeared completely. Subfebrile for 14 days, serous fluid discharge from wound; culture negative. Given antibiotics. Discharged on 24 April. The wound ultimately healed after application of compression dressing with gauze roll and figure-of-eight dressing for 14 days. No brachialgia symptoms since operation; 14 days previously left-sided attack of migraine cervicale; radiating pains in legs disappeared, as had tremors and attacks of paralysis. If neck unsupported for a time, a feeling of heaviness developed between back of neck over trapezius muscle and around left shoulder-blade. This was relieved on supporting the head or lying down. Extremely satisfied with results of operation; had become 'quite a different person' after some 10 years of constant pain. Because of erect posture the patient was asked whether she was a ballet dancer.

Distance from chin to suprasternal notch 11.5 cm; unable to see toes; also difficulty in going downstairs, or seeing plate if too near the body. Bed spectacles (Swift Instruments, Boston) ordered.

Follow-up examination, 28 August, 1972. Completely free from brachialgia; recurrent attacks of migraine cervicale over the previous week or so. No brachialgia for 6 months. One day, on flexing the upper trunk, felt something rupture in her neck, the head could be bent forward again. Immediately afterwards, radiating pains returned in left arm and up back of head left side. Re-operation at patient's request.

Re-operation (author), 8 June, 1973. Cervicolordodesis with Trevira ribbon.[3] (For technique, see p. 203). The Mersilene mesh, which had torn from its anchorages in the spinous processes and occipital bone, was removed. The prosthesis clamp was cemented into the deepened channel. The Teflon ribbon around the spinous processes T_2 and T_1 was tied above the latter; one end was cut off (no longer done) and the other end was led through a tunnel in the neck just above the cervical spinous processes to the clamp, where it was secured after the cervical spine had been extended.

Postoperative course. Following a week's intensive pain in right trapezius muscle no symptoms for 2 months. Then, intermittent, slowly increasing feeling of tension on left at back of neck, radiating pains on outside of left upper arm, anterior side of forearm and in all fingers, with paraesthesia. Relapse of migraine cervicale, with pains in bridge of nose and on left in both jaws, lachrymating left eye, pain in acoustic meatus and lobe of ear, alternating or simultaneously with brachialgia; globus sensation in throat and difficulty in swallowing.

Trevira ribbon tightened in the clamp (local anaesthesia), 26 September, 1973. Migraine cervicale disappeared, but brachial-

gia unchanged. Uncertain whether extension of rigid kyphosed cervical spine might have increased in spite of tightening of ribbon (which was, however, so taut as to cut through the unyielding skin near the occiput.) Relief of load by means of rotation flap contra-indicated by peristent brachialgia; neck part of the band therefore removed under local anaesthesia (29 October, 1973). Shortly afterwards neuralgia (migraine cervicale) returned.

A sleeve of connective tissue had formed round the ribbon and inhibited maximum flexion of the cervical spine. (No longer symptoms from long medullary pathways.)

Comments and discussion (Cases 1 and 2)

These two patients are of interest in connection with the chapter on spinal cord injury. Here, cervicolordodesis is recommended also in the case of high complete transverse lesions of the cervical cord, as a means of slackening the nerve-roots just above the lesion and hence safeguarding the conductivity of their fibres. No further surgical measures are then required.

In Case 2 the cervical spine had been immobilized in marked kyphosis after intercorporal spondylodesis by Cloward's method at two levels. Such kyphosis of the vertebral bodies invariably results in axial and transverse tension in the cervical cord and nerve-roots just at the level of the vertebra that projects most posteriorly. As shown in the section on pathodynamics, such tension in the spinal cord is always transmitted cranially and caudally. In this mechanical situation osteophytes in front of and below the nerve-roots inevitably produce bending tensile stress in the tissue of the involved nerve-roots. In the case in question it was therefore logical first to perform hemifacetectomy with removal of the part of the posterior articular process that, combined with the untouched anterior protrusion, might exert a pincer effect on the nerve-roots; this was followed by cervicolordodesis to slacken the nerve-roots enough for the anterior protrusions no longer to exert pressure on them and thus to set up bending tensile stress. Immediately after this the brachialgia disappeared completely and there were no longer sporadic symptoms from the long spinal pathways. In addition, there had been occasional pain in the hip region which may have been due to the stretching of a nerve-root over a pathological protrusion at the lumbar level. Before the actual operation on this patient the prospects of alleviating the pain were not rated high; for the preoperative radiographs showed that the slight degree of extension of the cervical spine that could be achieved produced only relatively little shortening of the cervical canal owing to the kyphosis.

The sensations radiating to the face in Cases 1 and 2 may be classed tentatively as migraine cervicale. A possible, formerly accepted explanation of the extent of these neurological manifestations is that the posterior cervical nerve-roots communicate with the descending

---

[3] 'Teflon'-type (p. 193).

tract of the fifth cranial nerve *via* the gelatinous substance in the posterior column. The irritative intermediate local impulses (226) evoked by bending tensile stress in any of these nerve-roots would then be transmissible to the Gasserian ganglion and be perceived as deriving from one or more receptor fields in the branches of the trigeminal nerve.

From the alleviation of pain obtained in these two patients through relaxing the nerve-roots by means of the cervicolordodesis operation, this would seem to be a beneficial form of treatment not only for cervical rhizopathies but also for rescuing the conductivity of the lowermost residual cervical nerve-roots after high-level transverse lesions of the cord.

Post-traumatic myelopathy

Case. Woman, aged 54 (in 1973).[1]

Neurological history. November, 1967, following an accident in which her car left the road and ran into the ditch the woman lost consciousness and woke up in hospital, where she lay for 2 weeks with a stiff and painful neck. While lying prone she was unable to turn her head to either side without severe pain and locking of the neck. Intense pain between shoulder blades, pain in hips and back.

January, 1968. While bending forward at the sink she sneezed and could not straighten again. Wore a surgical brace for about a year.

Summer, 1969. While sewing had difficulty in threading needles due to weakness of left fingers and unsteadiness on left side. Developed a fine tremor in left arm and tended to swing the arm to the right while walking. Normal movements of neck resulted in stiffness in both arms and hyperalgesia in both elbows and the joints of the hands. The tremor became worse in *1970;* began to develop weakness of the hand and tended to drop things. The arm, too, became increasingly weak; unable to shrug left shoulder effectively. Developed pain and prickling sensations, numbness down left arm radiating down medial side of arm and 3rd to 5th finger of left hand.

Autumn, 1971. Cervical fusion C_5–C_6. Immediately after the operation violent and continuous pain in the back and hips, worse in the right hip. Additional pain down outer aspect of right leg associated with prickling sensations and numbness as far as the knee.

Late 1971. Operation for a prolapsed lumbar disc (L_4/L_5). Afterwards, prickling and shooting pain down both lower limbs. Traction transferred most of the pain from right to left leg; constant numbness, tingling and pain in left leg from hip down to lateral aspect of leg, to the foot, and also the toes and sole.

Summer 1972. Another lumbar disc (L_5/S_1) removed and spinal nerves found to be inflamed. The left lower leg felt dead; burning ice-cold sensation in the skin. Touching elicited pain; aching pain along anterior and lateral sides of both legs. Improvement slow. There was some disorder of micturition after the lumbar disc operation. No desire to micturate when lying down, but on rising to seated or standing position there was urgency or leaking.

March, 1973. Chronic high neck pain with acute exacerbations, associated with prickling sensations radiating down the trapezius muscle to the left arm and ulnar two fingers. Continuous severe central low back pain, worse on movement; associated pain, numbness, prickling sensations in left

leg—particularly outer aspect—toes, and sole left foot. Right leg similarly affected down to knee.

September, 1973. Weakness of left arm and hands with tremor, some pain in left shoulder. Some weakness of left leg, which was dragged; a tendency to trip up and fall easily. Able to walk only with difficulty. Stress incontinence and little sensation from the bladder and urethra. Bladder function poor. Dyschezic constipation.

Neurological findings (National Hospital, Queen Square, London) September, 1973. Left eyelid sometimes droops; left corneal reflex very weak. Absence of tactile sensibility on left side of face and neck; diminished sensibility to pin-prick, cotton-wool, hot and cold. Constant marked tremor of left arm and hand increasing on performing finger–nose test. Deep reflexes of arm increased on left side. Deep and superficial leg reflexes normal.

Admitted to Department of Neurosurgery, Karolinska Hospital, Stockholm, 18 December, 1973.

Neurological findings. Neck stiff and painful. Severe pain in left side of face radiating to temple, forehead, eye and ear. General weakness on left side of face, most marked at left corner of mouth. Left-sided hemiparesis with slight but definite spasticity. Coarse power diminished in left arm and hand, arm and hand no longer used regularly. Left hand colder than right. Defective sensibility for all qualities on left side of body from face (left corneal reflex absent), arm, hand, trunk and leg. Pins and needles in left arm and leg. Gait stiff and dragging, especially left leg, with some circumduction of left leg. Totally unaware of bladder filling, complete incontinence. Pain in lower back and hips, radiating to legs, especially on back of right thigh. Paraesthesia and diminished sensibility along outer aspect of left leg and foot. Most of these symptoms increase on bending neck and spinal column; radiating paraesthesia and pain in both legs. Clear indication for the cervicolordodesis operation.

Radiographic examinations 17–19 December, 1973. Check of earlier films, heart and lungs, and encephalogram with technetium. Cervical spine: anteroposterior diameter of canal at level of osteosynthesis 13 mm.

Operation (author) 20 December, 1973. Cervicolordodesis with Trevira ribbon[2] (for technique see Fig. 153).

Postoperative course. Uneventful, except for some postoperative oedema and tenderness in left upper neck for some

[1] Not included in Table 5.
[2] 'Teflon'-type (p. 193).

days. Immediately after operation the left-sided tremor reappeared. Some 24 hours later, sensibility for all qualities on left side of body much improved. *24 December.* Sensibility of left side of body (face, trunk, arms and legs) normal again for all qualities. Coarse power in left arm and hand normal again and similar to that on right side. Temperature of left arm and hand normal. Pins and needles in left arm, hand and, especially, index finger reappeared for some hours. Tremor had diminished. Bladder function practically normalized. *29 December.* Transient pain radiating in left arm and hand on previous day now gone. Good power in left arm and hand, but frozen shoulder (elevation about 60°). On walking left arm swings less than right. Pain in low back region and hips diminished. Power in left leg and foot increased gradually. No longer any foot-drop or dragging of foot, though still some slight motor and coordination deficiency. Daily walks extended initially under supervision. Ultimately managed to climb several stairs without assistance.

Discharged 30 December, 1973, much improved.

Follow-up examination (National Hospital for Nervous Diseases, London) 12 March, 1974. "We have Mrs. X. in hospital again. I think her operation has been a great success, and so does she. The diminution in sensation in her face has disappeared; the tremor, she says, is a little better and it does seem to me so on most occasions; the pain in the upper left limb has all gone; and the disturbance of micturition is completely removed. Her control of her bladder is now back to normal. As she herself says, "the operation would have been worth-while for this alone". Dr X. saw the patient on 19 March, 1974, and also noted the improvement in facial numbness, neck pain, bladder control, and the slight improvement in the tremor of the upper limb. "This satisfactory picture has been spoilt, to a certain extent, by the fact that she still has a lot of analgesic drugs. When she was at home she slipped twice in the bathroom, perhaps when she was feeling dopey under these drugs, fell over the back of the bath, hyperextending her spine. This made her back and pain in the left lower limb much worse. She is taking a lot of analgesics for this. We are trying to get her off some of the analgesics, and are doing physiotherapy and trying a vibrator for the pain."

Comments (The patient's physician.) "It was considered that in the case of this patient the posttraumatic pathology that can result in over-stretching of the Vth nerve, the greater and lesser occipital nerves and greater auricular nerve, the nerves supplying either or both upper limbs and the nerves to the lower extremity, and particularly the nerves of the cauda equina, might account for the diminished corneal reflex and reduced sensation in the left side of the face, the dysaesthesia in the neck, aggravated by neck movements, perhaps the tremor due to pulling the inferior cerebellar peduncle on the left—though there is no nystagmus—the signs and symptoms in the left upper limb, the disturbance of micturition an defaecation and the signs and symptoms of the lower limbs."

Follow-up reports (extracts from letters)

11 March, 1974 (J. M. Robinson, G. P.). . . . When the patient first returned home she was amazingly well and had a general good improvement from most of her symptoms . . . her head-

ache became worse . . . she was taking large amounts of analgesics by mouth . . . and she began to have falls for no apparent reason. On one of these occasions she hit her neck on the edge of the bath . . .

14 April, 1974 (X.X., husband). . . . suffered a recurrence of the soreness from the operation and increased pain in the leg . . . all the head pains have gone and the bladder trouble has disappeared, as has the pain in the shoulder. All the doctors have been most impressed by the results of the operation . . .

2 June, 1974 (patient). . . . I am quite free from all the symptoms in the cervical area and head which were troubling me when I came to you, and it is a marvellous pleasure to be able to sit in a car and examine the view to the right, the left and almost to the rear on either side without any suggestion of pain or discomfort. The same is true of moving the head backward which was previously so painful . . . renewed crash against the corner of a desk . . . excruciating pain lumbar spine and left leg . . . left arm became very weak and useless again . . . bladder is not so (?) as it was before [after surgery] . . . I am almost certain that I am able to move my head forward much more than I could before . . . for instance, I can now look down and see my navel whereas before I couldn't . . . tendency for my left eyelid to droop when I am tired . . . Is it possible that I could have stretched either the tissues or the Teflon[3] when I fell? Is the weakness in my arm and the bladder discomfort attributable to this? Is is possible for the Teflon to be shortened? . . .

Re-operation (Mr. M. Sullivan & author) at Royal National Orthopaedic Hospital, Stanmore, England, *August 29,* 1974. The Trevira ribbon in the neck did not tighten until the chin had been lowered by about 3–4 cm. With the patient in the prone position on the operating table with the head and neck on a head-rest and brought into slight extension, a transverse incision was made some millimetres above the old scar in the occipital region. After removing a thin layer of connective tissue both Trevira ribbon and prosthesis clamp were found to be in place and quite unchanged. After loosening the 3 screws of the clamp this was removed from the baseplate (which was firmly anchored in the apparently sound occipital bone, just as it was after cementing 9 months previously). The Trevira was shortened and tightened sufficiently to hold the head and neck in the required extended posture.

It was concluded that as a result of the falls the ribbon had been pulled more tightly into contact with the upper thoracic spinous processes than it was just after the first operation.

Postopeative course uneventful.

24 September, 1974 (Mr M. Sullivan). . . . Mrs X. has done extremely well. There were no complications and her arm has increased function enormously. She is still complaining of pain in her back and leg . . .

15 October, 1974 (patient). . . . sciatic pain in my leg no better, on the other hand the feeling of tautness and that the heel is being drawn up is improved . . . my left arm is stronger . . . the bladder functions virtually normally again, which is a great blessing . . .

31 July, 1977 (patient). . . . postoperative improvement has stood up very well to the tests of time . . .

---

[3] Later identified as Trevira material (p. 193).

Thoracic myelopathy

Case. Man, aged 51.[1]

Occupation. Shipyard welder for more than 20 years, work entailing a stooped posture with trunk flexed.

Neurological history. Healthy until August, 1972, when particularly strenuous effort led to pain and stiffness in low back and buttocks, spreading to groin and inside of thighs, radiating down inside of legs to feet and toes. Both legs became stiff and weak, particularly in right ankle.

Early 1973, condition worse; right leg weaker, gait slowed; steps dragging and unsteady. Complained of increasing tenderness at back of knees and calves and on soles of feet on walking. Difficulty in sitting straight—leaning to one side or the other—and also in starting micturition.

Clinical findings. Marked forward thoracic curve with slight scoliosis convex to left; held neck flexed. Gait spastic and atactic, walking with legs wide apart. General weakness of muscles of both legs; foot-drop on right with paresis of dorsiflexors. Tendon reflexes exaggerated, clonus being elicited on tapping right ankle. Babinski's sign positive bilaterally. Sensibility to light touch subjectively diminished on outer side of right leg, and perianally.

Diagnosis. Thoracic kyphosis with progressive paraparesis.

CSF pressure. On performing Queckenstedt's test and recording CSF pressure, normal rise in pressure and pulsatile movements (87) when head and upper thorax extended; response limited in neutral posture; no response on flexing neck and trunk forward.

Radiographic examination. Cervical spine: minor osteophytes at posterior margins of C_4–C_7 vertebral bodies. Thoracic spine: wedge-shaped T_5–T_9 vertebral bodies with anterior osteophytosis. Lumbar spine: some osteophytes.

Gas myelogram. Indicative of narrowing of upper thoracic spinal cord.

Myelogram with positive contrast medium (Metrizamide). Angulation of spinal canal anteriorly at T_7/T_8 and T_8/T_9; obliteration of anterior subarachnoid space at the two intervertebral spaces. Cord at both levels apparently narrowed to almost half diameter. Whole dura displaced anteriorly, though posterior subarachnoid space remained well visualized.

Operation (author), 13 September, 1973. Cervicolordodesis using the prosthesis clamp cemented in a transverse channel drilled in the occipital bone 2 cm above the external occipital protuberance. Vertical skin incision, curved to left, from C_7 to T_3 level. The 2 cm wide Trevira ribbon[2] was laced round the spinous processes from T_3 to C_7, the ends being led to the clamp through a tunnel in the neck muscles just above the cervical spinous processes, where it was secured with the head in a predetermined degree of cervial extension.

Postoperative course. A few hours after operation patient able to sit on edge of bed, and the next day in a chair. Pain in buttocks, groins and thighs had disappeared. By 3rd day spasticity of lower limbs receded. On 5th day could sit straight and move more freely.

Two weeks postoperatively still some stiffness behind knees, and some weakness in right leg, but felt able to empty bladder at will. Gait still somewhat spastic, but improving steadily. Flexion of head arrested just forward of neutral position. Discharged 2 October with the wounds healed.

1 November, 1973. Reported walking several kilometres without discomfort. No pain, able to sit normally; bladder function further improved.

Comment. The significant points in this case were that there was a block to CSF pressure at mid-thoracic level when the head, neck and trunk were fully flexed. Simply by preventing cervical flexion it was possible to ameliorate the symptoms of spastic paraparesis arising from a thrust on the thoracic cord at T_7–T_9 (combined, during flexion of the cervical spine, with compression of the thoracic cord by the posterior aspect of the dura); 6 weeks later the patient was able to report a major improvement.

Follow-up examination (author), 28 October, 1974. Still at home waiting for lighter work. Slow but clear improvement of all symptoms. Can take somewhat longer steps, move quicker and easier. Right leg stronger, but still not so stable as left. Now able to walk up steps without gripping handrail and to lift right leg to next step, which was not possible before the operation. After a walk of 1 kilometer on even ground legs stiff and unstable, but recover after a few minutes' rest. Right ankle more stable, rarely stumbles. No longer lumbar pain, more upright posture. Stiffness in buttocks, radiating down inside of legs decreased. Tenderness in back of knee only after deep forward bending. Preoperative urgency of micturition (which he did not mention during stay in hospital) has disappeared. Was troubled by frequency of urination during daytime and difficulty of urination, and had to get up 6–7 times a night to void bladder. Now only once or twice a night.[3]

No symptoms referable to the cervicolordodesis operation. Can move head freely in all directions excepting flexion. When bending, the ribbon arrests movements about 6–5 cm above the jugular notch of sternum (ribbon lengthened by 4–5 cm since surgery). *Objective findings.* When rising after having been seated for about 20 minutes gait initially stiff and unsteady; after having walked a little, right-sided limp.

Follow-up report (local physician), May, 1975. Nearly total relapse of pre-operative neurological symptoms. Now able to flex neck much more than last autumn.

---

[1] Not included in Table 5.
[2] 'Teflon'-type (p. 193).
[3] Since making this report I had reason to suspect that the patient was dissimulating about the frequency.

Multiple sclerosis

Spinal cord manifestations

Case 1. Man, aged 38 (in 1961).

Neurological history. Diagnosis of multiple sclerosis confirmed on several occasions at the Department of Neurology, Serafimer Hospital, Stockholm.

One day in *1955* when the patient was using a heavy sledge-hammer, pains were suddenly felt in the upper thoracic spine, radiating to all the extremities. In the next few months these pains recurred in several other occupational contexts (flexion?) and generally disappeared after about 10 minutes. Occasionally when walking, piercing, boring pains felt between shoulder-blades and sacral region, and burning pains in knee regions; increasing heaviness of legs. Three months later, reduced sensibility in left foot and right forearm and hand, feeling of constriction around abdomen, difficulty in micturition and dizziness.

September, 1957. Pains still felt between shoulder-blades and in sacral region. Deep sensibility reduced in legs and vibratory sensation abolished. Increased tendon reflexes in legs; extensor plantar responses.

Since *January, 1960,* no further remissions. Spastic paralysis in both legs with increased tendon reflexes and inexhaustible clonus. Bilateral extensor plantar responses with shortening reaction. Sensibility abolished for all qualities below mamillary plane. Total urinary incontinence.

Admitted to a hospital for chronic diseases.

Treatment. 14 January, 1961. An attempt was made by the author to secure protective relaxation of the pons–cord tract by placing the patient's neck on a round bolster so as to obtain extension of the head and cervical spine. To prevent any change in the position of the cervical spine, Crutchfield's forceps were applied to the posterior part of the frontal bone in the temporal region and loaded with a weight of $\frac{1}{2}$ kg. The patient was informed that the object of the measure was to enable him to judge whether he could get accustomed to this position should his condition deteriorate and the need arise to immobilize the cervical spine in this position; care was taken to avoid giving the patient the impression that this technique was regarded as form of treatment.

Post-therapeutic course, 17 January. The patient volunteered that for the first time for 3 years he had recovered sensibility on the ulnar side of the right lower arm and hand; a check with the carefully kept records verified that for several years the sensibility had been totally extinguished in this region. A week later the patient could locate light pin pricks over the whole of the trunk correctly, though slightly less reliably in the thighs, quite weakly in the lower legs and not at all in the feet. A fortnight later the patient was able to perform barely visible movements of the legs and toes. They could be repeated 3 to 4 times on a single occasion.

4 February, 1961. The patient could distinguish between a sharp and a blunt pin prick between the mammillary and umbilical levels but not below the latter. The flow of urine was felt for the first time for several years. He could perform 4 or 5 barely visible adduction movements of the thigh at the temperature of the ward. The movements of the legs and toes were slightly more powerful (on the occasion of an attempt

to film them under the heat emitted by a high-power lamp the movements could no longer be made). At this time spasticity was clearly diminished; clonus was not longer elicited. The patient stated that he could move the diaphragm better and that breathing was easier (he had never mentioned these symptoms before).

27 February. During the author's absence for 3 weeks the Crutchfield's forceps were removed. The patient could no longer perform spontaneous movements. His relatives were reluctant to agree to the surgical immobilization of the cervical spine proposed by the author.

25 May. At the last personal check the patient stated that on his own initiative he had tried to maintain extension of the spinal column because he had the impression that he felt better in this position. Motility zero, as before. The sensibility was still improved almost to the same extent as during the time of permanent extension. Could control the bladder for about $2\frac{1}{2}$ and 3 hours; during this time he was able to start micturition voluntarily; however, the emptying started automatically if the patient had not passed urine for the last 3 hours. Euphoria. No further checks were made through the author at another nursing home for the chronically ill to which the patient was moved soon after.

The multiple sclerosis claimed the patient's life some years later.

Case 2. Woman, aged 29.

Neurological history. Since 1958, a general feeling of weakness; some time later paresis in both legs, more marked on left side. 1960: numbness and weakness in left arm (left-handed). 1961: difficulty in articulation. Symptoms stationary in the last 12 months.

Admitted to Centre of Neurosurgery, Cairo, November 1962. General condition deteriorated; no tendency for spontaneous remission; dysphoria; feeling of weakness in all extremities, more marked on left than right; unsteady spastic and atactic gait; able to take a few steps only with support; increased tendon reflexes, left more than right; bilateral patellar and Achilles tendon clonus. Bilateral extensor plantar responses. Abolition of sensibility for all qualities below T_8. Total urinary incontinence.

Radiographic examination of cervical spine (Ahmed Fouad El-Nadi). Normal.

Operation (author), December, 1962. Osteosynthesis of spinous processes C_4–T_1 in slight extension of cervical spine (acrylic cement).

Postoperative course uncomplicated, apart from retention of urine for 4 days, calling for catheterization; thereafter, improved bladder control and improved sensibility of lower part of the body. Improvement in general state and mobility of right arm and hand.

Radiographic examination. 16 December, 1962. Cervical spine immobilized in slight extension.

Discharged on 24 December, 1962. Patient did not appear for the important follow-up in the next few months.

Comments and discussion (Cases 1 and 2)

In spite of the theoretical foundation for the practical attempts to obtain relaxation of the spinal cord tissue it is still surprising that the sensibility and bladder control were improved to a fairly remarkable extent in the first 2 patients suffering from multiple sclerosis in which this method was used. The series is, of course, too small to permit any reliable conclusion on the value of the method in this disease. Nonetheless, the relatively modest improvement in the symptoms suggests that by relaxation of the pons–cord tract certain histodynamic stresses were reduced in spinal cord pathways still retaining some conductivity. In Case 1 where the improvement in motor function of the legs was extremely limited and of short duration it is probable that the demyelinization of the motor fibres was already far advanced. This statement is, of course, based on a coarse morphological view. The complicated dependance of the conductivity on interacting enzymes and intramedullary vascular factors (24)[1] in this disease is illustrated by the fact that when the legs were warmer than usual (see above) the patient was unable to perform any movement. (One of the first patients with multiple sclerosis that the author examined some 25 years ago stated that the legs felt stronger when he cooled them in ice-cold water.) Furthermore, that also the relief of the histodynamic stress in the fibres within the motor pathways of the cord can be beneficial is evident from the improvement in motor function in Case 2.

There can hardly have been any random coincidence between the relaxation of the cord and a spontaneous remission of the symptoms, since, to judge from the evidence in both these patients, the disease had obviously reached a stage where remission could no longer be expected. Though there might be some doubt about this in Case 2, the improbability of such a coincidence in Case 1, which had been most carefully examined, is confirmed by an authority in the field of multiple sclerosis.

In the above cases the relaxation of the cord resulted in some measure of benefit to the patients. This was hardly unexpected, for the method of treatment is based on verified biomechanical observations. The extent to which the neurological symptoms were reduced was, however, strikingly great, and in any case greater than expected. These favourable results, in their turn, prompted a still more thorough histological analysis of the action of unyielding intramedullary lesions and of the consequences of relaxation of the various components of the cord tissue, in an attempt to find an acceptable explanation of this improvement.

It is now known that in the case of foramen magnum tumours and spondylotic protrusions in the cervical canal the tension in the pons–cord tract is transmitted as far as the sacral nerve-roots. These roots are then exposed secondarily to pressure and bending tensile stress in the pedicle region. It is not known whether the bladder symptoms in multiple sclerosis are due to a similar mechanism, but it is more probable that the in-

tramedullary gliomatous scar foci exert local histodynamic effects on the surrounding nerve-fibres. It has been found experimentally that on stretching the pons–cord tract the nerve-fibres are bent in the form of 'tension spindles' over any unyielding structure in the cord tissue (Fig. 80); the gliomatous scar foci would presumably exert a similar effect on the fibres of the centrifugal micturition pathways. Spinal cord relaxation would appear to be the most logical way of eliminating the histodynamic tension that could give rise to these symptoms.

Case 3. Man, aged 51.

Neurological history. About 6 weeks before the onset of the disorder the patient had jumped from a first floor window of a burning building. There were no immediate sequelae. For previous 2 years, progressive spastic paraparesis in legs, spasticity and reduced power in right arm, worsening almost daily (grip unreliable, for instance, on raising a cup to the mouth); flexion of head elicited marked loss of power in right arm and hand and Lhermitte's sign radiating from the back of neck along the arms to his hands. Partial urinary incontinence. Rapid progress over previous 6 months. Often fell; could move only a step or two, with help of a crutch.

Admitted to Department of Neurology, Karolinska Hospital, March, 1972 (treated there previously in 1970 and 1971). Muscle relaxants without any objective effect on the spasticity.

The tentative diagnosis of multiple sclerosis was suggested by the relatively high age at onset, but supported by the changes in CSF electrophoretic picture, which resembled those in in demyelinization disorders.

Neurological findings. No cranial nerve symptoms. Weakness in right arm. Atrophy of muscles of right hand. Reduced sensibility to temperature on medial surface of forearms. Tetraspasticity; temporary paraspasticity in legs, especially right, which could not be bent at knee or hip. Ankle clonus; Babinski's sign positive bilaterally. Tremor in right leg when attempting to stand with heels together. Able to move 5–6 m with aid of two crutches, but only with difficulty. Unable to raise feet from ground (circumduction movements when walking). Abdominal reflexes abolished. Sensibility for all qualities reduced in both legs.

Radiographic examination and gas myelogram. Cervical spine slightly convex to right. C_5/C_6 disc lowered. Moderately large disc protrusions at C_4/C_5 and C_5/C_6 levels. Protrusions of soft tissues on anterior aspect of canal (C_3–C_6). At T_5/T_6 level, anteroposterior diameter of the thoracic cord reduced to 6 mm; local atrophy.

CSF pressure normal.

Neurophysiological and other findings. EMG on thumb and interossei muscles of right hand: Moderate reduction of voluntary activity.

Routine tests on blood and urine normal, likewise liver condition. Wassermann's reaction negative. Folic acid and B_{12} in serum normal. T_3 resin normal. Moderate changes in CSF as in

[1] Clark, S. L.: Innervation of blood-vessels of medulla and spinal cord. J Comp Neurol *48:* 247–265, 1929.

demyelinizing disease (barrier damage and immunopathy). Local cooling of legs had subjectively favourable effect on walking capacity.

Patient was offered treatment at a hospital for chronic diseases but chose operation.

Transferred from Neurological to Neurosurgical Department, Karolinska Hospital, 4 April, 1972.

Operation (author), 4 April. Cervicolordodesis (Mersilene mesh).

Postoperative course and neurological findings. Only a few hours after operation, subjective and objective increase in power in right arm and hand, though unchanged in legs. Bladder control improved little, if at all. On 5th postoperative day, *Staphylococcus aureus* infection of operation wound. During treatment at Department of Infectious Diseases (antibiotics and pressure dressings) wound healed in few days.

Readmitted 15 May. Results of operation judged unsatisfactory. X-ray follow-up of cervical spine showed that vertebrae had not the intended degree of lordosis.

Re-operation (author), 17 May. Mersilene mesh loosened from its anchorage in the spinous processes of T_1 and T_2 and was reattached with 8 Tycron no. 0.4 stutures in the bone and 4 in the fascia.

Postoperative course and neurological findings. Course uneventful. Antibiotic prophylaxis. Compression dressing just after removal of drain on 2nd day after operation.

Three hours after waking from anaesthesia the patient felt able to move his legs better than before. A day later normal bladder control recovered. Spasticity and spontaneous spastic tremor in the legs diminished very slowly without recourse to muscle relaxants. Physiotherapy with walking exercise introduced. Walked with 2 crutches; circumducted at first with spastically extended right leg. Some days later able to interrupt the extension spasm in both legs, and to rise almost normally from the seated position.

25 May. Eight days after re-operation able to walk without support for first time for 7 months, though very slowly, with circumduction of right leg. Seven days later able to walk on level floor and easy stairs without circumduction. Adductor spasm diappeared almost entirely; legs no longer tended to 'scissor' and patient able to move to either side without difficulty (film documentation). No longer a sensation of cold in right leg or reduced sensibility to temperature on inside of lower legs. Power in the right hand was now subjectively the same as in the left. Able to write and manage buttons, though still difficulty in strapping wrist-watch on left wrist.

Neurological findings, 31 May. Arms: muscle tone and power and sensation equal on the two sides; reflexes slightly more lively on right, Trömner's sign tentatively positive on right. Able to flex and extend right lower leg several times in succession. Gross power in flexion of right hip- and knee-joints considerably reduced. Sensibility normal for all qualities. Reflexes: no patellar clonus, though increased reflexogenic zone on both sides. Achilles clonus bilaterally. Babinski's sign positive, especially on right.

Admitted to the Red Cross Hospital, 1 June, 1972. Steady improvement (see above). Felt unwell during warm weather. Spasticity in legs reduced on cooling muscles.

Early August. Walking more difficult, increasing spasticity in

legs; *able to flex cervical spine more than just after operation.*

September. Great difficulty in moving; right arm worse, difficulty in combing hair and dressing. *November.* Back to wheel-chair. *January, 1973.* Discharged to home for handicapped.

Spring, 1973. Bronchopneumonia; thrombophlebitis in right leg.

Admitted, 18 May, 1973, to Rehabilitation Department, Danderyd Hospital. Unable to participate in gymnastics because of swelling of lower leg (following thrombophlebitis). Able to move unaided only between bed and wheel-chair.

Summer. Improved after taking Stesolid, papaverine and quinine; then able to move between bed and wheel-chair.

Admitted to Department of Neurosurgery, Karolinska Hospital, 8 September, 1973. Confined to the wheel-chair. Spastic paraparesis with spontaneous clonus in left leg; greatly reduced coarse power in right arm and hand; fumbling; unable to raise a cup to the mouth.

Preoperative evaluation. Insufficiency of cervicolordodesis (Mersilene mesh torn). Diagnosis of multiple sclerosis borne out by beneficial effect of cooling on spasticity. Reoperation with improved cervicolordodesis technique considered likely to lead to some improvement, but prognosis worsened by progress of the myelopathy and a 10 kg increase in weight through inactivity.

Re-operation (author), 10 September, 1973. Cervicolordodesis with Trevira ribbon technique. The mesh had torn away from the old groove in the occiput, where there was new bone; Mersilene mesh no longer identifiable in the scars. The prosthesis clamp was cemented in a new channel in the occipital bone. The Trevira ribbon[2] was anchored around the T_3, T_2 and T_1 spinous processes by the shoe-lacing technique. The strip was led through a muscle tunnel to the clamp, which was screwed tight with the cervical spine extended. Next day, a catheter à demeure introduced owing to total retention.

Postoperative course, 13 September. Neurological condition unchanged; infection of wound suspected. *16 September.* Felt better; able to clench right fist again. *18 September.* Catheter à demeure removed; able to pass water normally, but difficulty in arresting the flow. Cephalin therapy for the wound infection. *24 September.* Power in right arm and hand appreciably increased; able to eat and to write; able to flex the legs more easily in bed.

Transferred to Rehabilitation Department, Danderyd Hospital.

Comments and discussion (Case 3)

Follow-up examinations performed recently on large series of multiple sclerosis patients have shown that the course of the disease can vary still more than was formerly believed. The process can thus cease spontaneously at any stage—except the chronic one characterized by irreparable damage—or regress to a greater or lesser degree.

The patient in question had spondylotic changes of the cervical spine and changes in the CSF, as in a demyelinizing process. Though these had been relatively

---

[2] 'Teflon'-type (p. 193).

moderate, they led to invalidizing spasticity. The patient might thus be justifiably included in the multiple sclerosis group described by Brain & Wilkinson (30) with cervical spondylosis and disseminated sclerosis. Nothing seems to be known of the possible *spontaneous* regression of the symptoms in this group. Spondylosis is an extramedullary and sclerosis an intramedullary lesion and the neurological manifestations have different biomechanical origins (Figs. 98–100). Unlike the sclerosing foci, which are not always permanent, spondylosis remains unchanged, and spontaneous healing is therefore improbable. The intramedullary foci in multiple sclerosis—both pure and combined with spondylosis—are otherwise biomechanically equivalent since they give rise to neurological symptoms.

In the first cervicolordodesis operation in this patient the lordosis of the cervical spine was insufficient. Although the cord was therefore not as slack as intended, improved power and control in the right hand and arm were noticed only a few hours after the operation; but bladder insufficiency remained and the gross spasticity in the legs was more or less unchanged. This initial result, albeit inadequate, sufficed to prove that the degree of lordosis is the critical factor responsible for the neurological improvement.

The notable reduction in the patient's symptoms immediately after re-operation, in which the degree of extension of the head and cervical column was increased, constitutes clear evidence that it is the degree of relaxation of the cord that ultimately decides the effectiveness of the operation. The bladder insufficiency disappeared entirely within 48 hours of re-operation, and the spasticity in the legs then showed a definite tendency to regress, though very slowly.

The patient is the most recent of those in the multiple sclerosis group undergoing cervicolordodesis where the resulting relaxation of the spinal cord improved the conductivity of the pathways. Apart from Case 2, where the improvement could not be followed for non-medical reasons, this is the multiple sclerosis patient that, if all goes well, it will be possible to follow for a considerable period. The short observation time so far is not, of course, long enough for an assessment of the value of the relaxation operation for the average multiple sclerosis patient. While it might, of course, be objected that this case was not one of 'pure' multiple sclerosis, and therefore cannot be considered representative, it is notable that in 2 cases of 'pure' multiple sclerosis (nos. 1 and 2) a similar improvement in the conductivity of the spinal pathways was observed after relaxation of the cord. (In Case 3 the brake had to be removed subsequently because of infection.)

Histodynamic provocation of neurological symptoms. That Case 3 belongs to the mixed group of multiple sclerosis and cervical myelopathy (or rhizopathy) is indicated by the fact that prior to the operation flexion of the cervical spine evoked radiating paraesthesia in the right arm and hand. The responsible stress field is located either within the cervical cord (where the involved area will be the apex of the posterior column) or within the tissue of the posterior root (from the fila of the posterior nerve-root to the spinal nerve). In the former case it will probably be due to an inflammatory focus or gliosis which acts as an intramedullary impinging body (Fig. 100); and in the latter case to an osteophyte located outside the nervous tissue (extramedullary impinging body, Fig. 98). The mechanism responsible for the symptoms in the former case is in principle the same as that producing Lhermitte's sign. According to convention, however, this term relates to sensations that are intense and that are felt to radiate down the spinal column and to the extremities. The demyelinization manifested by the CSF changes in Case 3—which regularly lead to fragmentation fissures —suggests the presence of notch stress in the spinal cord tissue (for notch stress see, Fig. 68).

It is not only the preoperative signs and symptoms that show where in the pons—cord tract the stress has been concentrated but also, perhaps unexpectedly, the improvements after the operation. For instance, after relaxation of the cord had been secured one patient (Case 1) stated that his breathing was better than before; neither he nor his physician had previously been aware of any impairment of respiratory function.

General comments and discussion
(Case Reports pp. 214–31)

The sequence of the improvements in neurological function obtained by spinal cord relaxation has proved to follow a certain pattern. To begin with, as a result of an improvement in circulation the patient may notice a warm sensation in the arms and legs; this is followed by recovery of normal superficial and deep sensibility, caudalward from the level of primary impairment; at this stage bladder and colon sensibility may reappear; somewhat later arm and leg motor functions tend to improve and bowel control may be gradually recovered. Spasticity usually persists longest or may prove to be irreversible.

As spinal cord disorders are traditionally named according to début, epidemiology, acute or chronic nature, etc., the nomenclature does not reflect the histodynamic causation of the symptoms. The neurological symptoms in, for instance, cervical myelopathy and spinal cord injury are evoked by identical forces; these differ only in intensity, location, extent and rate of onset. The damage in paraplegia is the same whether it is caused by full extension of the head in the dentist's chair (cervical myelopathy) or by hyperextension of the neck due to a fall (spinal cord injury). In these examples the same functional surgical countermeasures are required to eliminate the pathological tension. It would be useful if the origin of the tension were stated in the diagnosis, for then the patient is more likely to receive the appropriate treatment.

Spinal cord injury

There can be little doubt that in all six patients to whom the following Case Reports relate the cord trauma was a result of rapid and violent extension of the cervical spine. These Case Reports illustrate the development of post-traumatic neurological manifestations against the background of the histodynamic effects of the cord trauma and the secondary damage produced by physiological stretching of the pons–cord tract and skull traction. The course of the neurological symptoms after spinal cord relaxation secured by the cervicolordodesis operation is also reported.

It is customary to divide spinal cord damage into total and partial cross-sectional lesions (14, 115, 225). Spinal cord lesions that have led to abolition of all neurological functions, with no evident tendency for their recovery, are classed as *total lesions*, and those where the loss of function is initially restricted to a few pathways and where the neurological functions show improvement in a matter of weeks are classed as *partial lesions*.

In the light of our knowledge of the effect of histodynamic tension set up in the compressed medullary tissue, it is logical to give the same spinal cord relaxation treatment for both partial and total cross-sectional lesions; for the tensile stress generated is the same, there being only a difference in its magnitude, and hence its destructive potential.

The patients to which Case Reports 1–3 refer were by chance ones with partial lesions, while nos. 4–6 were total lesions. All six patients were operated upon with the same protective technique, which produces effective relaxation of the damaged axis-cylinders and blood-vessels. Axons that had been damaged at the instant of compression by over-stretching and fissuring of the cord can then no longer be exposed to tension.

The first and second groups of three patients are discussed separately because the emphasis lies on different aspects of the cord damage.

Case 1. Man, aged 67.

Admitted to the Department of Neurosurgery, Karolinska Hospital, Stockholm. End of June, 1970, thrown over the handlebar of his bicycle on to his face. Immediate paraparesis in the legs and paraplegia in the arms and hands.

Objective findings. Reduced power in knee flexors and extensors. Marked reduction of power in extension of the feet but less so in flexion. A few centimetres' abduction and adduction of right arm at the shoulder joint; right elbow flexed so as to move forearm a centimetre or so when supported; no extension. Immobility of hands and fingers. Sensibility to pain greatly reduced below knee level. Babinski's reflex positive on right side. Complete urinary incontinence.

Preoperative evaluation. Typical central spinal cord injury, possibly with rupture of cervical cord parenchyma due to intramedullary tension at level between osteophytes C_6/C_7 and upper rim of C_7 vertebral arch. Possibly oedema in the cord

with increase in thickness of axis cylinders and consequent tendency for their contraction and shortening.

Cervicolordodesis indicated for relief of stress in any unimpaired nerve-fibres. Since the increase in the diameter of the cord on extension of the cervical spine may be greater than normal owing to the oedema, also C_7 arco-cristectomy was decided on.

Operation (author), 3 July, 1970. Skin incision from C_6 to T_1, C_7 protective arco-cristectomy and cervicolordodesis with fascia lata graft. For procedure see Fig. 150. The operation was modified by making a 4 cm transverse incision in the skin at the level of the external occipital protuberance and a sagittal incision at the T_1 spinous process; between these two sites the fascia lata graft was placed beneath the skin.

Postoperative course. After 4 uneventful days there was difficulty in swallowing. Right-sided recurrent nerve paresis. Aspiration pneumonia in right middle lobe. Prophylactic tracheostomy. Penicillin. No evidence of postoperative epidural haematoma (motor power in arms slightly improved; able to extend left arm and move left thumb feebly).

Patient could not be mobilized owing to severe orthostatic lowering of the blood pressure. *ECG.* Atrial fibrillation. Marked coronary insufficiency; signs of myocardial failure in left ventricle.

Decannulation after 7 days. Neurological improvement. Able to flex and extend right elbow slightly; weaker on left side. Feeble flexion of fingers of both hands.

On discharge from hospital on 6 August, 1970, the power in the legs had recovered appreciably, and the patient was able to walk short distances. The mobility of the arms had also improved and there was a considerable increase in the abduction and adduction in the right shoulder joint, good flexion and extension in the right elbow, and some mobility of the fingers of the right hand. The mobility of the left arm and hand was only slighty improved. Extremely feeble movement in the fingers of both hands could be performed.

Follow-up check at Nynäshamn Hospital, January 16, 1971. Indwelling catheter removed October, 1970. Full control of the bladder recovered. Good return of power in both arms and hands. Marked atrophy of small muscles of hands, more on right than left (dynamometer: 4 and 12 kg, respectively) and right hand remained clumsy. All modalities of sensation reduced in finger-tips and toes of left foot. Walked without impediment. Reflexes slightly exaggerated in both arms and left ankle (with unsustained clonus). The wounds had healed well.

Comments. To what extent the nerurological improvement can be ascribed to the operation cannot be judged, since some spontaneous regression invariably follows purely conservative treatment for such injuries. Only after more extensive experience of this operation in a large number of patients will it be possible to assess its merits. There is, however, little doubt that cervicolordodesis, preceded by arco-cristectomy, is a logical and beneficial measure, with a sound biomechanical background.

To judge from the events of the accident there was 'hyperextension trauma' with neurological signs typical of central spinal cord injury. Radiographs visualized osteophytes on the lower border of the C_6 and upper border of the C_7. In slight extension of the cervical spine the osteophyte at C_6 approached the upper rim of the C_7 arch. This was apparently the narrowest site in the generally shallow cervical canal, and probably the level of a pincer action on the cervical spinal cord. The resulting tension probably led to over-stretching and rupture of nerve-fibres—especially those in the central pyramidal pathways to the arms; the tension set up in the fibres of the peripheral pathways to the legs was probably lower. The simultaneous over-stretching of the blood-vessels probably led to central oedema, if not to rupture and haemorrhage. These in turn would presumably have accentuated the tension in the nerve-fibres of the adjacent pathways.

Because it has been recognized that it is the narrowing of the cervical canal that is responsible for cord compression, it has been the practice to keep the cervical spine in the neutral or even flexed position, so that the cervical canal is widened. However, flexion subjects the conducting nerve-fibres and blood-vessels in the cord to tension, although less pronounced than that to which these structures would have been exposed as a result of a pincer action.

In the case in question it was inferred that the axis-cylinders of the cervical cord were subjected to pathological tension.

The fact that the post-traumatic oedema is not only interstitial but also intracellular will enhance their tendency to retract (35, 59). Accordingly, in order to bring the surfaces of the wound fissure in the cord together and to achieve at least a gliotic repair, the cord was slackened by inducing extension, thus relieving the tension in the nerve-fibres that were still conducting and saving them from further mechanical damage.

It is now known (to some extent through surgical experience) that post-traumatic oedema can lead to a significant increase in the thickness of the cervical cord. So as to be able to relax its conducting nerve-fibres without risk of further compression of the cervical cord, it is necessary first to remove the osseous structure that in the prospective cervicolordodesis might give rise to a pincer action. The first surgical measure was therefore C_7 arco-cristectomy. Because of a lack of space owing to the relatively short skin incision the upper border of the C_7 spinous process was also removed (Fig. 147). The cervicolordodesis by the fascia lata graft could then be performed. This operation was carried out on the third day after the trauma; Decadron had not been administered and the operation was the only treatment given. From the very slight but definite neurological improvement observed as early as the second and the third days after the operation in this patient, where the cord was particularly susceptible to any maltreatment, it may be concluded that this type of operation, whereby the tension in the cervical cord is reduced, is the most beneficial measure.

Case 2. Man, aged 18.

Synopsis from files. (For data: see below.)
Neurological history. When diving in shallow water the patient sustained a compression of the C_5 vertebral body, a fracture of its arch and dislocation of the left lower articular facet. Immediately after admission to hospital a pair of Winkelmann's forceps with a load of 5 kg had been applied in the conventional manner. This was apparently followed by aggravation of the neurological symptoms. When the traction had been applied there was in any case tetraplegia with extinction of most functions below the C_5 segment. The patient could manage only to lift the shoulders and abduct the upper arms slightly; the other functions in the arms were abolished and the forearms and hands were totally paralysed. The sensibility was reduced for all qualities, increasing distally from a level three fingers above the mammillary plane. There was total urinary incontinence. Confusional state for several days.

Transferred to the Department of Neurosurgery eleven days after the accident. The traction was removed immediately and the cervical spine reclined over a round bolster. The radiograph taken immediately afterwards showed lowering of all the intervestebral spaces compared with their widening during skull traction. As expected, the C_5 vertebral body protruded again 2–3 mm into the cervical canal (Fig. 69 B).

Twenty-four hours after the spinal cord relaxation had been introduced the sensibility to touch was normal above the nipple level. The next day the level for normal sensation had fallen 5–6 cm below this plane, and the progress continued throughout the next few days. Only a week after the relaxation was begun there was sensibility to light touch with cotton wool even in the sacral dermatomes. The sensation for filling of the bladder and rectum was also normalized. On completion of bladder training 14 days after the spinal cord relaxation had been effected the catheter was removed. The range of movement of the left arm, left hand and left leg had increased appreciably.

Operation (author). Cervicolordodesis was performed, a fascia lata graft being anchored between the external occipital protuberance and the spinous processes T_1 and T_2. Ten weeks after the accident the patient was able to use the left arm and hand (for instance, in writing, buttoning and manoeuvring the wheel-chair), although there was still some weakness. The thumb of the right hand could be approximated to the little finger.

The spasticity in the legs had diminished. The left leg recovered its full range movement and the power was satisfactory. With the aid of a pelvic support the right thigh could be raised almost to horizontal. The patient was able to walk short distances between the bars with the aid of a splint for the right knee and a crutch-handled stick.

Clinical data relating to the above extract.

Admitted Nacka Hospital, 17 July, 1971, at 23.00.

Transferred to Department of Neurotraumatology, Karolinska Hospital, 18 July.

Radiological examination. 17, 18 July.

Operation (Levander), 18 July, 1971. Winkelmann's calipers for skull traction applied with 5 kg load.

Transferred to Department of Neurosurgery, Karolinska Hospital, 28 July, 1971. Traction discontinued. Cervical spine instead placed on a round bolster, held slightly extended by means of a pair of Crutchfield's forceps anchored in frontal bone with a 500 g load.

Operation (Körlof & author), 16 September, 1971. Cervicolordodesis by fascia lata graft.

Postoperative course. Operation wound infected with *Staphylococcus aureus.*

Transferred to Department of Rehabilitation, Karolinska Hospital, 20 October, 1971.

Follow-up examination (author), 29 October, 1974. Largely rehabilitated. Has clerical work which he can manage without help. But still prefers to write with left hand. Still has two symptoms, which no longer disturb him, viz. right-sided limp and slightly impaired function of right hand, whose fingers are slightly flexed and relatively weak. Left hand more serviceable than right: can, for example, undo, but not do up, buttons; can cut bread and meat, provided meat is not too tough. Swims for at least half an hour every week, using rubber foot-fins. Finds bakstroke easiest.

Objective findings. Right arm slightly spastic. Fairly strong biceps, hand flexors and extensors; right triceps muscle weakest. Gross functional strength of right hand considerably reduced. Sensibility of arm and hand normal. Left arm and hand: normal strength of all muscle groups. Sensibility impaired in patches, especially on the ulnar surface of the forearm and hand. Abdominal muscles weaker on right side than on left. Right leg: generally weaker, wears Camp bandage round right knee, which is apt to bend backwards. Gross strength reduced, especially of foot extensors. Sensibility: normal everywhere. Left leg: normal strength everywhere, but impaired sensibility, especially to heat and normally painful stimuli. Strength normal. Gait: slight right-sided limp. Normal but somewhat robot-like sequence of movements. Locomotion much better in afternoon—can then walk several kilometres without getting tired.

Comments. To judge from the neurological picture the tension set up on compression had torn fibres of, for example, the right lateral spinothalamic and pyramidal tracts; the ruptures here obviously occurred first of all in the fibres to the arms and hands. Fibres of the right posterior column, too, were involved, as well as part of the medial area of the left pyramidal tract. The neurological picture and the dislocation of the left intervertebral joint thus indicate an oblique course of the pincer action—from the right front to the left back, or conversely. The time between the relaxation of the spinal cord and the distinct improvement in conductivity for sensibility, motor power and bladder control was remarkably short (Table 5, pp. 214–5).

This elucidation of the histodynamic events in the cord tissue in spinal cord injury would seem to indicate a new logical and practical approach to our task of achieving better results of treatment of patients with spinal cord injury.

Case 3. Man, aged 58.

Neurological history. Following a fall indoors on 23 March, 1971, there was weakness in the arms and legs and slurred speech (confusional state). After 2 days in bed, the patient was admitted to St. Erik's Hospital, Stockholm, 25th March. Diagnosis of cerebral stroke; total paresis of right arm and leg, increasing neurological deficit. 27 March. Total paresis in arms and right leg, only slight movements in left leg.

Admitted, 27 March, to Department of Neurology, Karolinska Hospital.

Radiographic examination. Anteroposterior diameter of cervical canal reduced from C_4 to C_7. Disc degeneration with osteophytes at several levels. C_3 vertebral body dislocated posteriorly, maximum narrowing (8 mm) between lower border of C_3 and arch of C_4.

Gas myelogram. Considerable thickening of soft tissues between C_3 and C_7.

Transferred to Department of Neurosurgery, Karolinska Hospital, 28 March.

Neurological findings. Marked dyspnoea at rest. Complete paresis in both arms and right leg, subtotal in left leg. Babinski's sign positive bilaterally. Below C_4 slight reduction in sensibility, below T_1 loss of all qualities. Total urinary incontinence (indwelling catheter).

Operation (author), 28 March. Protective bilateral laminectomy C_4, C_5, C_6, arco-cristectomy C_7 and cervicolordodesis (Mersilene mesh).

Postoperative course and neurological findings. Definite improvement on day after operation. Respiratory difficulty experienced prior to operation disappeared (according to patient). Practically normal mobility of left leg but considerable reduction in power. Mobility of right leg improved, range much reduced; extension easiest. Could elicit muscle twitches in left arm. Complete paresis in right arm persisted. Spasticity in both legs. Babinski's sign positive bilaterally. Normal sensibility for slight touch and pain over whole body. Proprioception normal in left foot, reduced in right, absent in arms and hands. Able to sit up in bed. More or less dazed; wished to get up and had to be strapped to bed. Sensation of bladder filling normal on 3rd postoperative day. Catheter removed on 4th day, able to pass water in bottle. Could sit up in a chair on 6th postoperative day. Disturbed and anxious at night.

Radiographic examination showed basal atelectasis in right lung in regress. Seventh postoperative day: bladder management normal whole day with bottle. *7 April.* Urinary tract infection; epididymitis on right side. Urine passed in bed. Uridom; sulphonamide therapy. *14 April.* Left hand recovered some mobility, able to grasp objects and clench fist, though with reduced power. *14 April.* Fainting sensation on sitting up in chair. Haemoglobin level 6.9. Weber's test checked. *19 April.* Vomited blood; melaena. Tired and weak; blood transfusion. *7 June.* Improved mobility of *left* hand; able to grasp objects, now with improved power. Slight movements of fingers of *right* hand. Mobility and gross power in legs improved. *12 June.* Able to stand and to walk with support. Walking capacity increased towards end of month.

Patient died on 3 July following operation for gastric carcinoma. Autopsy (cervical cord) refused by relatives.

Discussion (Cases 1–3)

As is well known from experience of injury to peripheral nerves, any trauma that produces tearing of the nervous tissue results not only in immediate interruption of the conductivity of the involved nerve-fibres but also in elastic retraction of all those whose surrounding connective tissue has also been damaged. A gap will thus form that sooner or later fills with glial or connective scar tissue, thereby ultimately preventing any contact between the torn surfaces of the nervous tissue. The isolated parts of torn nerve-fibres then undergo degeneration.

Trauma of the spinal cord is, in principle, followed by a similar sequence of events, but separation of any torn fibres of the cord is still more likely to occur here than in a peripheral nerve. The extent to which the torn ends separate on flexion of the spinal column will be determined by (i) the stretching of the whole pons–cord tract and (ii) the lengthening of part of the spinal canal in the vicinity of the cord lesion, including the dura, to which the upper and lower ends of the torn part of the cord are anchored by the nerve-roots and attachments of the dentate ligaments (Fig. 67). If the gap is not too great—and, as can happen, it is filled by avascular débris from torn cord tissue—the traumatic defect will usually be repaired by formation of a glial or connective tissue scar, a process that will be promoted by organization of the haemorrhage that often accompanies such an injury (161).

In the treatment of spinal cord injury in man no practical efforts have so far been made to prevent separation of the edges of the ruptured nervous tissue and the consequent formation of the scar. In recent animal experiments conducted with the purpose of analysing the mechanism of trauma in spinal cord injury and of evolving methods of minimizing its untoward neurological effects, the separation of the cut ends at the level of the trauma was largely disregarded. Bassett & Campbell, 1962, however, used a stabilizing device inserted through skin, paraspinal muscles and T_6 to T_{12} spinous processes prior to cord transection or to grafting procedures at the T_9 level (13).

In radiographs of the living dog's spinal column in extreme functional positions the author found some years ago that, as in man, the cervical section of the column and the canal was elongated and shortened more than the rest (Fig. 67 D). Thus, if stretching of the spinal cord is to be prevented it is the *cervical* column and canal that must be immobilized.

As has been shown both in the living patient and the cadaver, any forward bending of the head from the neutral position of the cervical spine leads to an increase in tension in the pons–cord tract, and hence in further traumatization of the tissue, wherever the lesion of the spinal cord is located. Accordingly, when a fresh spinal cord injury is to be treated, it would seem to be logical and mandatory first to *immobilize the cervical spine in extension*, so as to slacken the whole pons–cord tract. The need for such immobilization at an early stage is born out by now well established facts. About 10 per cent of patients receiving spinal cord injuries suffer further damage during transport to hospital (123). There is general agreement that conservative treatment by suitable positioning of the patient has yielded the best results; but even when this measure is taken in the hospital bed, measures to obtain adequate immobilization of the spinal cord tissue and thus prevent tension are all too frequently neglected. Any

forward bending movements of the cervical spine inevitably lead to an increase in tension in the cord tissue, and thus aggravation of the injury. The conservative methods practised today are thus, in fact, by no means conservative enough (47).

The orthopaedic measures for preventing the untoward effects of tension in the spinal cord tissue must be centred in the first place on the axial component. To minimize this the cervical spinal canal must be shortened by extension. As shown in biomechanical experiments on the cadaver, this position reduces the separation of the torn ends of the spinal cord at any level. Both astroglial and connective scar tissue will then be thinner and possibly spread over a smaller area (Fig. 70 F) (161). If the formation of a large scar is prevented in this way the pressure and tension to which the intact nerve-fibres in its vicinity are exposed will be minimized.

Besides the purely biomechanical reasons, there are physiological ones for bringing about early contact of the ruptured surfaces in the cord tissue, for tissue cultures have shown that the uptake of nutritive substances, including oxygen, that promote cell growth increases with the area of contact between living cells.

From the histodynamic observations it is evident that besides the complicating effects of a scar—whether superficial or intramedullary—this can exert an outward thrust on uninvolved nerve-fibres, thereby overstretching them to the point where their conductivity is impaired. It may be re-established when the tension has been relieved by relaxing the spinal cord (Fig. 70 H).

The amelioration of the neurological symptoms obtained by the relaxation technique in the actual 3 patients with cord injury and in 3 cases of multiple sclerosis (see above) suggests that this treatment might well be effective also in other partial, and even total, cord lesions. Following myelotomy at the T_9–T_{12} level in 2 other patients with multiple sclerosis there was recovery of some mobility of the legs which may well have been concealed by the spasticity (168). If residual function can appear in such apparently hopeless cases after destructive surgery, there would seem to be even greater reason to expect a recovery of masked residual capability of neurological function after spinal cord relaxation in cases of partial cord lesions and multiple sclerosis. As has been shown earlier, there is a certain parallel between these two quite distinct pathological conditions; in both cases there is intramedullary oedema or glial or connective tissue scarring that overstretches adjacent blood-vessels and nerve-fibres and blocks the conductivity of the latter.

It is generally accepted that in high-level spinal cord lesions it is of the greatest importance to retain the function of the nerve-roots belonging to the lowermost intact spinal cord segment, and this is the prime object of any surgical method; it is usually achieved by the removal of bone. However, no account has been taken of the stretching of the spinal cord and nerve-roots that inevitably results from the lengthening of the spinal canal accompanying any forward bending of the cervical spine. In the case of high-level lesions the nervous parenchyma of the cord does not tolerate the slightest elongation; those axis-cylinders which have been so greatly over-stretched that they are liable to rupture ultimately do so if relaxation is not effected immediately. Others that have ruptured partially, but whose ends are still in contact, retract as soon as the fissure between the ends is enlarged by oedema and/or haemorrhage during skull traction, thereby promoting the growth of glial or connective tissue and hence preventing recovery of conductivity. In high-level cross-sectional lesions in particular, therefore, it is of prime importance to perform cervicolordodesis as soon as possible after the trauma has been sustained.

Nor, in the case of a trauma to a caudal section of the spinal cord that is apparently, if not certainly, isolated from its cranial section, can the tension set up in the former due to lengthening of the canal be disregarded, especially when rupture is incomplete. For even at a level where a pincer action has led to an apparently total or subtotal rupture of the cord tissue the pia cylinder may still be intact and transmit tensile forces caudalward to the possibly isolated section of the cord. It remains to be seen whether also in such cases—where a cervicolordodesis operation is indicated primarily to relieve the tension in the intact *cranial* cord section and its *nerve-roots*—there is anything to be gained from relaxation of the apparently isolated *caudal* section of the spinal cord, for example, a reduction in spasticity.

In the case of incomplete and apparently complete cross-sectional lesions protective relaxation should *always* be performed, since in both cases the neurological symptoms may be due in some degree to tension in the cord tissue set up by the pressure of scars rather than to total rupture; for if there is a neurological improvement in respect of nerve-fibres whose anatomical continuity is retained, their conductivity must have been blocked by the tension in the intact nerve-fibres around an intramedullary fissure (Fig. 68).

The evidence suggests that this surgical measure can be beneficial in more or less any form of spinal cord injury that has produced a neurological deficit. The relaxation eliminates the tension in the most important parenchymal elements of the damaged cord tissue, namely, the nerve-fibres and blood-vessels.

General conclusions

In any patient with a spinal cord injury that has resulted in a partial or total cross-sectional lesion of the cord, whatever the level, it is advisable to perform cervicolordodesis at the earliest opportunity so as to secure the best conditions for transmission of the action potentials, glial repair at the level of the lesion, and even axonal regeneration (65, 121, 141, 268–270). Prior to this a thorough radiological examination should be made to exclude the possibility of a persistent pincer action on the cord tissue. Any such mechanism should be

eliminated by protective arco-cristectomy or protective bilateral laminectomy before the cervicolordodesis is undertaken.

Case 4. Man, aged 19.[1]

2 July, 1973. Late in the evening the patient dived into water of unknown depth. Friends pulled him to the shore unconscious and he lay thus for 20–25 minutes until the ambulance arrived.

Admitted to the Emergency Department, Karolinska Hospital, at 23.50 Mentally lucid. Minor bruise near vertex. Pain in back of neck, dry throat, difficulty in swallowing. *Transferred* to Department of Neurosurgery.

Neurological findings. Abdominal breathing, only. Paraplegia and areflexia in legs. Abdominal wall reflexes absent. Priapism. Reduced gross power, numbness and paraesthesia in arms. Paraplegia in hands. Abolished sensibility bilaterally up to nipple level.

Radiographic examination. Compression fracture of C_5 vertebral body with 1 cm long tear-drop fracture anteroinferiorly; C_5 body displaced 2–3 mm posteriorly in relation to C_4, 1 cm in relation to C_6; resulting in severe narrowing of spinal canal at level of inferior posterior border of the C_5 body. No rotation.

Treatment. Skull traction applied immediately, with 12 kg load.

Course, 3 July, 9.30. More pronounced numbness in arms (more paretic?), hands paraplegic, 'almost tetraplegic'. Periodical confusion for several days. Traction removed (date?).

Pre-operative evaluation. The traumatic pincer action on the cervical cord was probably located between the posterior, inferior border of the C_5 vertebral body and the upper part of the C_6 arch. Arco-cristectomy and relaxation of the spinal cord were considered indicated; the former operation on the C_6 vertebral arch would remove one of the pincer components, while slackening the spinal cord would tend to approximate the wound margins in the cord rupture, and provide a 'tissue reserve' to eliminate any thrust due to the displacement of the vertebra.

Operation (author), 6 July, 1973. Protective arco-cristectomy on C_6 and cervicolordodesis. Prosthesis clamp (26 by 6 by 4.5 mm) cemented in a transverse groove in occipital bone about 1.5 cm above external occipital protuberance. Vertical skin incision (curved to left) from C_7 to T_4. Short sagittal incisions in the erector trunci muscles at level of interspinous ligaments. Trevira ribbon[2] 2 cm wide anchored below the ligaments around T_3 to T_1 spinous processes. In tunnel through neck muscles just above cervical spinous processes two ends of ribbon drawn up to the clamp where, with cervical spine extended to predetermined degree, they were secured by the screws. (See Fig. 153 A–C.)

Radiographic examination, 7 July. Upper anterior part of arch of the C_6 vertebra removed. Anterior compression of the C_5 body increased; its upper posterior part had slipped 1–2 mm, its lower part 5 mm, into the cervical canal. Lordosis of cervical

---

[1] Not included in Table 5.
[2] 'Teflon'-type (p. 193).

spine had straightened. *17 July.* Kyphosis increased with anterior angle of about 10° at level of compression. Vertebral body displaced 2 mm or so posteriorly. *24 July.* Angle increased to 20°.

Postoperative course and neurological findings, 7th July. Level of sensibility to touch had fallen one hand-width below nipple level. *8 July.* Sensibility to touch now also in legs, better on left side. *12 July.* Limit for normal thermaesthesia 2 finger widths above nipple level, for vibratory sensation at level of lowermost rib on both sides, for light touch (with cotton-wool) just below umbilical plane. *19 July.* During last few days weak contractions in extensor carpi radialis muscles (especially left); slight but definite opposing movements of thumb and index finger (especially left). Limit for normal sensibility to touch, unchanged for some days, about 3 finger widths below umbilical level; distal to this level sensibility reduced; anaesthesia one hand-width above symphysis. Sensibility to touch from feet up to knees (left better than right); able to locate somewhat uncertainly, but for most part correctly. No positional proprioception in feet or legs. Paraesthesia in feet and legs in form of numbness and, priodically, of pins and needles. Arm reflexes lively, areflexia in legs. *23 July.* Tilting training (begun a few days after trauma): now able to tolerate 50° for 30 min without orthostatism; *24 July.* Tilting evoked pain in shoulders, and had to be stopped at 35°. Sensibility to touch on right pelvic crest. Perceived pain stimulus in S_3 dermatome bilaterally. Aware of incipient passage of faeces. *25 July.* Plaster cast for Minerva plastic neck support. *26 July.* Radiographic check showed increase in anterior angle of cervical spine in the fracture plane (20°) and in the backward displacement of the vertebral body (see above).

Preoperative evaluation. In spite of relaxation of the spinal cord, the thrust and compression exerted by the greatly displaced C_5 vertebra appeared to be affecting the conductivity of the cord and nerve-roots. The shoulder pain was attributable to tension in the cervical nerve-roots due to stretching over the vertebra; the relatively slow and modest neurological improvement could have been due in some measure to residual tension in the cord from the same causes. Removal of the vertebra in question was therefore indicated; to avoid increasing the compression of the cervical cord, protective bilateral laminectomy was planned and the clamp had therefore to be opened. This would presumably afford an opportunity to examine whether the ribbon permitted, and even contributed to, the displacement of the vertebra.

Operation (author), 27 July, 1973. Revision of cervico-lordodesis. In prone position, placing of head on self-adjusting head-rest immediately produced marked lordosis of the cervical spine. Radiographs showed that part of spinal column containing fracture was practically straight. Positional correction achieved with Trevira ribbon in place. Prosthesis clamp opened (clamp and ribbon well integrated; no gross evidence of foreign body reaction). Because of unforseen extraneous circumstances operation discontinued without planned measures being carried out or Trevira ribbon being replaced in clamp. Patient placed on back in posterior part of plastic support before waking.

Postoperative course. Uneventful. *28 July.* Complained of increased intensity and frequency of spastic twitches in legs and pain in shoulders. Recommended to lie either in prone position in anterior half of support or on back in posterior half. Before turning, and in seated position, both halves assembled.

Increasing mental depression, manifested in aggressiveness and negative attitude. Unwilling to undergo any further surgical treatment. (Parents, however, still favoured removal of vertebra, although warned that chance of any improvement rapidly decreased as time passed.) Transferred to Department of Rehabilitation, South Stockholm Hospital, 23 August, 1973.

Readmitted, 27 September, 1973, to the Department of Neurosurgery, Karolinska Hospital. Since previous discharge both arms had recovered weak triceps function. Recently aware of abdominal muscle function. Arm and leg reflexes brisk and equal on each side; Babinski's sign negative bilaterally.

Re-operation (author). *First séance,* 2 October, 1973. Bilateral protective laminectomy C_5; Trevira ribbon clamped with cervical spine extended.

Postoperative course. Uneventful. *3 October.* Patient aware of reduction of spasticity in legs. Attitude to next operation remained negative, but parents still persistent.

Second séance, 22 October, 1973. Extirpation of displaced C_5 vertebral body by anterior access, and spondylodesis on C_4 and C_6 bodies using steel-frame prosthesis and tibial bone graft. (See Figs. 154 A and B.)

Postoperative course uneventful.

Radiographic examination, 29 October. Prosthesis anchored in C_4 and C_6 vertebral bodies. Anterior angle at level of fracture increased by one or two degrees.

Urological examination, 5 November. Marked tendency for contraction of bladder, with increased tonus; erythema and irritation of mucosa; sensibility abolished. Reflexes: bulbocavernosus muscle and anal reflexes positive; autonomic hyperreflexia. Catheter removed; micturition induced with carbacholine and throbbing.

Follow-up examination (Bergman) Treklöverhemmet, Ljungskile, 24 September, 1974. Still bound to wheel-chair, but drives it himself and manages thresholds and lifts. Able to brush his teeth, comb his hair, wash his face and upper body, put on shirt, but not draw it down back or do up buttons; able to eat and drink without help, turn over pages of newspapers and books and can telephone. Can get up from prone position on carpet with aid of elbows and can turn over from prone to supine position in bed. Able to help a little when moved with davit. Almost normal function of shoulder muscles, both biceps and extensor muscles of hand, but no active wrist or finger function (passive digital function with aid of extension of wrists). Able to approximate right thumb and index finger. Can extend arms completely, but with reduced power. Can contract abdominal muscles, somewhat more in upper than in lower part and sit upright without support. No mobility of legs. Sensibility normal on radial side of right hand (finger–thumb grip); impaired on index finger and ulnar surface of left hand; normal above wrists. Good sensibility to touch on back and posterior surface of legs; impaired on anterior surface below umbilical plane. Sensibility to pain and temperature lost below T_2; joint proprioception, sensitivity to touch and vibratory sensation normal in legs. Bladder sensation now partly restored. Urgency of micturition—urine retention for only half a minute, otherwise spontaneous evacuation. Induces urination at certain hours of the day by throbbing area over bladder. Spasticity of legs, which had decreased somewhat already in March despite reduced doses of antispasmodic (Lioresal), now practically disappeared without further medical treatment.

Radiographic examination, 18 November, 1974. Position of steel-frame prosthesis unchanged. C_4, C_5 and C_6 vertebral bodies fused with an anterior open obtuse angle of about 166°.

Case 5.   Man, aged 22.[3]

On 7 July, 1973, dived into shallow water; got up on hitting the bottom, but collapsed and was pulled out by friends. Cyanotic, arms and legs paralysed. Conveyed to South Stockholm Hospital.

Admitted to Emergency Department, Karolinska Hospital.

Objective findings. A muscular young man; apprehensive, oriented. Diaphragmatic respiration. Loss of sensibility on thorax below C_4 dermatome, on arms and ulnar aspects of forearms, total on hands (normal sensibility only in C_5 dermatome). Minor head lesions. *Tentative diagnosis:* High cross-sectional lesion with poor prognosis.

Preliminary treatment. Skull traction introduced immediately with 5 kg load.

Transferred to Department of Neurosurgery, Karolinska Hospital.

Radiographic examination, 7 July. Compression fracture of C_5 with anterior tear-drop fracture and posterior fragment displaced 4 mm into cervical canal (in relation to C_6). Axial length of C_4/C_5 and C_5/C_6 intervertebral spaces greater than normal due to skull traction. No pathological features in lungs observed in supine position. *8 July.* (Fracture and displacement of C_5 probably reduced at previous examination.) On removal of traction, lower margin of C_5 protruded 3 mm into canal; distance from there to upper edge of arch of C_6 was 11.5–12 mm. Manifest reduction of distance between lower lamina of C_5 and upper of C_6. Tear-drop fracture unchanged.

Clinical observation. Respiratory difficulties, rhonchi in right half of thorax. Lung radiographs showed patchy infiltrations. Tracheostomy performed. Catheter *à demeure,* plugged for bladder training with emptying at three-hourly intervals. Laxatives required.

Pre-operative evaluation. Relaxation of spinal cord and nerve-roots indicated to approximate intramedullary rupture surfaces and to save as much as possible of arm and hand function.

Operation (author), 8 July, 1973. Cervicolordodesis.[4] Prosthesis clamp cemented in occipital bone. Vertical skin incision (curved to left) comprising T_1 to T_3. Trevira ribbon[5] anchored with shoe-lacing technique around T_2 and T_1 spinous processes, ends of ribbon being led to clamp through tunnel just above cervical spinous processes. Head and cervical spine placed in predetermined extension position and ribbon screwed tight in clamp.

Postoperative course, 8 July. Radiographic check of cervical spine: no change. *9 July* (report by nurse). Able to move arms but not legs; respiration poor. Radiographic check of lungs: diffuse areas of infiltration in middle and basal parts of right lung. Pneumonia, right lung.

10 July. Basal, partly confluent infiltration of parenchyma on right side, disappearing by 16 July.

10 July. Respiration improved; sensibility to touch approximately at level of 10th rib, slightly lower on left side, elevated temperature in the anaesthetic areas. Tilting training begun.

14th July. Cannula removed; spotted exanthema around tracheostoma on chest, extending to back. Secretion from stoma cultured *Staphylococcus aureus;* treatment with potassium permanganate, Ecomytrin hydrocortisone.

16 July. Able to tolerate 30 minutes' tilting without orthostatism; trained energetically and diligently; recovered slight but reasonable function in biceps and triceps of both arms; feeble extension and flexion of hands had begun to advance; weak opposing movement of thumb and index finger indicative of innervation of carpi radialis muscles. Diffuse sensibility to touch in hands and volar and dorsal aspects of hands and fingers. Vibratory sensation normal in upper arms and forearms, greatly reduced distal to wrists. Propriception in ankles? Increasing extensor spasticity and foot clonus, especially right.

19 July. During isometric exercise of neck muscles patient suddenly and vigorously pressed chin and cervical spine forward (no definite neurological damage discerned, but this was, of course, masked by deficit symptoms).[6]

20 July. Radiographic check of the cervical spine. Slightly increased displacement of posterior fragment of C_5 into cervical canal; kyphosis in the fracture region, with anterior angle of 30°.

23 July. Plaster cast for Minerva plastic neck support. Urine culture: moderate growth of *Klebsiella* and enterobacteria. *24 July.* Radiographic check showed the kyphosis to have disappeared; C_5 displaced 4–5 mm in relation to the C_6. *28 July.* Lay in posterior part of the support, position comfortable. Now tolerates 60–70° tilting for 30 minutes. *31 July.* Able to sit up in a wheel-chair for first time.

Transferred to Department of Rehabilitation, Karolinska Hospital. *Diagnosis,* 31 July. Fracture of C_5 with probably total transverse lesion just below C_5 segment.

Radiographic check of cervical spine, 2 August. Reduction of fracture satisfactory; 10 August. In seated position without neck support kyphosis in region of fracture, disappearing in supine position and on extension of cervical spine.

Neurological findings, 3 August. Elbows: flexion 2, extension 1; wrists: radial flexion right 1, left 2; hand: opposition thumb and index finger 0–1; left hand: kinaesthesia dig I–II, partly (20 November much) improved in all fingers. Vibratory sensation to costal arch bilaterally, absent distal to this level. Reflexes: Biceps, right and left, +; triceps, right and left, (+); brachioradialis, right and left, +; quadriceps, right and left, ++; calf, right and left, +++, with inexhaustible foot clonus; Babinski's sign negative bilaterally. Severe spasticity; related attacks of cramp.

6 August. Two finger-widths below prosthesis clamp a fistula from formerly infected pressure sore in back of neck. *7 August.*

---

[3] Not included in Table 5.
[4] In prone position on self-adjusting head-rest pressure sore observed on back of neck.
[5] 'Teflon'-type (p. 193).
[6] 'Masked intramedullary tearing'?

Incision in erythematous skin at level of T_2 spinous process disclosed no communication with fistula, no secretion. Antibiotic therapy continued.

7 August. Depressed to point of nervous collapse. *13 August.* Catheter removed; able to pass water after injection of carbacholine and throbbing; still considerable incontinence, some ischuria paradoxa with about 150 ml of residual urine. Troublesome extensor spasms; antispastic medication ineffective. *22 August.* Difficulty in breathing. *23 August, Urological examination.* Bladder calculus removed, inflamed mucosa. *30 August.* Mobilization continued steadily; tired easily on sitting up; with aid to support arms, able to use typewriter, electric shaver and to eat. Kyphosis of cervical spine returned to 25° without collar.

Analysis of level of lesion (Normell), 5 October. Sensibility to pain in arms and hands completely recovered: right to C_6, left to C_8; tactile sensibility: right hand to C_6 (incompletely to C_7), left to C_7 (incompletely to C_8). Subjective: Cold, burning, aching sensations in legs, scrotum; (no sensibility in legs or heels; phantom pains).

16 October. Fracture of cervical spine now reliably healed.

19 October. Greatly irritated urinary bladder with marked tendency to contraction (autonomous hyperreflexia), strongly positive anal reflex; cutano-anal and bulbocavernosus reflexes absent.

25 October. Slight recovery of voluntary mobility in both quadriceps muscles.

1st November. Voluntary innervation of adductor muscles present, especially on left side, where some sensibility definitely recovered on medial and anterior aspects of thigh (Lindblom). Recovery of voluntary mobility and sensibility seen as indicative of some sort of regeneration.

8 November. For the previous week headache during filling of bladder and associated increase in spasticity. Blood pressure rose from 120 to 150 mmHg; sweating (typical late development in damage to sympathetic nervous system). Trevira ribbon visible in fistula, which was surrounded by granulations; no infected secretion (antibiotics). Surgery strongly indicated; considered that spasticity might diminish on removal of ribbon.

Operation (Nylén, author), 14 November, 1973. Trevira ribbon removed under local anaesthesia. Relaxation of spinal cord had thus been maintained for 4 months.

Postoperative course, 19 November. Wound healing satisfactorily. Flexing of head revealed tense, string-like elevation beneath the skin (connective tissue scar along tunnel formed around Trevira ribbon, this tension restricted flexion from the neutral position to about 50 per cent.

Patient's bed consisted of 2 equally long plane sections, the head end inclined at about 50°; a bolster was placed on sloping plane. This resulted in flexion of cervical spine, neck and hip-joints and extension of legs, and hence stretching of the spinal cord with potential impairment of conductivity after removal of cervicolordodesis (Figs. 131–4). A different bed was recommended.

Follow-up examination (Physiotherapist's report 6 March, 1974). Voluntary contraction of muscles of both thighs; after relaxation of the quadriceps able to draw both knee-caps upwards; in the seated position the patient can contract his left

quadriceps and extend the knee against gravity. Voluntary contraction of adductor muscles on both sides; feeble contraction of extensor muscles of the left thigh; this faculty is occasional and transient and cannot be reproduced at will. Voluntary flexion of both big toes. All these movements easier and more powerful on left side. Clear but diminished sensibility to touch and pain on left anterior surface of body below the C_4 level to a hand breadth above knee-cap; same applies to left side of back, including L_2 dermatome, where pain stimuli are clearly felt; some diffuse sensibility on anterior side of lower leg. Sensibility to touch on right side of abdomen diffuse and very weak; weak sensibility to touch on right side of thigh, none on lower leg. No kinaesthesia in either hip- or knee-joints.

Follow-up examination (author) 24 September, 1974. Steady but slight improvement in function of various muscles including neck and shoulder muscles. Able to contract both triceps muscles powerfully with no resistance; some increase in power in hand muscles (only those already functioning earlier). Distinctly more powerful contraction of abdominal muscles (rectus and obliquus abdominis); able to straighten upper trunk from 45° plane with aid of arms. With flexed thigh and knee and the feet held able to turn the body from right or left lateral to supine posture. Able to contract quadriceps muscles against relatively great resistance—right more than left; in attempts to contract the dorsal thigh muscles sometimes feels weak vibrations on the right side. Slight adductor function. Since August 1974 able to stand upright in the bars about one minute without bandage. Able to eat, shave, light a cigarette, etc., with effort. Sensibility unchanged; no perception of cold or warmth below T_4. Coarse positional perception on pulling hairs on anterior and posterior surfaces of lower leg. Spasticity in legs increased since removal of Trevira band. Renewal of cervicolordodesis is contemplated to avoid proposed intrathecal injection of phenol.

Case 6. Man, aged 20.[7]

On 16 July, 1973, the man dived into shallow water, floated up in a curious manner and was pulled ashore by friends. At 17.00 admitted to Norrtälje Hospital where tetraplegia, air hunger, abdominal respiration and presence of normal cough reflex noted. No mention of external injuries.

Transferred immediately to Department of Neurotraumatology, Karolinska Hospital.

Neurological findings. Able to move right and left shoulders, and slightly flex and extend right elbow and fingers of right hand. Almost total absence of sensibility below C_4, except for arms; for an hour or so no mobility or sensibility at all.

Diagnosis. Transverse lesion at C_4–C_5 level.

Radiographic examination. Compression fracture of C_5; vertebral body C_5 lowered and fractured in several places. Vertebral body of C_4 slipped forward along sloping anterior aspect of C_5 to form an anterior angle of 10°. Corresponding compression on the anterior aspect, intervertebral joints open posteriorly (rupture of joint capsules). When round bolster was placed under neck, and head and cervical spine were extended, C_4 immediately slipped backwards again and angle

---

[7] Not included in Table 5.

between C_4 and C_5 decreased to 1–2°. Lower lamina of C_4 and upper one of C_5 approximated; disc appeared to be completely crushed.

Treatment. Because, for extraneous reasons, immediate operation could not be performed that evening, head and cervical spine immobilized in reclined position by means of Crutchfield's forceps applied to frontal bone with 500 g load. In this position, distance between posterior inferior margin of C_4 and arch of C_5 was 17 mm (enlargement factor not subtracted). Catheter *à demeure* introduced.

Pre-operative evaluation. The trauma had probably been caused by the posterior inferior margin (edge) of the C_4 rotating backwards over the compressed vertebra and approaching the superior margin of the C_5 vertebral arch to pinch the cervical cord. As seen from the radiograph, on compression the bone of the C_5 body was displaced mainly in transverse directions. Most of the crushed C_4/C_5 disc will presumably have moved laterally with it. However, in the relatively spacious cervical canal, fragments of this disc may have remained. This is no contraindication to spinal cord relaxation (which may actually eliminate any thrust exerted by a small body on the cord). Since all neurological functions were abolished below C_4, immediate slackening of the cervical nerve-roots was indicated in order to rescue as much of their conductivity as possible.

Operation (author), 17 July, 1973. Transverse incision over external occipital protuberance. Prosthesis clamp cemented in a transverse groove drilled in occipital bone. Vertical skin incision, curved to left, from C_7 to T_3 level. Erector trunci fascia dissected on each side of spinous processes. Short sagittal incisions bilateral to supra- and interspinous ligaments of T_3–T_2, T_2–T_1 and T_1–C_7. Trevira ribbon[8] 2 cm wide anchored between muscle and bone by lacing around spinous processes. Neck muscles over cervical processes tunneled and two ends of ribbon led through and clamped, with cervical spine in the pre-determined extension posture.

Postoperative course. Uneventful. Radiographs showed that forward displacement of C_4 and anterior angle between C_4 and C_5 were eliminated. Uppermost section of cervical spine now greatly extended (occipital squama almost in contact with arch of atlas; the C_2 and C_3 and the C_3 and C_4 spinous processes had moved together, reducing posterior angle of plane between clivus and axis; cervical spine as a whole only slightly lordosed.[9]

18 July. Tilted to 35° for 10 minutes (Camp collar provided). Difficult to cough up mucus and to breathe; occasionally a sensation of suffocation (paresis of diaphragm). Capable of only slight contraction of deltoid muscles; normal sensibility within C_5 dermatome; level of sensibility on thorax unchanged. Three days later sensibility recovered in right C_6 dermatome to proximal joint of thumb. Severe numbness in hands and feet (especially right) and temporary tingling sensation, increased on rubbing skin. Knock against bed elicited tingling sensation throughout body to legs; tapping of tibia (reflex check) produced shock radiating to back of neck and head (Lhermitte's sign). Phantom sensations: Feeling of legs being separated widely, either curved or elevated; toes of both feet bent toward soles.

23 July. To increase mobility of patient without disturbing

fracture, plaster cast taken for a Minerva plastic neck support. Radiographic check next day showed C_4 vertebral body to have slipped forwards 2–3 mm on C_5 body.

2 August. Radiographic check of cervical spine in Minerva neck support. Convex neck part of support had slipped upwards and was acting as a pivot under the neck. Increased forward displacement of C_4, and C_4 and C_5 pressed closer together. Angle between C_4 and C_5 now 17–18°. Patient should now lie either supine in the anterior part of support, or on his back in posterior part; but this was difficult to manage.

4 August. Malposition in fracture reduced a couple of degrees. Patient still tilted 55–60° twice a day for 30 minutes.

Mid-August (one month after accident). Tetraplegia persisted, moderate spasticity in legs since end of July. Much disturbed sleep at nights; still difficult to breathe deeply. Able to sit up in wheel-chair for 1–5 hours a day. Sensibility to touch improved slightly in arms, upper trunk, legs and gluteal region; now present in right hand, on radial aspect of forearm, on both buttocks (on rubbing perineum), back of right thigh, in right popliteal fold and lower leg and on dorsal and plantar sides of toes of both legs. No sensibility to pain below C_5 dermatome. Vibratory sensation present on sternum to xiphoid process, on chest to middle ribs, on both hands and fingers and on legs. Still marked numbness from toes to halfway up lower legs, from finger-tips to forearms. On rubbing dorsal side of right middle finger a burning pain, felt as a shock-like pain in arm.

24 August. Suddenly able to flex right forearm. Power steadily increasing; 4 days later arm could be raised from extended position to chest.

Indications for re-operation. Reoperation desirable since fracture was disturbed through displacement of Minerva neck support.[10] For reduction and stabilization of fracture osteosynthesis was required. Traction of cervical spine contraindicated. Delivery of new design of prosthesis awaited.

Since 9 August twitching, felt in left shoulder muscles and also in left biceps, similar to that experienced on right side before recovery of contraction function in right biceps. Able to sit up in wheel-chair for 3–8 hours.

Operation (author), 24 September, 1973. Osteosynthesis by anterior access on C_4 and C_6 vertebral bodies, using steel-frame prosthesis and bone graft from right tibia. Only narrow frontally compressed part of C_5 body visible. After removing fragments of totally crushed C_4/C_5 disc and callus in C_4/C_5

---

[8] 'Teflon'-type (p. 193).

[9] Check in biomechanical experiment on cadaver showed that when the uppermost section of the cervical spine is extended as much as it was in this patient, the whole cervical cord slackens appreciably. The purpose of the operation was thus probably achieved in spite of the limited extension of the cervical spine.

[10] If the partial lordosis of the upper section of the cervical spine had not produced sufficient relaxation, the posterior margin of the C_5 might still have exerted a thrust on the cervical cord, and set up tension in the medullary tissue (possibly causing the prolonged paraesthesia, Lhermitte's sign, muscle twitching, and the like). Reduction of the kyphosis was therefore considered highly desirable.

space this could be widened when cervical spine was extended. Steel-frame prosthesis cemented in transverse grooves drilled in C_4 and C_6 bodies. Bone defect in compressed vertebra filled with graft from right tibia; anchored to prosthesis frame with fine steel wire.

Postoperative course. Uneventful. Radiographs show prosthesis with dislocated vertebral body reduced and graft in place (Fig. 154 g–i). Difficulty in swallowing for 3 days (radiographs showed oesophagus to be about 1 cm from prosthesis). Felt fit. Voluntary contraction of right deltoid, pectoralis major, teres major and minor subscapular, infra- and supraspinatus and brachioradialis muscles.

Transferred to Department of Rehabilitation, Sahlgrenska Hospital, Göteborg.

Follow-up examination (Bergman) Treklöverhemmet, Ljungskile, 3 July, 1974. After training urinary continence, able to manage voiding without catheter since spring 1974. Can drink and eat by himself, but needs help with everything else. Flaccid paralysis of trunk and legs. Left arm: can abduct the arm a little from the shoulder and contract biceps muscle, and supinate forearm with aid of biceps muscle (function of biceps muscle and abduction of shoulder recovered only during the last few weeks). Right arm: can raise arm to 90°; fairly good strength of biceps and brachioradialis muscles, can contract against moderate resistance, supinate with good strength, pronate only feebly. Triceps muscle: only very weak contractility. Not able to move any fingers of right hand. Sensibility to touch normal on surface of upper trunk. Below the T_2 level sensitive to pin-prick, but not able to locate exact site of stimulus. Normal passive mobility of neck; contraction of muscles in certain postures causes pain in right semispinalis capitis muscle.

General evaluation (Bergman). Subtotal lesion, thus no total transverse lesion as was supposed from the outset. Not yet possible to say whether neurological restitution can be expected. Recent course suggests steady recovery of neuronal functions.

Follow-up examination (Olanders) Treklöverhemmet, Ljungskile, 18 September, 1974. Continued urinary infection with fairly resistant mixed flora of ordinary type (had previously had bladder stones). Some increase in strength of earlier functioning muscles. Further recovery of motor function. Sensibility somewhat better: Right arm and hand: can sometimes exactly say where upper arm, forearm and hand have been touched. Trunk: impaired sensibility to touch on left side. Left arm and hand: sensibility to touch of skin of upper and forearm fairly good but poor on hand. Right leg: diffuse sensibility to touch over entire leg, best in toes and posterior surface of leg. Left leg: impaired sensibility of heel and toes, can locate touch of big toe. Good balance of trunk. To be examined at Department of Orthopaedics in Göteborg because of neck pain. Travelling to Tenerife on September 25th, 1974.

Radiographic examinations (Sahlgren's Hospital, Göteborg). 12 October, 1973; 29 January, 4 June and 24 September, 1974. Position of steel-frame prosthesis in C_4 and C_6 largely unchanged since last follow-up on 25 September, 1973 at Karolinska Hospital, Stockholm. (N.B. The transverse channels in the vertebral bodies for receiving lugs of prosthesis are filled with radiolucent cement which can readily be misinterpreted as resorption.)

Comments and discussion (Cases 4–6)

In skull traction treatment for fractures of the cervical spine the intervertebral spaces are widened, but they are normalized again when the tractive force is removed; this is clearly depicted in spinal radiographs (Fig. 69 B). When the cervical spinal cord is compressed by a dowel from anteriorly in the fresh cadaver, and then exposed by bilateral laminectomy, transverse fissures appear in the tissue (Table 1). If tension is applied to the cervical spine by loading a pair of forceps with a weight equivalent to the force used in traction therapy, the transverse fissures in the cord are widened (Fig. 69 A). Since the intervertebral discs of the living patient are separated in traction therapy and since the artficial fissures widen on applying traction to the cadaveric skull, there is every reason to suppose that the fissures in the patient's cord behave similarly. So long as these surfaces remain apart no union is possible without incorporation of glia and connective tissue (161, 218); for subsequent recovery of the functional capacity of the damaged nervous tissue, however, the wound surfaces must be approximated so that the severed axon ends make contact with each other and regenerative growth will be promoted (65, 221, 268–70). In traction therapy tension is set up around the ends of such a fissure (Fig. 68); and this can block the conductivity even of the undamaged nerve-fibres in this tissue.

To judge from the extent of the neurological deficit symptoms of the 3 patients considered here, there must have been fissures over a large cross-sectional area of the cord. (The secondary role of oedema and haemorrhage in the histodynamic picture is dealt with on p. 58.) The specific purpose of relaxing the spinal cord was to bring these intramedullary wound surfaces into contact with each other and to maintain that contact. This was accomplished by keeping the cervical spine slightly extended, thereby slackening the cervical cord and normalizing its contour. To achieve this and at the same time to normalize the repair of the cervical spine fracture the following technique and aids were used:

(a) *Cervicolordodesis* with a Trevira ribbon[11] (Fig. 153).

(b) *Plastic shell* (Minerva) for the back of the neck and the chin, cervical spine and thorax, with removable anterior and posterior parts (Fig. 107).

(c) *Steel-frame prosthesis* (author's design) for spondylodesis, which bridges the fracture in the cervical spine when it is in the extended position (Fig. 154 A).

The results obtained with these aids in these three patients may be summarized as follows:

Cervicolordodesis. *Effect on the fracture.* In Cases 5 and 6 cervicolordodesis at first apparently helped to reduce the respective fractures, but later on, when there was renewed and unforeseen loading, there was an inevitable relapse, with displacement. In Case 4 cervicolordodesis at first had no effect at all in reducing the

[11] See p. 193.

fracture and correcting the displacement; there was even a further displacement of the bone fragments. (Even though the Trevira ribbon keeps the cervical spine extended constantly, it can rotate about its fixed thoracic anchorage, and thus permit forward and backward slipping of the unstable vertebra or bone fragments.)

Effect on the cervical spinal cord. The cervicolordodesis has constantly kept the cervical spinal cord relaxed. However, especially in Case 6, it has not prevented renewed dislocation of the C_4 vertebra and the formation of a hump, which in certain body postures exerted a thrust on the anterior aspect of the slackened cord, and thus possibly reopened the fissures.

Plastic shell. The *plastic shell* was used too late in all the patients. It has been extremely uncomfortable and has not provided a sure safeguard against renewed displacement of bone fragments. In Case 6 the posterior part of the support, which had slipped upwards, had pressed the head forwards and hence promoted forward slipping of the vertebra C_4.

Prosthesis. The *steel-frame prosthesis* was for various reasons also used too late in Cases 4 and 6. The frame is intended to be anchored or cemented in the vertebral bodies while the cervical spine is extended. To achieve this, continuous X-ray monitoring is required during the operation. The unsatisfactory result in both these cases must be ascribed in some measure to the fact that this equipment was not available for long enough.

General practical conclusions

From the observations in these three cases it would seem justfied to draw the following inferences:

Traction as a method for treating fractures of the cervical vertebrae is unsuitable because it sets up tension in the nervous tissue and prevents proper healing of any intramedullary lesion. For the use of Crutchfield's forceps loaded with a weight of $\frac{1}{2}$ kg or so, as a means of stabilizing the extended cervical spine transiently, see p. 250.

Cervicolordodesis can prevent the separation of the wound surfaces in the axial direction but not their displacement by a shearing action; nor can it prevent a renewed thrust or pincer action on the cord.

On the other hand, cervicolordodesis has proved to be an effective measure in preventing the generation of intramedullary tension; it leads to relaxation of the spinal cord so that the intramedullary wound surfaces are approximated, thus promoting their union. It reduces or eliminates tension in the intact nervous tissue around the ends of the fissures. Since cervicolordodesis alone is clearly insufficient for preventing displacement of a loosened vertebra or bone fragments, it would seem logical to combine it with another technique for stabilizing the spine in the region of the fracture.

Osteosynthesis by a *steel-frame prosthesis* can be re-

garded as the method of choice. It has been incorporated without complications in Cases 4 and 6 and has stabilized the fractures; the results are promising. This method might, of course, be replaced by a bone graft (67); but then the vertebral column would have to be immobilized for at least 8–10 weeks with the patient supine. Here, too, external stabilization must be provided by other means than skull *traction*. One conceivable though not fully reliable alternative is to use a pair of Crutchfield's forceps anchored in the frontal bone to hold the cervical spine reclined over a round bolster; a load of 500 g would suffice.

To prevent displacement similar to that in the present patients, immediate internal stabilization of the cervical spine with the steel-frame prosthesis is indicated; since reliable stabilization is obtained immediately the prosthesis is in place, the patient is able to sit up in bed only a day or so after the operation. Rehabilitation potentials are then greatly improved.

Another future method probably with similar prospects is an *adaptable* halo-pelvic splint to hold the cervical spine in slight extension without exerting traction (see p. 183, footnote 6).

Prior to healing of the intramedullary lesion due to a compression injury there is a risk that secondary tension will be generated in the cervical cord during positional changes of the spine—for instance, during conveyance of the patient to hospital and during admission. From the observations made during the treatment of the 3 patients in question it would appear that renewed tension can be set up in the traumatized cervical cord in the following situations:

(a) *Renewed pincer action* on the cord through displacement of vertebrae or bone fragments; see Cases 4 and 5.

(b) *Flexion of the cervical spine;* see Case 6.

(c) *Skull traction;* see Cases 4 and 5 (treated with skull traction by the duty physician immediately after admission to the Emergency Department).

Neurological deterioration in these traumatizing situations may be due to extension of the fissures. In a renewed pincer action and flexion of the cervical spine such extension of the fissures will probably be immediate; but in skull traction it may be delayed; in this case the ischaemia produced by the increase in tension in the blood-vessels will also impair conductivity. The development of permanent disability in the case of secondary tension may have its explanation in total rupture of the axoplasm. (Electron microscopic examinations provide a closer insight into these structural changes in axons so damaged that render them particularly sensitive to secondary tension.)

The analysis of the forces to which the cervical cords of the patients were exposed suggests that they could probably be avoided in the future when the technical shortcomings of the method have been eliminated.

The slight improvement in the neurological functions —which had been expected to be permanently abolished—in one of these patients (Case 5) would seem to indicate that this therapeutic approach is a promising one. Five months after the cord trauma that resulted in total interruption of all afferent and efferent pathways at the level of the lesion, there were definite, though admittedly very weak and diffuse, signs of recovery of sensibility on the anterior surface of both thighs and also on the outer aspect of the left thigh, and an ability to perform weak voluntary contractions of the quadriceps and adductor muscles on both sides, accompanied a week or so later by a weak voluntary movement of the abdominal muscles. After a further 5 months the contractile function had improved and toe movements were possible. In the patient's opinion the function of the abdominal muscles was good enough to help in emptying the bladder and in guiding trunk movements, position control and the like. Rehabilitation experts regarded these movements as indicative of 'some kind of regeneration'. This is probably one of the first occasions on which signs of a slight degree of true physiological recovery have been recorded in patients with spinal cord lesions of the type and severity of those in Case 5.

"Immobilization and realignment with skeletal or similar traction has been an undisputed therapeutic regimen since Hippocrates" (26, 181)—such arguments are still advanced in defence of skull traction therapy today. In the light of the above observations it would seem difficult to avoid the conclusion that skull traction unbeknown can expose the area of a lesion in the spinal cord to chronic excess tension of a potentially harmful, albeit relatively low, intensity. Even the small separation of the wound surfaces in the spinal cord that may be produced by skull traction is sufficient to prevent the intended healing of the spinal cord tissues under optimal conditions for axonal regeneration; in addition, this traction obviously aggravates the damage to the nerve-fibres and blood-vessels already involved.

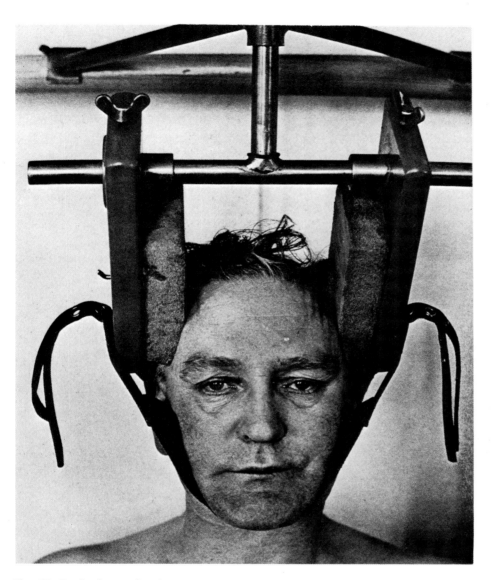

Fig. 160. Device for traction therapy.

In the light of the results of this research traction therapy can no longer be considered an acceptable measure in spinal cord disorders. When traction is applied with the spine in the neutral position or, especially, flexed, there is a real risk of over-stretching the cord together with the nerve-roots and the blood-vessels, with resulting neurological manifestations—even if there are only minor pathological changes of the spine or nervous structures. This is particularly true in the case of post-traumatic interlocking of the articular facets or transverse tearing of the nervous tissue, and in the presence of extra- or intra-medullary firm structures (lesions).

Courtesy of G. Högberg, Stockholm.

Comprehensive abstract

This book deals with a new area of neurology, namely, the fundamental causes, the sequelae and the relief of adverse mechanical tension generated in the central nervous system by external or internal dynamic forces acting on the nervous tissue. The resulting deformation of the nerve-cells, nerve-fibres and blood-vessels is ultimately responsible for a wide range of familiar neurological symptoms. The forces in question have their origin in a variety of pathological conditions and mechanical situations in different parts of the central nervous system, and they give rise to specific functional disorders.

This chain of cause and effect has been analysed on the basis of simple mechanical principles; the insight gained from this analysis has pointed to methods for eliminating the adverse tension, and hence the deformation of tissue elements and the resulting neurological manifestations.

An important feature of this book is the ample illustration of the mechanical analysis and the principles underlying the therapeutic methods. Supported by detailed captions, the photomicrographs, diagrams and radiographs enable a survey of the subject-matter to be obtained independently of the more thorough treatment presented in the body of the text.

Part One of the book deals with the experimental reproduction and analysis of the pathological forces acting on the brain, spinal cord and nerve-roots, and the tensile stress set up in these structures. *Part Two* concentrates on the neurological, radiological, neurosurgical and orthopaedic aspects of this tension. In *Part Three* descriptions are given of new methods of functional neurosurgery designed to reduce, if not eliminate, the adverse tension by applying the technique of spinal cord relaxation developed and described by the author in 1957.[1] The promising and sometimes early beneficial results obtained with this technique in thirty or so patients with various acute and chronic lesions of the pons–cord tract are presented in detail.

Pathological tension set up in the pons–cord tract by pressure mechanisms differs in its origin and effects from *physiological* tension generated by flexion of the spine. Whereas the latter increases as the cervical spine or the whole column are flexed from their neutral position, it is only when some part of the stretched pons–cord tract is pressed against, and stretched over, a firm extra- or intramedullary pathological structure that symptom-producing tension is set up.

Micromanipulatory experiments on spinal cord tissue have disclosed that under tensile stress the visco-elastic cytoplasm of the nerve-cells and axis-cylinders is deformed. Just prior to the ultimate rupture of the medullary tissue in the case of excessive tension this cytoplasm is drawn out into filaments—presumably consisting of myelin fibres. This suggests that the cause of the neurological symptoms experienced when the pons–cord tract is subjected to acute and chronic pressure, and also of a number of the still puzzling chronic afflictions of the central nervous system (including multiple sclerosis), might ultimately lie in the pathological distortion of the nerve-fibres and the associated rheological phenomena in their cytoplasm.

According to the results of analyses in patients suffering from these diseases, pathological pressure occurs chiefly as *bilateral compression* of slack nervous tissue, and as a *uni-* or *multilateral thrust* on the physiologically stretched spinal-cord tissues. The effect of these two distinct dynamic mechanisms has been examined by various methods using cadaveric brains and spinal cords fixed *in situ* under conditions of loading. It was found that the resulting pathological tensions appear in three-dimensional stress fields in the tissues. Nerve-fibres and blood-vessels running parallel to the direction of a tensile field were found to be elongated; the cross-sections of the axis-cylinders and the lumina of the vessels were reduced to an extent dependent on the magnitude of the tension in the nervous tissue. The function of these structures would thus be reduced, if not completely blocked; this would obviously lead to neurological signs and symptoms of excitation or deficit.

A knowledge of the principles governing the generation and distribution of the tensile stress in the brain, spinal cord and nerve-roots is an important aid to the interpretation of the symptoms, and, so long as no irreversible damage has been inflicted, to their elimination. The fund of experience accumulated in this investigation opens up new perspectives in neurology, neurosurgery and neuropathology. *Intracerebral tension* evokes neurological symptoms in the case of all expanding intracranial lesions—such as hydrocephalus, subdural haematoma and cerebral tumour; *intramedullary tension* can give rise to neurological symptoms in, for example, cervical myelopathy and in those cases of multiple sclerosis where the cord is chiefly involved; and *intraradicular tension* can generate symptoms ranging from trigeminal neuralgia to sciatica.

The long-obscure traumatizing effect of compression of nervous tissue can now be explained. As the visco-elastic cytoplasm of the nerve-cells and axis-cylinders and the intercellular fluid are incompressible, when the

---

[1] Breig, A.: Biomechanics of the Central Nervous System. Almqvist & Wiksell, Stockholm, 1960. (Out of print.)

The author has shown here that during flexion and extension of the vertebral column the tissues of the pons–spinal cord tract undergo deformation. When the spinal canal is shortened on extension the nerve fibres go into folds and spirals whereby they slacken, and when the canal is elongated—by about 7 cm—on full flexion, they are first drawn out smooth, and then stretched. This discovery renders obsolete the long-standing conception of a static state of the tissues of the central nervous system.

isolated axis-cylinder is subjected to a pincer action the cytoplasm flows towards the ends of the axon membrane, causing them to bulge. This deformation is accompanied by a powerful local axial tension in the cohesive cytoplasm, which is then stretched into fine filaments. The greater the compressive force the finer will the residual filaments become, and they will eventually rupture. The same stretching of the cytoplasm perpendicular to the plane of compression also takes place in the axis-cylinders of the medullary tissue *in situ*. Once the yield limit is reached in a large number of adjacent axons, transverse fissures occur at the level where the cord is pinched or clamped. In sagittal sections through the cervical cord of the fresh cadaver where the anteroposterior diameter has been reduced by more than one fifth through compression, transverse fissures are produced in the over-stretched tissue. These experimental results clearly suggest that it is such intramedullary fissures that are responsible for interruption of the conductivity of the affected pathways.

In traction therapy the intervertebral discs are stretched and the vertebral bodies are separated; the cervical spinal canal may then be elongated by up to 10 mm with a load of only 5 kg or so. If there are transverse intramedullary fissures in the spinal cord they will open to produce wound surfaces in the nervous tissue; for the pons–cord tract is firmly anchored at its cranial and caudal extremities.

Animal experiments have shown that, just as the axons of a partly severed peripheral nerve display a distinct tendency to grow out towards each other, so do axons of the severed cord tissue. For this approximation and regeneration of the axons to occur the wound surfaces must be kept in contact, and tension in the cord must therefore be avoided. Flexion of the cervical spine results in powerful physiological tension throughout the pons–cord tract, though under normal conditions this is, of course, not harmful. From the fact that if a transverse incision is made in, for example, the thoracic or lumbar cord in this posture the ends separate more than one centimetre, it is clear that the surfaces of intramedullary fissures at any level may well separate far enough to prevent regeneration.

As has been demonstrated in histological sections of canine and human spinal cord that has been damaged by compression, the presence of wedge-shaped glial and connective tissue scars in the wound gap con-stitutes a barrier to axonal regeneration. For this reason, too, the spinal cord must be kept slack after any injury resulting in tissue rupture. One logical implication of this is that the conventional skull traction therapy must be abandoned. The author has designed surgical procedures for approximating the wound surfaces as soon as possible after the injury, and for keeping them in contact.

A number of methods of functional surgery, with appropriate instruments, have also been developed for eliminating the tension produced by pathological extra- and intramedullary structures and lesions (such as osteophytes, glial scars and localized oedema).

Stretching of the pons–cord tract, whether by pathological structures, normal flexion of the cervical spine or both, can be prevented or relieved by restricting the range of movement of the cervical spine and head. For this purpose the author has designed a brake, which consists of a woven ribbon of polyester fibre anchored in the occipital bone and the three uppermost thoracic spinous processes; it passes through a tunnel in the neck muscles. This operation has been designated 'cervicolordodesis'. As a means of keeping the cord relaxed and preventing separation of possible intramedullary wound surfaces the brake is indicated in practically all types of spinal cord trauma, irrespective of their level.

The author has also designed methods of protective surgery to replace the conventional bilateral laminectomy; for in the case of a pre-existing subcritical spinal cord compression even pressure of fairly short duration on the dura, and thus on the cord, exerted by, say, the jaws of a rongeur can produce a sudden potentially harmful increase in tension in the axis-cylinders.

The beneficial results obtained in patients so far with the new surgical methods bear witness to the great therapeutic potential of functional neurosurgery; these fundamental advances are bound to have important implications for neurological thinking.

For these reasons the subject-matter of this volume is of topical interest not only to workers in the fields of neurology, neurosurgery, traumatology, neuroradiology, neurophysiology and functional anatomy, but also to the orthopaedic and paediatric surgeon and to the physiotherapist and other paramedical personnel concerned with rehabilitation of the patient suffering or recovering from, for example, spinal cord injury.

Summary

Certain pathological conditions of the central nervous system can result in excessive stretching of nerve-fibres and impairment of their conductivity. Through the development of a discharging lesion this stretching can give rise to both centrifugal and centripetal impulses (266). If the stretching has not resulted in rupture or damage to the nerve-fibres there are good prospects for a partial, if not complete, restoration of their conductivity by methods of functional neurosurgery. These are designed to relieve the tension in both blood-vessels and nerve-fibres, thereby alleviating the neurological signs and symptoms.

Basic biomechanics

When the vertebral column moves within its normal range the tissues of the pons–cord tract, from the mesencephalon to the filum terminale, undergo extensive external and internal physiological deformation. The basic phenomenon here is the folding and drawing out of the medullary tissue that takes place with extension and flexion of the spinal column, respectively. The axoplasm and membranes of the nerve-fibres and the myelin sheaths are likewise relaxed and stretched. The nerve elements and the blood-vessels are then protected from harmful elongation by various mechanisms.

Basic histodynamics

Under the topographical and functional conditions outlined below, pathological extra- and intramedullary structures and lesions impinging on the nervous tissue from outside or within can exert one or more of the following types of mechanical action; *1,* a unilateral thrust from without; *2,* a multilateral thrust from within; *3,* pinching or clamping, and *4,* concentration of tension in intact nerve-fibres around an intramedullary (intraradicular) fissure (notch stress).[1]

A *unilateral thrust* is usually exerted by a structure located anterior or anterolateral to the pons–cord tract; the force is generated by stretching of the tract during *flexion* of the spine.[2] A *multilateral thrust* from within is exerted by a firm intramedullary lesion or structure, especially during stretching of the tract on flexion. In a bilateral *pincer* or *clamping action* on the cord one of the contact surfaces is either a pathological structure in the spinal canal, such as a herniated disc, an osteophyte or a fractured bone; or as in spinal cord injury, it may be the lower margin of a posteriorly displaced vertebral body; the other surface is the canal wall. The pincer and clamping actions tend to occur during extension of the spine. They are intensified by the normal protrusion of the soft tissues into the canal, and the increase in the cross-section of the spinal cord accompanying extension.

As has been demonstrated by photoelastic experiments on a methacrylate model, a pincer action sets up a high local tensile stress. When the cord is exposed to a pincer or clamping action *in situ* the resulting tension can be great enough to produce tearing and fissuring; this will occur for the most part centrally in the cord. In the case of any intramedullary fissure due to tearing, even physiological stretching of the pons–cord tract will tend to separate these wound surfaces and to set up tension in the intact nerve-fibres and blood-vessels around the end of the fissure.

Similarity of the histodynamic effects of the four adverse mechanical situations[3]

Histological and microangiographical examinations of spinal cords and nerve-roots exposed to the above four mechanical situations in the cadaver and fixed *in situ* in formaldehyde while under load have shown that in all four cases the nerve-fibres, blood-vessels and their supporting tissues in the various sections of the pons–cord tract can be over-stretched. Unilateral and multilateral thrust give rise to a transverse as well as an axial tensile component. As has been demonstrated in experiments on peripheral myelinated nerve-fibres in the frog and in man, the forces acting in all four situations result in a constriction (reduction of the cross-sectional area) of the nerve-fibres and ultimately in an impairment of their conductivity (117). This reduction was found to occur not, as might be expected, at a Ranvier's node, but at the point between two such nodes where the cross-section is smallest (232).

Extent of the stress fields and their histodynamic effects

Pincer action. The stress field set up in the cord tissue by a pincer action has a limited cranial and caudal range. The axial component of the field is of the greatest

---

[1] The mechanical action of type 4 does not necessarily imply that the fissure-producing impinging structure is still retaining its place.

[2] So long as the tract is *slack*, it will usually not be exposed to a thrust from any structure protruding into the spinal canal. Besides the large and firm intraspinal tumour, there are only a few lesions that can exert a symptom-producing thrust on the *stretched* tract, from either the *lateral* or *posterior* direction. An example of a lateral thrust is that produced on the over-stretched tract by a kyphotic deformation of the spine; an otherwise harmless inward convex scoliotic curvature can then exert a thrust and produce neurological symptoms. Again in kyphosis, the wedge formed by the arches C_2 and C_3 might possibly exert a thrust from the posterior direction (2). This is a common result of flexion injury to the spine due to a fall on the neck (trampoline, pole-vaulting (209), where bone from a fractured vertebral arch enters the elongated canal, from the posterior direction.

[3] The force situation is different but the type of stress may be the same.

pathological significance, since it is this that is largely responsible for the damage in the nerve-fibres and blood-vessels. When the anteroposterior diameter of the spinal cord has been compressed to about a fifth or a fourth of its normal value the axial tension in these structures is so great that rupture of the nerve-fibres (and blood-vessels) will probably occur—at first in the centre of the cord. The number of nerve-fibres involved, and hence the potential neurological impairment, will depend on the magnitude of the pincer force.

Uni- and multilateral thrust and notch stress. The forces involved in uni- and multilateral thrusts and in notch stress around intramedullary fissures are considerably weaker than the pincer and clamping forces, and the resulting stress fields have a different configuration. In contrast to the limited range of the pincer action, in the two former situations the forces are transmitted through the pons–cord tract and can therefore produce neurological manifestations remote from the actual source of the tension. In the case of unilateral thrust the neurological symptoms are due in the first place to the axial tension in the nervous tissue; it is this component that constricts the nerve-fibres and myelin sheaths, and distorts the axoplasm.

The axial and transverse tensile forces to which the nervous and vascular elements are subjected in the case of unilateral or a multilateral thrust and the tensile forces around the end of a fissure can be eliminated by slackening the cord.

Origin of the adverse forces

The presence of excessive tension in the nervous tissue can evoke neurological symptoms regardless of whether it is acting in the brain, the pons–cord tract or the trigeminal or sacral nerve-roots. Among the sources of adverse tension in the central nervous system are: tumours, cysts, hydrocephalus, haemorrhage, an elevated asymmetric petrous bone, a fractured and dislocated odontoid process, an osteophyte or a herniated intervertebral disc, calcified tissues, intraparenchymal oedema, glial scar, arachnoid adhesions, intramedullary fissures or fragmentation of the myelin sheaths of axis-cylinders.

Techniques in functional spinal cord surgery

Protective arco-cristectomy and protective bilateral laminectomy. According to the results of an analysis of compressive stress, a structure that impinges on the spinal cord from the anterior, lateral or posterior direction and subjects it to a pincer action sets up a local axial tension in the tissue. Effective methods of eliminating this tension are protective arco-cristectomy and protective bilateral laminectomy, in which one of the responsible pincer or clamping structures is removed.

Cervicolordodesis. The tension produced by uni- or multilateral thrust and an intramedullary fissure can be relieved by relaxing the pons–cord tract. Permanent slackening can be secured by cervicolordodesis, in which the forward movement of the head and cervical spine is arrested in slight extension by means of a brake—consisting originally of a *fascia lata* graft and now of a ribbon of a synthetic material.

The degree of relaxation of the cord, and hence of extension of the cervical spine, required to avoid adverse effects of intramedullary tension can be ascertained radiographically.

Relaxation of the dura, which accompanies spinal extension, is also of special therapeutic significance, since tension in it may be partly responsible for compression of the spinal cord.

Improvement of cord circulation by functional spinal cord surgery

Besides the nerve-fibres, the blood-vessels of the spinal cord are subjected to tension in the four mechanical situations specified above. The potentially great axial tension in the part of the tract exposed to a pinching or clamping action can lead to such severe stretching of the vessels, especially those located centrally in the medullary tissue, that they, too, may be ruptured. Less extreme tension may result in narrowing of the vessels, especially the small descending and ascending branches of the central arteries; the detrimental effect of this will be aggravated if their lumina are already reduced by fibrosis (148, 255). The consequent reduction of the blood supply to the nerve-fibres may further impair their conductivity.

The tension set up in the vessels in any of the four mechanical situations should be released by appropriate functional measures—the tension due to the pincer action by protective arco-cristectomy or protective bilateral laminectomy, and that due to the uni- and multilateral thrust by cervicolordodesis. Cervical myelopathy due to spondylosis often produces both these adverse mechanisms—a pincer action on extension of the cervical spine, and a unilateral thrust on flexion. Thus, the optimal beneficial effect on the central and peripheral arterial circulations of the spinal cord can be attained only by a combination of either protective arco-cristectomy or protective bilateral laminectomy with cervicolordodesis.

Pons–cord tract relaxation in spinal cord surgery

Indications and methods
A résumé

Temporary spinal cord relaxation

Relaxation in acute spinal cord injury

Indication

Spinal cord injury manifested by neurological deficit.

Methods

The cervical spine should be kept slightly extended and lateral flexion and rotation prevented by reclining the head over a round bolster or by some other means to avoid potentially aggravating spinal movements prior to and during examination of the patient. This measure should be taken from the moment at which the injury is first recognized or suspected. Great care is essential to ensure that the neck is not accidentally flexed when inserting the bolster under the head: first-aid workers must be taught accordingly.[1]

Relaxation in brain-stem and spinal cord surgery

Indications

In any operation calling for access to the anterior and anterolateral aspects of the pons–cord–cauda equina tract. Such operations include:

Removal of tumours at all levels:

Solitary tumours such as acoustic neurinoma, and subpontine expanding lesions (including clivus tumours and tumours located anterior to the medulla oblongata). *Invasive tumours* and other lesions such as tumours within the medulla oblongata and spinal cord, and intrapontine haemorrhage. Open cordotomy (visualization of the anterior aspect of the cord prior to the incision).

Vascular surgery, including aneurysms.

Excision of parts of the pedicles for transposition of the dural theca and spinal cord.

Extirpation of osteophytes and spurs of bone in diastematomyelia.
Removal of large intracerebellar tumours where pressure exerted by the spatula on the already compressed pons may result in deleterious over-stretching of the mid-brain.

Methods

The head is placed on the self-adjusting head-rest (Fig. 141) by means of which the head and cervical spine can be extended during the operation to relax the pons–cord tract and afford access to the offending lesion.

Long-term or permanent spinal cord relaxation

Relaxation in acute spinal cord surgery

Indication

Spinal cord injury *at all levels* manifested by neurological deficit.

Methods

Methods [A] Stable injury ('hyperextension injury') with no apparent vertebral fracture or dislocation

Stage 1 (if the canal lumen is reduced by spondylotic spurs or osteophytes):
 Protective bilateral laminectomy or arco-cristectomy performed to remove one of the pincer or clamping surfaces (Figs. 147 and 148).
Stage 2: Either Cervicolordodesis (Fig. 153).
 Or Application of *adaptable* halo-pelvic splint to hold cervical spine in slight extension without exerting traction. This measure can be considered only when relaxation needs not to be permanent.

[1] The patient should be transported with the entire vertebral column immobilized in a slightly extended position by means of, e.g., a Vacuum immobilizer (Camp).

Methods [B] Stable injury at cervical level with vertebral fracture but no gross dislocation

Stage 1 (if there is reduction of the canal lumen):
Protective bilateral laminectomy or arco-cristectomy; if necessary removal of bone or disc fragments by anterior or anterolateral access.

Stage 2: As for Methods [A].

Methods [C] Unstable injury at cervical level with vertebral fracture or dislocation

Stage 1: As for Methods [B].

Stage 2: Reduction of fracture or fracture/dislocation; fusion of vertebrae in the extended posture by:
(i) steel-frame prosthesis, (ii) bone graft or (iii) acrylic prosthesis (139). The choice of method will depend on the type of fracture or dislocation. (See *Surgical techniques*, p. 195.)

Stage 3: In the event that the fracture has not been completely reduced and there is instability, the head and cervical spine must be held in slight extension by using, for example, halo-pelvic splint adapted for the extended posture, or by nursing the patient on a Stryker frame, a Circ-O-lectric bed or similar apparatus (with a head-rest and neck support) to keep the cervical spine slightly extended in either prone or supine postures.

Methods [D] Stable and unstable injuries at thoracic or lumbar levels with vertebral fracture or dislocation

Stage 1: Reduction of fracture or dislocation by surgical methods (excluding traction) or possibly by postural reduction. (See p. 134.)

Stage 2: As for Methods [A].

Relaxation in disorders of the brain-stem, spinal cord and nerve-roots

Indications

1. Cervical myelopathy.
2. Cervical rhizopathy.[2]
3. Trigeminal neuralgia (tic douloureux).[3]
4. Post-traumatic myelopathy.
5. Multiple sclerosis.[4]
6. Intramedullary cyst formation.[5]
7. Thoracic myelopathy.
8. Conus-cauda lesion; sacral rhizopathy.
9. Congenital spinal, meningeal and medullary malformations (including diastematomyelia and myeolomeningocele).
10. Amyotrophic lateral sclerosis.
11. Cerebral palsy.[6]
12. Painful spasticity.[7]
13. Urinary incontinence due to extra- or intramedullary lesions of various origins.
14. Respiratory insufficiency (failure) due to extra- or intramedullary lesions of various origins.

Methods

Relaxation is obtained by placing the spine in slight extension and maintaining this position by means of a brake—the operation of cervicolordodesis.

Cervicolordodesis is preceded by supplementary measures in:

1. Cervical myelopathy: Protective arco-cristectomy or protective bilateral laminectomy is performed in order to eliminate the pincer or clamping action exerted on the cord by the osteophytes when the spine is extended.
2. Cervical rhizopathy: Protective hemifacetectomy is performed to eliminate the pincer or clamping action exerted on the nerve-roots by the osteophytes when the spine is extended.

Skull traction in damage to the spine and possibly the spinal cord

The application of traction to the skull and cervical spine for the purpose of reducing a dislocation, fracture, etc., incurs a risk of over-stretching and tearing damaged nerve-fibres and blood-vessels, and hence of further neurological impairment (219, 220). For this reason traction therapy should be avoided in the case of any spinal injury in which there may be damage to the cord or the nerve-roots.

Skull traction is also *contraindicated* in forward displacement of a cervical vertebra (especially in young persons with intervertebral discs of normal height), when the upper articular processes are interlocked in front of the lower ones. The unilateral thrust exerted by the upper margin of the subjacent vertebra produces axial *and* transverse bending tensile stress in the cord tissue (nerve-fibres) and a corresponding narrowing of the lumina of the blood-vessels at this level. When skull traction is applied this tension is increased and this may aggravate the neurological symptoms. The alternative measure here is exposure and reduction of the dislocation(s). This can be achieved without damage to the nervous tissue when the head and the 2 uppermost vertebrae are kept in the extended position, while the rest

---

[2] Moreover, sequelae of arachnoiditis in the posterior cranial fossa, migraine cervicale, etc.

[3] If conventional measures of neurosurgery are useless and drug therapy or destructive physical measures (radiosurgery [175], etc.) have proved ineffective.

[4] All stages where there are invalidizing spinal cord manifestations.

[5] Where puncture or permanent drainage have proved ineffective.

[6] Where stereotaxic surgery has proved ineffective.

[7] Before destruction of nervous tissue is considered.

of the cervical spine is in the neutral posture (p. 239). The dislocated intervertebral joint(s) can then be levered into place (69); if this proves difficult, levering may be facilitated by removing a small part of the upper border of the lower articular process(es). Calipers supporting the head during this measure should be loaded just enough to keep the head immobile in the extended position.

Skull traction with a load not exceeding 500 g may be used as a temporary measure in a number of situations where uncontrolled movements of the spine must be avoided—for example, in fracture of the odontoid process and during and after any kind of osteosynthesis; traction with, preferably, Crutchfield's forceps, anchored in the frontoparietal region of the skull is required in order to keep the cervical spine extended and thus to obtain reduction, to maintain the position and, eventually, to promote consolidation (Fig. 107 A).

References

These 276 entries are a selection from more than 700. Those having special relevance are marked by an asterisk *.

1. Abbott, K. H.: Foramen magnum and high cervical cord lesions simulating degenerative disease of the nervous system. Ohio St Med J 46: 645–651, 1950.
2. Aboulker, J., Metzger, J., David, M., Engel, Ph., Ballivet, J.: Les myélopathies cervicales d'origine rachidienne. Neuro-chirurgie 11 (2): 89–198, 1965.
3. Adams, C. B. T., Logue, V.: Studies in cervical spondylotic myelopathy. I. Movement of the cervical roots, dura and cord, and their relation to the course of the extra-thecal roots. Brain 94: 557–568, 1971.
   II. The movement and contour of the spine in relation to the neural complications of cervical spondylosis. Ibid. 569–586.
   III. Some functional effects of operations for cervical spondylotic myelopathy. Ibid. 587–594.
4. Aho, A. J., Aurenen, A., Pesonen, K.: Analysis of cauda equina symptoms in patients with lumbar disc prolapse. Preoperative and follow-up clinical and cystometric studies. Acta Chir Scand 135: 413–420, 1969.
5. Albin, M. S., White, R. J., Acosta-Rua, G. et al.: Study of functional recovery produced by delayed localized cooling after spinal cord injury in primates. J Neurosurg 29: 113–120, 1968.
*6. Allen, A. R.: Remarks on histopathological changes in the spinal cord due to impact: an experimental study. J Nerv Ment Dis 41: 141–147, 1914.
7. Allen, K.: Neuropathies caused by bony spurs in the cervical spine with special reference to surgical treatment. J Neurol Neurosurg Psychiat 15: 20–36, 1952.
8. Arutiunov, A. I., Baron, M. A., Majorova, N. A.: The role of mechanical factors in the pathogenesis of short-term and prolonged spasm of the cerebral arteries. J Neurosurg 40: 459–472, 1974.
9. Austin, G.: The Spinal Cord. Thomas, Springfield, Ill., 1961.
10. Baddeley, H., Roberts, G. M.: Unpublished data, 1973.
11. Bakke, S. N.: Röntgenologische Beobachtungen über die Bewegungen der Wirbelsäule. Acta Radiol Suppl 13, 1931.
12. Bärtschi-Rochaix, W.: Migraine cervicale. Huber, Bern, 1949.
13. Bassett, C. A. L., Campbell, J. B.: Spinal cord regeneration within microfilter sheaths. In French, J. D., Porter, R. W. (eds.): Basic research in paraplegia. Thomas, Springfield, Ill., 1962.
14. Bastian, H. C.: On the symptomatology of total transverse lesions of the spinal cord; with special reference to the condition of the various reflexes. Med Chir Transact 73: 151–217, 1890.
15. Beaver, D.: Electron microscopy of the Gasserian ganglion in trigeminal neuralgia. J Neurosurg, Suppl 26: 138–150, 1967.
16. Bell, H. S.: Paralysis of both arms from injury of the upper portion of the pyramidal decussation: "cruciate paralysis". J Neurosurg 33: 376–380, 1970.
*17. Bellamy, R., Pitts, F. W., Stauffer, E. S.: Respiratory complications in traumatic quadriplegia. Analysis of 20 years' experience. J Neurosurg 39: 596–600, 1973.
18. Bellman, S.: Microangiography. Acta Radiol, Suppl 102, 1953.
19. Berthold. C. H.: Ultrastructural and light-microscopical features of postnatally developing and mature feline peripheral, myelinated nerve fibres. Brogenhart Tryckeri AB, Stockholm, 1968.
20. Bischoff, A.: The node of Ranvier. Sandorama: The Physician's Panorama 8–9, December, 1968.
21. Bischoff, A.: Unpublished data, June, 1969.
22. Blackwood, W.: Unpublished data, June, 1973.
23. Blau, J. N., Logue, V.: Intermittent claudication of the cauda equina: an unusual syndrome from central protrusion of a lumbar intervertebral disc. Lancet 1: 1081–1086, 1961.
24. Blau, J. N., Rushworth, G.: Observations of the blood vessels of the spinal cord and their responses to motor activity. Brain 81: 354–363, 1958.
25. Blom, S., Ekbom, K. A.: Early signs of meningiomas of the foramen magnum. A new syndrome. J Neurosurg 19: 661–664, 1962.
26. Blume, H. G.: Surgical management of the cervical fracture dislocation with neurological deficit in conjunction with hypothermia to the spinal cord. Proceedings of the Fourth European Congress of Neurosurgery. Prague, June–July 1971.
27. Bohm, E., Franksson, C., Petersén, I.: Sacral rhizopathies and sacral root syndromes (S II–S V). Experience and results of posterior rhizotomy and radicolysis in the treatment of pelvic pain. Acta Chir Scand, Suppl. 216: 1956.
*28. Braakman, R., Penning, L.: Injuries of the cervical spine and cord. Excerpta Medica, Amsterdam, 1972.
29. Braakman, R., Penning, L.: Mechanisms of injury to the cervical cord. Paraplegia 10: 314–320, 1973.
*30. Brain, R., Wilkinson, M.: The association of cervical spondylosis and disseminated sclerosis. Brain 80: 456–478, 1957.
31. Breig, A.: Om centrala nervsystemets biomekanik. A paper read at the Herbert Olivecrona Society. Stockholm, November 1958 (unpublished data).
32. Breig, A.: The mechanical effect of head movements upon cranial nerves in the posterior fossa. A paper read at the 14th Annual Meeting of the Scandinavian Neurosurgical Society. Stockholm, September 1959a (unpublished data).
33. Breig, A.: Zur Biomechanik des Zentralnervensystems. Fortschr Neurol Psychiat 27: 3–7, 1959b.
34. Breig, A.: Ryggmärgens och hjärnstammens biomekanik och dess betydelse för uppkomsten av neurologiska symptom. A paper read at the XVI. Annual Meating of the Swedish Neurological Society. Stockholm, December 1959c (unpublished data).

*35. Breig, A.: Biomechanics of the central nervous system. Almqvist & Wiksell, Stockholm, 1960a.

36. Breig, A.: Biomechanics of the cervical spinal cord in diagnosis of and operation on tumours at the anterior aspect of the foramen magnum. Stockholm, 1960b (unpublished data).

37. Breig, A.: Biomechanics of the dura and the spinal cord. A paper read at the 4th Annual Congress of the Middle East Neurosurgical Society. Alexandria, December 1962 (unpublished data).

38. Breig, A.: A theoretical basis for the treatment of multiple sclerosis by functional surgery. Stockholm, 1963 (unpublished data).

39. Breig, A.: Biomechanics of the spinal cord in kyphosis and kyphoscoliosis. A paper read at the 17th Annual Meeting of the Scandinavian Neurosurgical Society. Helsinki, September 1963. Acta Neurol Scand 40: 196, 1964a.

40. Breig, A.: Dehnungsverschiebungen von Dura und Rückenmark im Spinalkanal. Fortschr Neurol Psychiat 4: 195–208, 1964b.

41. Breig, A.: Die Biomechanik des Rückenmarks und seiner Häute im Wirbelkanal. Verh Anat Ges (Jena) 115: 49–69, 1965.

42. Breig, A.: Trigeminusneuralgi. A paper read at the Staff Meeting, Karolinska Hospital. Stockholm, September 1966 (unpublished data).

43. Breig, A.: Biomechanical and pathological basis of the cervical syndromes. A paper read at the 4th Annual Meeting of the Federation of Western Societies of Neurological Science. San Diego, March 1968 (unpublished data).

44. Breig, A.: The thrust effect of pre-, epi- and intramedullary lesions on the pons–cord tissue tract under tension. A preliminary report. 1969 (unpublished data).

*45. Breig, A.: Overstretching of and circumscribed pathological tension in the spinal cord. A basic cause of symptoms in cord disorders. J Biomech 3: 7–9, 1970a.

46. Breig, A.: A model for biological simulation and measurements of the effects of high-speed impact on the fluid in the subarachnoid space and the cord tissue. 1970b (unpublished data).

47. Breig, A.: The therapeutic possibilities of surgical bioengineering in incomplete spinal cord lesions. Paraplegia 9, 4: 173–182, 1972.

48. Breig, A.: Kompressionsstressens effekter på nervfibrer och blodkärl inom ryggmärgsvävnaden. Läkartidn 17: 1765–1766, 1973a.

49. Breig, A.: Pathological stress in the pons–cord tissue tract and its alleviation by neurosurgical means. Clin Neurosurg 20: 85–94, 1973b.

50. Breig, A.: Effect of histodynamic tension on the function of the central nervous system; with special reference to its analysis in spinal cord injury and skull traction. Mod Asp Neurosurg 3: 36–54, 1973c.

51. Breig, A., Ekbom, K., Greitz, T., Kugelberg., G.: Hydrocephalus due to elongated basilar artery. Lancet 1: 874–875, 1967.

52. Breig, A., El-Nadi, A. F.: Biomechanics of the cervical spinal cord. Relief of contact pressure on and over-

stretching of the spinal cord. Acta Radiol (Stockh.) 4: 602–624, 1966.

53. Breig, A., Marions, O.: Biomechanics of the lumbosacral nerve roots. Acta Radiol (Stockh.) 1: 1141–1160, 1963.

54. Breig, A., Turnbull, I. M., Hassler, O.: Effects of mechanical stresses on the spinal cord in cervical spondylosis. A study on fresh cadaver material. J Neurosurg 25: 45–56, 1966.

*55. Brodal, A.: Neurological anatomy in relation to clinical medicine. Oxford University Press, London, 1969.

56. Brodkey, J. S., Richards, D. E., Blasingame, J. P., Nulsen, F. E.: Reversible spinal cord trauma in cats. Additive effects of direct pressure and ischemia. J Neurosurg 37: 591–593, 1972.

57. Brody, A., Wilkins, R. H.: The signs of Kernig and Brudzinski. Arch Neurol (Chic.) 21: 215–218, 1969.

58. Carlsson, C. A.: Regeneration of spinal ventral roots. An experimental study in cats. Erlanders Boktryckeri AB, Kungsbacka, 1973.

*59. Causey, G.: The effect of pressure on nerve fibres. J Anat (Lond.) 82: 262–270, 1948.

*60. Causey, G.: The effect of pressure on conduction and nerve fibre size. J Anat (Lond.) 84: 65 (P), 1950.

61. Charnley, J.: Acrylic cement in orthopedic surgery. Williams & Wilkins, Baltimore, 1970.

62. Charnley, J.: Postoperative infection after total hip replacement with special reference to air contamination in the operating room. Clin Orthop 87: 167–187, 1972.

63. Charnley, J.: Clean air in the operating room. Clean air symposium. Part I. Cleveland Clin Quart 40: 99–114, 1973.

64. Clarke, E., Bearn, J. G.: The spiral nerve bands of Fontana. Brain 95: 1–20, 1972.

65. Clemente, C. D.: Structural regeneration in the mammalian central nervous system and the rôle of neuroglia and connective tissue. In Windle, W. F. (ed.): Regeneration in the central nervous system, pp. 147–161. Thomas, Springfield, Ill., 1955.

66. Cloward, R. B.: The anterior approach for removal of ruptured cervical disks. J Neurosurg 15: 602–617, 1958.

67. Cloward, R. B.: Treatment of acute fractures and fracture-dislocations of the cervical spine by vertebral body fusion. A report of eleven cases. J Neurosurg 18: 201–209, 1961.

68. Cloward, R. B.: Unpublished data, March 1968.

69. Cloward, R. B.: Reduction of traumatic dislocation of the cervical spine with locked facets. J Neurosurg 38: 527–531, 1973.

70. Cobb, C., Ehni, G.: Herniation of the spinal cord into an iatrogenic meningocele. Case report. J Neurosurg 39: 533–536, 1973.

*71. Cohen, F. L.: Effects of various lesions on crossed and uncrossed descending inspiratory pathways in the cervical spinal cord of the cat. J Neurosurg 39: 589–595, 1973.

72. Croft, T. J., Brodkey, J. S., Nulsen, F. E.: Reversible spinal cord trauma: a model for electrical monitoring of spinal cord function. J Neurosurg 36: 402–406, 1972.

*73. Cushing, H., Eisenhardt, L.: Meningiomas. Thomas, Springfield, Ill., 1938.

*74. Dandy, W. E.: Surgery of the brain. Prior Company Inc., Hagerstown, Md., 1945.

75. D'Angelo, C. M., Van Gilder, J. C., Taub, A.: Evoked cortical potentials in experimental spinal cord trauma. J Neurosurg *38:* 332–336, 1973.

76. Day, M. H.: The anatomy of the lumbosacral plexus with particular reference to the blood supply. Ph.D. Thesis, University of London, 1962.

*77. Denny-Brown, D., Brenner, C.: Paralysis of nerve induced by direct pressure and by tourniquet. Arch Neurol Psychiat (Chic.) *51:* 1–26, 1944.

*78. Denny-Brown, D., Doherty, M. M.: Effect of transient stretching of peripheral nerve. Arch Neurol Psychiat (Chic.) *54:* 116–129, 1945.

*79. Denny-Brown, D., Brenner, C.: Lesion in peripheral nerve resulting from compression by spring clip. Arch Neurol Psychiat (Chic.) *52:* 1–9, 1955.

80. De Palma, A. F., Rothman, R. H.: The intervertebral disc, pp. 154–170. The intervertebral disc. Saunders, Philadelphia, 1970.

*81. Dodge, H. W., Love, J. G., Gottlieb, C. M.: Bengin tumors at the foramen magnum: surgical considerations. J Neurosurg *13:* 603–617, 1956.

82. Dohrman, G. J., Wagner, F. C., Jr, Bucy, P. C.: The microvasculature in transitory traumatic paraplegia. An electron microscopic study in the monkey. J Neurosurg *35:* 263–271, 1971.

83. Dohrman, G. J., Wagner, F. C., Jr, Bucy, P. C.: Transitory traumatic paraplegia: electron microscopy of early alterations in myelinated nerve fibers. J Neurosurg *36:* 407–415, 1972.

*84. Dohrman, G. J., Wick, K. M., Bucy, P. C.: Spinal cord blood flow patterns in experimental traumatic paraplegia. J Neurosurg *38:* 52–58, 1973.

85. Doppman, J. L., Ramsey, R., Thies, R. J.: A percutaneous technique for producing intraspinal mass lesions in experimental animals. J Neurosurg *38:* 438–447, 1973.

*86. Drooglever Fortuyn, J.: Structure and orientation of cells and fibres in the nervous system of vertebrates. Nature (Lond.) *198:* 398–399, 1963.

87. Du Boulay, G. H.: Pulsatile movements in the cerebrospinal fluid pathways. Brit J Radiol *39:* 255–262, 1966.

88. Ducker, T. B., Kindt, G. W., Kempe, L. G.: Pathological findings in acute experimental spinal cord trauma. J Neurosurg *35:* 700–708, 1971.

89. Ehni, G., Clark, K., Wilson, Ch., Alexander, E., Jr.: Significance of the small lumbar spinal canal: Cauda equina compression syndromes due to spondylosis. Parts 1–5. J Neurosurg *31:* 490–519, 1969.

90. Emmet, J. L., Love, J. G.: Vesical dysfunction caused by protruded lumbar disk. J Urol (Baltimore) *105:* 86–91, 1971.

*91. Epstein, J. A., Carras, R., Epstein, B. S., Levine, L. S.: Myelopathy in cervical spondylosis with vertebral subluxation and hyperlordosis. J Neurosurg *32:* 421–426, 1970.

92. Epstein, J. A., Epstein, B. S., Levine, L. S. et al.: Lumbar nerve root compression at the intervertebral foramina caused by arthritis of the posterior facets. J Neurosurg *39:* 362–369, 1973.

93. Evarts, C. M.: Trends in the management of scoliosis. Cleveland Clin Quart *36:* 23–34, 1969.

94. Fager, C. A.: Results of adequate posterior decompression in the relief of spondylotic cervical myelopathy. J Neurosurg *38:* 684–692, 1973.

*95. Fairholm, D. J., Turnbull, I. M.: Microangiographic study of experimental spinal cord injuries. J Neurosurg *35:* 277–286, 1971.

*96. Fernández-Morán, H.: Sheath and axon structures in the internode portion of vertebrate myelinated nerve fibres. An electron microscope study of rat and frog sciatic nerves. Exp Cell Res *1 (2):* 309–340, 1950.

97. Fernández-Morán, H.: Membrane ultrastructure in nerve cells. (Intensive study program in the neurosciences, Boulder, Colorado. Summer 1966.) To be published by the Rockefeller University Press.

98. Frankel, H. L., Hancock, D. O., Hyslop, G., Melzak, J., Michaelis, L. S., Ungar, G. H., Vernon, J. D. S., Walsh, J. J.: The value of postural reduction in the initial management of closed injuries of the spine with paraplegia and tetraplegia. Part 1. Paraplegia *7:* 179–192, 1969.

99. Fredzell, G., Greitz, T., Grepe, A., Holmström, L.: Mimer III and rotating chair. Acta Radiol (Stockh.) *7, 6:* 543–552, 1968.

100. Freebody, D., Bendall, R., Taylor, R. D.: Anterior transperitoneal lumbar fusion. J Bone Jt Surg *53 B:* 617–627, 1971.

101. Fried, L. C., Goodkin, R.: Microangiographic observations of the experimentally traumatized spinal cord. J Neurosurg *35:* 709–714, 1971.

102. Friede, R. L., Martinez, A. J.: Analysis of the process of sheath expansion in swollen nerve fibres. Brain Res *19:* 165–182, 1970*a*.

103. Friede, R. L., Martinez, A. J.: Analysis of axon–sheath relations during early Wallerian degeneration. Brain Res *19:* 199–212, 1970*b*.

104. Frykholm, R.: Cervical nerve root compression resulting from disc degeneration and root sleeve fibrosis. Acta Chir Scand, Suppl. 160, 1951.

105. Garceau, G. J.: The filum terminale syndrome (the cord traction syndrome). J Bone Jt Surg *35 A:* 711–716, 1953.

106. Gardner, W. J.: Meningeal tumor in the foramen magnum and upper cervical region of the cord. Arch Neurol Psychiat (Chic.) *39:* 1302–1307, 1938.

*107. Gardner, W. J.: Trigeminal neuralgia. Clinical neurosurgery. Proc. Congress of Neurological Surgeons, San Francisco, Calif., 1967.

108. Gardner, W. J.: The dysraphic states from syringomyelia to anencephaly. Excerpta Medica, Amsterdam, 1973.

109. Goddard, M. D., Reid, J. D.: Movements induced by straight leg raising in the lumbo-sacral roots, nerves and plexus, and in the intrapelvic section of the sciatic nerve. J Neurol Neurosurg Psychiat *28:* 12–18, 1965.

110. Golub, B. S., Silverman, B.: Transforaminal ligaments of the lumbar spine. J Bone Jt Surg *51 A:* 947–956, 1969.

111. Gooding, M. R.: A study of some aspects of the blood supply to the spinal cord. M.Sc. Thesis, University of London, 1964.

112. Goodman, S. J., Becker, D. P.: Vascular pathology of the brain stem due to experimentally increased intracranial pressure, noted changes in the micro- and macrocirculation. J Neurosurg 39: 601–609, 1973.

113. Gortvai, P., Fairburn, B.: Kyphoscoliosis with paraplegia. J Neurosurg 33: 60–66, 1970.

114. Gosch, H. H., Gooding, E., Schneider, R. C.: Cervical spinal cord hemorrhages in experimental head injuries. J Neurosurg 33: 640–645, 1970.

115. Gowers, W. R.: A manual of diseases of the nervous system. Vol. I. Diseases of the spinal cord and nerves. Churchill, London, 1886.

*116. Granit, A. R., Leksell, L., Skoglund, C. R.: Fibre interaction in injured or compressed region of nerve. Brain 67: 125–140, 1944.

*117. Gray, J. A. B., Ritchie, J. M.: Effects of stretch on single myelinated nerve fibres. J Physiol (Lond.) 124: 84–89, 1954.

118. Gray's anatomy. Descriptive and Applied. 32nd ed. Longmans, London, 1958.

*119. Greitz, T.: Effect of brain distension on cerebral circulation. Lancet 1: 863–865, 1969.

120. Greitz, T., Ekbom, K., Kugelberg, E., Breig, A.: Occult hydrocephalus due to ectasia of the basilar artery. Acta Radiol (Diagn) (Stockh.) 9: 310–316, 1969.

121. Guth, L., Windle, W. F.: The enigma of central nervous regeneration. Exp Neurol, Suppl. 5: 1–43, 1970.

122. Guttmann, L.: Initial treatment of traumatic paraplegia and tetraplegia. In Harris, Ph. (ed.): Spinal injuries, pp. 80–92. Morrison & Gibb, London, 1963.

123. Guttmann, L.: Spinal injuries. Initial treatment of fractures and dislocations in traumatic paraplegia. Folia Traumatologica Geigy 1–16, 1972.

*124. Guttmann, L.: Spinal cord injuries. Comprehensive management and research. Blackwell, Oxford and Adlard & Son, Dorking, Surrey, 1973.

125. Hadley, L. A.: Intervertebral joint subluxation, bony impingement and foramen encroachment with nerve root changes. Amer J Roentgenol 65: 377–402, 1951.

126. Halldin, M.: Narkos och bedövning. Svenska Bokförlaget Bonniers, Stockholm, 1964.

127. Hammon, W. M., Kempe, L. G.: The posterior fossa approach to aneurysms of the vertebral and basilar arteries. J Neurosurg 37: 339–347, 1972.

*128. Hansson, H. A.: Unpublished data, September 1971.

129. Harris, Ph.: Some neurosurgical aspects of traumatic paraplegia. In Harris, Ph. (ed.): Spinal injuries, pp. 101–112. Proceedings of a symposium held in The Royal College of Surgeons of Edinburgh 7 and 8 June, 1963. Morrison & Gibb, London, 1964.

130. Harris, Ph.: New methods of treating acute spinal injuries: (a) a cranio-spinal splint; (b) halo cranio-trunk immobilization. A paper read at the 5th International Congress of Neurological Surgery, Tokio, Japan, October 1973.

*131. Hassler, O.: Angioarchitecture in hydrocephalus. An autopsy and experimental study with the aid of micro-angiography. Acta Neuropath (Berl.) 4: 65–74, 1964.

132. Hassler, O.: Calcifications in the intracranial arachnoid. Microradiological and histological study of the occurrence and appearance of calcifications with special reference to the trigeminal nerve. J Neurosurg 27: 336–345, 1967 a.

*133. Hassler, O.: Arterial pattern of human brainstem. Normal appearance and deformation in expanding supratentorial conditions. Neurology (Minneapolis) 17: 368–376, 1967 b.

134. Hassler, R., Walker, A. E.: Trigeminal neuralgia. Pathogenesis and pathophysiology. Thieme, Stuttgart, 1970.

*135. Heilbrun, M. P., Davis, D. O.: Spastic paraplegia secondary to cord constriction by the dura. Case report. J Neurosurg 39: 645–647, 1973.

136. Heyl, H. L.: Research on regeneration in the central nervous system. Editorial. J Neurosurg 37: 127–128, 1972.

137. Hirsch, C., Lewin, T.: Lumbosacral synovial joints in flexion-extension. Acta Orthop Scand 39: 303–311, 1968.

138. Hitchcock, E.: Initial management of head injuries. Folia Traumatologica Geigy 1–6, 1971.

139. Hoppenstein, R.: R.: Immediate spinal stabilization using acrylic prosthesis. Bull Hosp Jt Dis (N.Y.) 23: 66–75, 1972.

140. Hughes, J. T.: Pathology of the spinal cord. Lloyd & Luke, London, 1966.

141. Hughes, J. T., Brownell, B.: Aberrant nerve fibres within the spinal cord. J Neurol Neurosurg Psychiat 26: 528–534, 1963.

142. Hukuda, S., Wilson, C. B.: Experimental cervical myelopathy: effects of compression and ischemia on the canine cervical cord. J Neurosurg 37: 631–652, 1972.

143. Humphreys, R. P.: Unpublished data, December 1972.

*144. Hyndman, O. R.: Transplantation of the spinal cord. The problem of kyphoscoliosis with cord signs. Surg Gynec Obstet 84: 460–464, 1947.

145. Iwayama, T. et al.: Dual adrenergic and cholinergic innervation of the cerebral arteries of the rat. An ultrastructural study. Circulat Res 26: 635–646, 1970.

146. Idanov, D. A.: Unpublished data (University of Moscow), 1969.

147. Jefferson, G.: Concerning injuries of the spinal cord. Brit Med J 2: 1125–1130, 1936.

148. Jellinger, K.: Pathomorphical aspects of the biomechanics of the CNS. Mod Asp Neurosurg 3: 27–35, 1973.

149. Jirout, J.: Studies in the dynamics of the spine. Acta Radiol (Stockh.) 46: 55–60, 1956 a.

150. Jirout, J.: Changes in the size of the subarachnoid spaces after the insufflation of air. Acta Radiol (Stockh.) 46: 81–86, 1956 b.

151. Jirout, J.: Pneumographic investigation of the cervical spine. Acta Radiol (Stockh.) 50: 221–225, 1958.

152. Jirout, J.: Myelographic syndrome of caudal dislocation of the brain stem. Brit J Radiol 32: 188–192, 1959 a.

153. Jirout, J.: The mobility of the cervical spinal cord under normal conditions. Brit J Radiol 32: 744–751, 1959 b.

154. Jirout, J.: Mobility of the thoracic spinal cord under normal conditions. Acta Radiol (Stockh.) 1: 729–735, 1963.

155. Jirout, J.: Mobility of the spinal cord under abnormal conditions. Acta Radiol (Stockh.) 5: 1042–1046, 1966a.

156. Jirout, J.: Fehldiagnostik in der Pneumomyelographie. Radiologe 12: 469–472, 1966b.

*157. Jirout, J.: Dynamics of the spinal dural sac under normal conditions. Brit J Radiol 40: 209–213, 1967.

158. Jirout, J., Fischer, J., Nadvornik, F.: Anatomische und pneumographische Studien des hinteren Arachnoidalraumes der normalen Brustwirbelsäule. Fortschr Röntgenstr 101: 391–399, 1964.

159. Jones, R. A. C., Thomson, J. L. G.: The narrow lumbar canal: a clinical and radiological review. J Bone Joint Surg 50 B: 595–605, 1968.

160. Kahn, E. A.: The rôle of the dentate ligaments in spinal cord compression and the syndromes of lateral sclerosis. J Neurosurg 4: 191–199, 1947.

161. Kao, C. C., Shimizu, Y., Perkins, L. C., Freeman, L. W.: Experimental use of cultured cerebellar cortical tissue to inhibit the collagenous scar following spinal cord transection. J Neurosurg 33: 127–139, 1970.

162. Kemp, H. B. S., Jackson, J. W., Jeremiah, J. D., Cook, J.: Anterior fusion of the spine for infective lesions in adults. J Bone Jt Surg 55 B: 715–734, 1973.

*163. Kerr, F. W. L.: Pathology of trigeminal neuralgia: light and electron microscopic observations. J Neurosurg, Suppl. 26: 151–156, 1967.

*164. Key, A., Retzius, G.: Studien in der Anatomie des Nervensystems. Folio 166: 1. Norstedt & Söner, Stockholm, 1875.

165. Kontury, M.: Investigations into bladder dysfunction in prolapse of lumbar intervertebral disc. Ann Chir Gynaec Fenn 57, Suppl. 162, 1968.

166. Krenz, J., Troup, J. D. G.: The structure of the pars interarticularis of the lower lumbar vertebrae and its relation to the etiology of spondylosis. J Bone Jt Surg 55 B: 735–741, 1973.

167. Kuhlendahl, H.: Unpublished data, April 1974.

168. Laitinen, L. V.: Severe spasticity relieved by myelotomy. Medical Tribune, September 30, 1971.

*169. Lanz, T.: Über die Rückenmarkshäute. I. Die konstruktive Form der harten Haut des menschlichen Rückenmarks und ihrer Bänder. Archiv Entwickl Mech Org 118: 211–307, 1929.

170. La Torre, E., Fortuna, A.: Syndrome of anterior spinal artery from cervical spondylosis relieved by surgery. A case report. Minerva Neurochir 15: 22–23, 1971.

171. Lausberg, G.: Behandlung von Wirbelsäulenverletzungen mit Rückenmarksbeteiligung. Actuelle Chir 3: 289–296, 1968.

172. Law, W. A.: Lumbar spinal osteotomy. J Bone Jt Surg 41 B: 270–278, 1959.

173. Leaver, R. C., Loeser, J. B.: Lhermitte's phenomenon after high velocity missile injuries of the brain. J Neurosurg 34: 159–163, 1971.

*174. Lehmann, H. J.: Die Nervenfaser. Handbuch der Mikroskopischen Anatomie, Bd. IV, pp. 513–701. Springer, Berlin, 1959.

175. Leksell, L.: Stereotaxic radiosurgery in trigeminal neuralgia. Acta Chir Scand 137: 311–314, 1971.

176. Lewin, T.: Foramen intervertebrale und Wirbelbogengelenke im Lendenabschnitt der Wirbelsäule. In Junghanns, H. (ed.): Die Wirbelsäule in Forschung und Praxis, Vol. XL, pp. 74–82. Hippokrates-Verlag, Stuttgart, 1968.

*177. Lhermitte, J.: Multiple sclerosis. The sensation of an electric discharge as an early symptom. Arch Neurol Psychiat (Chic.) 22: 5–8, 1929.

178. Liliequist, B.: Gas myelography in the cervical region. Acta Radiol (Stockh.) 4: 79–92, 1966.

*179. Lindquist, C., Nilsson, B. Y., Skoglund, C. R.: Observations on the mechanical sensitivity of sympathetic and other types of small-diameter nerve fibres. Brain Res 49: 432–435, 1973.

180. List, C. F.: Multiple meningiomas. Removal of four tumors from region of foramen magnum and upper cervical region of the cord. Arch Neurol Psychiat (Chic.) 50: 335–341, 1943.

181. Loeser, J. D.: History of skeletal traction in the treatment of cervical spine injuries. J Neurosurg 33: 54–59, 1970.

182. Lubin, A. J.: Adhesive spinal arachnoiditis as a cause of intramedullary cavitation. Arch Neurol Psychiat (Chic.) 44: 409–420, 1940.

183. MacNab, I.: Negative disc exploration: an analysis of the causes of nerve root involvement in sixty-eight patients. J Bone Jt Surg 53 A: 891–903, 1971.

184. Malmcomb, D. S.: Method of measuring reflex times applied in sciatica and other conditions due to nerve root compression. J Neurol Neurosurg Psychiat 14: 15–24, 1951.

185. Malmros, R.: Compression of the spinal cord in kyphosis and kyphoscoliosis. Motion picture. Third International Congress of Neurological Surgery, Copenhagen, August 1965.

186. Manelfe, C.: Contribution à l'étude de la vascularisation artérielle de la dure-mère rachidienne chez l'homme. Étude anatomo-radiologique et histologique. Considérations pathologiques. Imprimerie Fournie, Toulouse, 1969.

*187. Maxwell, J. A., Kahn, E. A.: Spinal cord traction producing an ascending reversible, neurological deficit. Case report. J Neurosurg 26: 331–333, 1967.

*188. Mayer, E. T., Peters, G.: Pathologische Anatomie der Rückenmarkverletzungen. In Kessel, E. K., Guttman, L., Maurer, G.: Handbuch der Neurotraumatologie, pp. 39–61. Urban und Schwarzenberg, München, 1971.

*189. McVeigh, J. F.: Experimental cord crushes with a special reference to the mechanical factors involved and subsequent changes in the areas of the cord affected. Arch Surg 7: 573–600, 1923.

190. Meinecke, F. W.: Early treatment of traumatic paraplegia. Paraplegia 1: 262–270, 1963.

191. Metzger, J., Engel, P., Dilenge, D., Aboulker, J.: La myélobulbographie gazeuse dans les myélophathies chroniques. Acta Radiol (Diagn) (Stockh.) 5: 1079–1089 1966.

192. Millen, J. W., Wollam, D. H. M.: On the nature of the pia mater. Brain 84: 514–520, 1961.

*193. Mixter, W. J.: Rupture of the lumbar intervertebral disk. An etiologic factor for so-called 'sciatic pain'. Ann Surg *106*, 777–787, 1937.

194. Morgan, T. H., Wharton, G. W., Austin, G. N.: The results of laminectomy in patients with incomplete spinal cord injuries. Paraplegia *9:* 14–23, 1971.

195. Motavkin, P. A. et al.: Histochemical characteristics of the acetylcholinesterase of the nerve innervating the brain vessels. Acta Morph Acad Sci Hung *19:* 159–173, 1971.

196. Murphey, M. G.: Successful evacuation of acute pontine hematoma. Case report. J Neurosurg *37:* 224–225, 1972.

197. Nachemson, A.: Intradiscal measurements of pH in patients with lumbar rhizopathies. Acta Orth Scand *40:* 23–42, 1969.

198. Nagashima, C.: Cervical myelopathy due to ossification of the posterior longitudinal ligament. J Neurosurg *37:* 653–660, 1972.

199. Nathan, P. W.: Results of antero-lateral cordotomy for pain in cancer. J Neurol Neurosurg Psychiat *26:* 353–362, 1963.

*200. Nathan, P. W., Smith, M. C.: The centrifugal pathway for micturition within the spinal cord. J Neurol Neurosurg Psychiat *21:* 177–189, 1958.

*201. Nauck, E. T.: Bemerkungen über den mechanisch-funktionellen Bau des Nerven. Anat Anz m Erg Heft *73:* 260–275, 1931/32.

202. Negrin, J.: Spinal cord hypothermia to relieve muscle spasticity and rigidity. Proceedings of the Fourth European Congress of Neurosurgery, Prague, June–July 1971.

203. Newman, P. H.: The etiology of spondylolisthesis (including "The mechanism of slipping in degenerative spondylolisthesis" by Stone, K. H.). J Bone Jt Surg *45 B:* 39–59, 1963.

204. Nurick, S.: The natural history and the results of surgical treatment of the spinal cord disorder associated with cervical spondylosis. Brain *95:* 101–108, 1972*a*.

205. Nurick, S.: The pathogenesis of the spinal cord disorder associated with cervical spondylosis. Brain *95:* 87–100, 1972*b*.

*206. Obrador, S., Queimadelos, V. G., Soto, M.: Trigeminal neuralgia secondary to asymmetry of the petrous bone. Case report. J Neurosurg *33:* 596–598, 1970.

207. Ochoa, J., Danta, G., Fowler, T. J., Gilliat, R. W.: Nature of the nerve lesion caused by a pneumatic tourniquet. Nature (Lond.) *233:* 265–266, 1971.

208. O'Connell, J. E. A.: The place of surgery in the treatment of cervical spondylosis. Proc Roy Soc Med *49:* 201–208, 1956.

209. O'Hanlan, J. T.: Schools warned about spinal injuries from "Fosbury flop". Med Trib Med News (N.Y.) *1:* 3, 1969.

*210. Olivecrona, H.: Die Trigeminusneuralgie und ihre Behandlung. Nervenarzt *14:* 49–57, 1941.

211. Osterholm, J. L., Mathews, M. B.: Altered norepinephrine metabolism following experimental spinal cord injury. Part 1: Relationship to hemorrhagic necrosis and post-wounding neurological deficits. J Neurosurg *36:* 386–394, 1972*a*.

212. Osterholm, J. L., Mathews, M. B.: Altered norepinephrine metabolism following experimental spinal cord injury. Part 2: Protection against traumatic spinal cord hemorrhagic necrosis by norepinephrine synthesis blockade with alpha methyl tyrosine. J Neurosurg *36:* 395–401, 1972*b*.

213. Parkinson, D., Shields, C.: Treatment of protruded lumbar intervertebral disc with chymopapain (Discase). J Neurosurg *39:* 203–208, 1973.

214. Peerless, S. J., Yasargil, M. G.: Adrenergic innervation of the cerebral blood vessels in the rabbit. J Neurosurg *35:* 148–154, 1971.

215. Pennal, G. F., Schatzker, J.: Stenosis of the lumbar spinal canal. Clin Neurosurg *18:* 86–105, 1971.

*216. Penning, L.: Functional pathology of the cervical spine. Excerpta Medica, Amsterdam, 1968.

217. Perelson, H. N.: Occipital nerve tenderness; a sign of headache. South Med J (Bgham, Ala.) *40:* 653–656, 1947.

218. Perkins, L. C., Solow, E., Freeman, L. W.: The effect of enzymatic debridement on scar formation and cavitation in experimental spinal cord transection. Neurology (Minneapolis) *20, 12:* 1185–1187, 1970.

219. Prolo, D. J., Hanbery, J. W.: Cervical stabilization-traction board. A new device for immediate stabilization of the injured cervical spine. JAMA *224:* 615–616, 1973.

220. Prolo, D. J., Runnels, J. B., Jameson, R. M.: The injured cervical spine. Immediate and long-term immobilization with the halo. JAMA *224:* 591–594, 1973.

*221. Ramon y Cajal S.: Degeneration and regeneration in the nervous system, Vol II, May, R. M. (ed). Oxford University Press, London, 1928.

*222. Reid, J. D.: Ascending nerve roots and tightness of dura mater. N Z Med J *58:* 17–26, 1958.

223. Rexed, B.: Arachnoidal proliferations with cyst formation in human spinal nerve roots at their entry into the intervertebral foramina. J Neurosurg *4:* 414–421, 1947.

224. Rexed, B., Wennström, K. G.: Arachnoidal proliferation and cystic formation in the spinal nerve-root pouches of man. J Neurosurg *16:* 73–84, 1959.

225. Riddoch, G.: The reflex functions of the completely divided spinal cord in man, compared with those associated with less severe lesions. Brain *15:* 264–272, 1917.

*226. Rosenblueth, A., Alvarez Buylla, R., García Ramos, J.: The responses of axons to mechanical stimuli. Acta Physiol Lat Am *3:* 204–215, 1953.

*227. Rosomoff, H. L., Johnston, J. D. H., Gallo, A. E., Ludmer, M., Gimens, F. T., Carney, F. T., Kuehn, C. A.: Cystometry as an adjunct in the evaluation of lumbar disc syndromes. J Neurosurg *33:* 67–74, 1970.

228. Rossier, A. B., Berney, J., Rosenbaum, A. E., Hachen, J.: Value of gas myelography in early management of acute cervical spinal cord injuries. J Neurosurg *42:* 330–337, 1975.

*229. Rushton, J. G., Olafson, R. A.: Trigeminal neuralgia associated with multiple sclerosis. Arch Neurol (Chic.) *13:* 383–386, 1965.

*230. Sachs, E.: Diagnosis and treatment of brain tumors and care of the neurosurgical patient. 2nd ed. Mosby, St. Louis, Ill., 1949.

231. Scheier, H.: Prognose und Behandlung der Skoliose. Thieme, Stuttgart, 1967.

*232. Schneider, D.: Die Dehnbarkeit der markhaltigen Nervenfaser des Frosches in Abhängigkeit von Funktion und Struktur. Z Naturforsch 7: 38–48, 1952.

*233. Schneider, R. C., Cherry, G., Pantek, H.: The syndrome of acute central cervical spinal cord injury with special reference to the mechanisms involved in hyperextension injuries of cervical spine. J Neurosurg 11: 546–577, 1954.

234. Schneider, R. C., Schemm, G. W.: Vertebral artery insufficiency in acute and chronic spinal trauma with special reference to the syndrome of acute central cervical spinal injury. J Neurosurg 18: 348–360, 1961.

235. Schneider, R. C., Gosch, H. K., Norell, H., Jerva, M., Combs, L. W., Smith, R. A.: Vascular insufficiency and differential distortion of brain and cord caused by cervicomedullary football injuries. J Neurosurg 33: 363–375, 1970.

236. Scoville, W. B.: Cervical spondylosis treated by bilateral facetectomy and laminectomy. J Neurosurg 18: 423–428, 1961.

*237. Skoglund, C. R.: Unpublished data, October 1969.

*238. Smith, C. G.: Changes in length and position of the segments of the spinal cord with changes in posture in the monkey. Radiology 66: 259–266, 1956.

239. Smolik, E. A., Sachs, E.: Tumors of the foramen magnum of spinal origin. J Neurosurg 11: 161–172, 1954.

240. Sunderland, S.: Nerves and nerve injuries. Livingstone, Edinburgh, 1968.

*241. Tarlov, I. M.: Acute spinal cord compression paralysis. J Neurosurg 36: 10–20, 1972.

*242. Tarlov, I. M., Klinger, H., Vitale, S.: Spinal cord compression studies. I. Experimental techniques to produce acute and gradual compression. Arch Neurol Psychiat (Chic.) 70: 813–819, 1953.

243. Tarlov, I. M., Klinger, H.: Spinal cord compression studies. II. Time limits for recovery after acute compression in dogs. Arch Neurol Psychiat (Chic.) 71: 271–290, 1954.

244. Tarlov, I. M.: Spinal cord compression studies. III. Time limits for recovery after gradual compression in dogs. Arch Neurol Psychiat (Chic.) 71: 588–597, 1954.

*245. Taylor, A. R.: The mechanism of injury to the spinal cord in the neck without damage to the vertebral column. J Bone Jt Surg 33 B: 543–547, 1951.

246. Taylor, A. R.: Vascular factors in the myelopathy associated with cervical spondylosis. Neurology (Minneapolis) 14: 62–68, 1964.

*247. Taylor, A. R., Blackwood, W.: Paraplegia in hyperextension cervical injuries with normal radiographic appearances. J Bone Jt Surg 30 B: 245–248, 1948.

*248. Teng, P., Shapiro, M. J.: Arterial anomalies of the spinal cord: myelographic diagnosis and treatment by section of the dentate ligaments. Arch Neurol Psychiat (Chic.) 80: 577–586, 1958.

249. Thulin, C. A., Carlsson, C. A.: Regeneration of transected ventral roots submitted to monomolecular filter tubulation (Millipore). An experimental study in cats. J Neurol Sci 8: 485–586, 1958.

*250. Torkildsen, A.: Lesions of the cervical spinal roots as a possible source of pain simulating sciatica. Acta Psychiat Scand 31: 333–344, 1956.

251. Towbin, A.: Latent spinal cord and brain stem injury in newborn infants. Develop Med Child Neurol 11: 54–68, 1969.

252. Troup, J. D. G.: The problem of assessing internal stresses in the human body, with particular reference to the spine. Paper read at the Conference on Materials for Biomedical Use, in the session "Forces in biomedical systems", held by The Institute of Physics and The Physical Society, London, November 1970 (unpublished data).

253. Troup, J. D. G., Chapman, A. E.: The strength of the flexor and extensor muscles of the trunk. J Biomech 2: 49–62, 1969.

254. Turnbull, I. M.: Microvasculature of the human spinal cord. J Neurosurg 35: 141–147, 1971.

255. Turnbull, I. M.: Blood supply of the spinal cord. In Vinken, P. J., Bruyn, G. W. (eds.): Handbook of clinical neurology, Vol. XII. North Holland Publishing Company, Amsterdam, 1972.

*256. Turnbull, I. M., Breig, A., Hassler, O.: Blood supply of cervical spinal cord in man: a microangiographic cadaver study. J Neurosurg 24: 951–965, 1966.

257. Unterharnscheidt, F., Higgins, L.: Traumatic lesions of brain and spinal cord due to non-deforming angular acceleration of the head. Tex Rep Biol Med 27: 127–166, 1969.

258. Verbiest, H.: A radicular syndrome from developmental narrowing of the lumbar vertebral canal. J Bone Jt Surg 36 B: 230–237, 1954.

*259. Verbiest, H.: Anterior operative approach in cases of spinal cord compression by old irreducible displacement or fresh fracture of cervical spine. Contribution to operative repair of deformed vertebral bodies. J Neurosurg 19: 389–400, 1962.

260. Verbiest, H.: Surgery of the cervical vertebral body in cases of traumatic deformity or dislocation. In Harris, P. (ed.): Spinal injuries, pp. 112–120. Morrison & Gibb, London, 1963.

261. Verbiest, H.: Unpublished data, August 1973.

262. Wagner, F. C. Jr, Dohrman, G. J., Bucy, P. C.: Histopathology of transitory traumatic paraplegia in the monkey. J Neurosurg 35: 272–276, 1971.

263. Waldron, H. A.: Cholinergic fibres in the spinal cord of the guinea pig. Brain Res 12: 250–252, 1969.

264. Weisl, H., Osborne, G. V.: The pathological changes in rats' nerves subjected to moderate compression. J Bone Jt Surg 46 B: 297–306, 1946.

265. Weiss, P., Hallowell, D.: Pressure block in nerves provided with arterial sleeves. J Neurophysiol 6: 269–286, 1943.

266. Wennerstrand, J.: Unpublished data, February 1973.

267. Williams, J. G. P.: Sport Injuries. Folia Traumatologica Geigy 1–16, 1973.

268. Windle, W. F.: Regeneration in the central nervous system. Thomas, Springfield, Ill., 1955.

*269. Windle, W. F.: In French, J. D., Porter, R. W. (ed.): Basic research in paraplegia. Thomas, Springfield, Ill., 1962.

270. Windle, W. F.: Unpublished data, 1974.

271. Wolff, J. R.: The astrocyte as link between capillary and nerve cell. Triangle Sandoz J Med Sci *9:* 153–164, 1970.

*272. Wolman, L.: The neuropathology of traumatic paraplegia. A critical historical review. Paraplegia *1:* 233–251 1963.

273. Woodhall, B., Hayes, G. J.: The well-leg-raising test of Fajerstajn in the diagnosis of ruptured lumbar intervertebral disc. J Bone Jt Surg *32 A:* 786–792, 1950.

*274. Wretblad, G.: Spätschädigungen des Rückenmarks bei Wirbelsäulenverkrümmungen besonders solchen vom Typus der juvenilen Kyphose Scheuermann. Acta Psychiat Scand *14:* 617–647, 1939.

*275. Yakovlev, P. I.: Paraplegias of hydrocephalics (clinical note and interpretation). Amer J Ment Defic *51:* 561–576, 1947.

276. Yamada, H., Ohya, M., Okada, T., Shiozawa, Z.: Intermittent cauda equina compression due to narrow spinal canal. J Neurosurg *37:* 83–88, 1972.

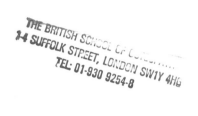

Index

Italic arabics relate to Figure Numbers.
Roman numerals relate to the Tables.

A

Anterolisthesis,
  intramedullary tension set up by, *108 A*, *146*, 197, 195
Arco-cristectomy,
  protective *147*, *148*, *152*, 12, 194–5, 248
  (*See* also Functional neurosurgery)
Artificial synapse,
  histodynamic stress possibly giving rise to, 41
Axis-cylinder,
  deformation of, setting up tension in cytoplasm *45*, 178, 186, 206
  causes of changes in conductivity of, *See* Neural conductivity.

B

Biomechanics & pathodynamics
  of thoracolumbar cord, cauda equina and pelvic plexus, *122–9*, *133–4*, 140, 141–2, 152–6
  of sympathetic plexus and ganglia *130–2*, 117
Blood-vessels, intramedullary,
  change in shape of, due to stretching and relaxation of cord *19*, *24–5*, 16, 140
'Brachiogenic sciatica', biomechanical phenomena evoking, 111
Brain stem, impaired function of pathways in,
  due to bilateral compression of, *82–3*, *84 A*
  due to squeezing in craniocaudal direction *82*, 180
Brain tissue,
  histodynamic stress in, *Frontispiece*, *87*, *97*, 122

C

Cementing procedures in anchoring of prosthesis clamp & steel-frame prosthesis *153–4*, 191
Central spinal cord injury,
  histodynamic events giving rise to,

59, 217, 223, 232–4
Cervical myelopathy,
  intramedullary tension as the cause of, *77 A, B*, 140, 248
Cervicolordodesis
  fascia lata graft, *150–3*, V, 12, 191, 203, 205, 248
  synthetic ribbon, *153*, V, 191–3, 203
Clamping action on cord and nerve-roots,
  histodynamic effects of, *77 A, B*, *135 B*, II, 178, 189, 195
Cloward's procedure,
  biomechanical effects of, *32 B*, *33 C, D*, 184
Coiling of blood-vessels after cord rupture due to compression *59*, *65*, 178
Compression,
  analysis of physical effects of,
    on a body (Araldite model), *77 A, B*, 54
    on spinal cord, *45–66*, I, II, 54
    on nerve-fibres, *73–4*, I, II, IV, 54, 178, 248
    on blood-vessels, *65*, 178, 248
Conductivity of axis-cylinders,
  change in, due to tension *97*, 122, 248
Confusional state,
  histodynamic sources of, 180, 189, 233, 236
Cord circulation,
  improvement of, induced by cord relaxation V, 188–90, 248
Cord retraction
  resulting from flexion of spine
    after transverse incision in medullary tissue *26*, *67 A–D*, *69*, *70*, 182
    after fissuring of medullary tissue *69 A*, 54–60
Cord (slackened),
  displacement of, due to changes of posture *5*, *6*, *8–10*, *102–3*, 184–5
Crenation of myelin sheath,
  possible biomechanical causation of, *14*, *15*
Cytoplasm,
  visco-elastic property of, flow of, *45 C*, 178, 195, 245–6

D

Diastematomyelia,
  histodynamic stress in cord-halves due to, *109–10*, 142–3

Displacement layer
  39, *38–9*
  See also: Epidural displacement layer.
Dura mater,
  physiological changes in tension in, *2–6*, *28*, *142*, 38, 129–30
  pathological tension in, (a contributory cause of cord compression) *119*, *142 B*, 39, 130

E

Elastic deformation,
  Elasticity
  See Definitions: 12
Epidural displacement layer,
  pathological displacement of fibres in, *28*, *39*, 38
Erector trunci spasm,
  clinical diagnosis of, 162
  kymographic registration of, *127*

F

Fascia lata graft
  See Cervicolordodesis
Fissure,
  intramedullary, transverse, *41*, *46–8*, *56–60 A*, *61–2*, *69 A*, *69 C*, I, IV, 27, 55–7, 59
  histodynamic cause of, *44*, *77 A, B*
  growth of glia and connective tissue into, *70–1*, 192, 234–6
Foramen magnum tumour,
  remote histodynamic effects of, 116, 155, 207, 210
Forces exerted on a nerve-root
  in thrust, I, II, III, 115
  in clamping or pincer actions, *135*, II
Fragmentation of nervous tissue,
  neurological effects of, *97*, III, 41, 111
Functional neurosurgery,
  definition of, 12
  measures of, *See* Arco-cristectomy, protective; Laminectomy, protective bilateral; Cervicolordodesis; Spondylodesis, using steel-frame prosthesis

G

Ganglionic chain, lumbar,
  causes of tension in, *Frontispiece*, 117
Gas myelography,
  diagnosis of tension in medullary